Veterinary Infections: Diagnostic and Management Techniques

Veterinary Infections: Diagnostic and Management Techniques

Edited by Alexis Bradshaw

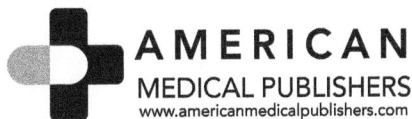

AMERICAN
MEDICAL PUBLISHERS
www.americanmedicalpublishers.com

American Medical Publishers,
41 Flatbush Avenue,
1st Floor, New York,
NY 11217, USA

Visit us on the World Wide Web at:
www.americanmedicalpublishers.com

ISBN: 978-1-63927-527-4

Cataloging-in-Publication Data

Veterinary infections : diagnostic and management techniques / edited by Alexis Bradshaw.
    p. cm.
Includes bibliographical references and index.
ISBN 978-1-63927-527-4
1. Communicable diseases in animals. 2. Communicable diseases in animals--Diagnosis.
3. Communicable diseases in animals--Treatment. 4. Veterinary medicine. I. Bradshaw, Alexis.
SF781 .V48 2022

636.089 69--dc23

Table of Contents

Preface

The infections that affect animals are known as veterinary infections. The most common of such diseases are anthrax, foot and mouth disease, black quarter, tetanus and listeriosis. Anthrax is caused by the bacterium named as Bacillus anthracis. It usually occurs in four forms – lungs, skin, intestinal and injection. The symptoms of anthrax include blister, fever, chest pain, abdominal pains, nausea and vomiting. Black quarter, also known as blackleg disease, is commonly caused by the bacteria Clostridium chauvoei. It is often seen in livestock such as cattle, goats and sheep. Foot and mouth disease is a highly infectious veterinary disease that is caused by a virus. It affects the cloven-hoofed animals and causes fever, blisters on the feet and inside the mouth, and causes lameness. This book provides comprehensive insights into the area of veterinary infections. It presents researches and studies performed by experts across the globe. Coherent flow of topics, student-friendly language and extensive use of examples make this book an invaluable source of knowledge.

This book is the end result of constructive efforts and intensive research done by experts in this field. The aim of this book is to enlighten the readers with recent information in this area of research. The information provided in this profound book would serve as a valuable reference to students and researchers in this field.

At the end, I would like to thank all the authors for devoting their precious time and providing their valuable contribution to this book. I would also like to express my gratitude to my fellow colleagues who encouraged me throughout the process.

Editor

In vitro antimicrosporidial activity of gold nanoparticles against *Heterosporis saurida*

Mona Saleh[1], Gokhlesh Kumar[1], Abdel-Azeem Abdel-Baki[2,3], Saleh Al-Quraishy[2] and Mansour El-Matbouli[1*]

Abstract

Background: Worldwide, there is a need to expand the number of drugs available to treat parasitic infections in aquaculture. One of the new materials being tested is metal nanoparticles, which have unique chemical and physical characteristics owing to their extremely small size and high surface area to volume ratio. We examined the effectiveness of gold nanoparticles against the microsporidian parasite *Heterosporis saurida*, which causes severe economic losses in lizard fish, *Saurida undosquamis* aquaculture.

Results: We synthesized gold nanoparticles by chemical reduction of tetrachloroauric acid as a metal precursor. We assessed the antimicrosporidial efficacy of the nanoparticles against *H. saurida* using an in vitro screening approach, which we had developed previously using the eel kidney cell line EK-1. The number of *H. saurida* spores produced in EK-1 cells was reduced in a proportional manner to the dosage of gold nanoparticles administered. A cell metabolic activity test (MTT) indicated that the gold nanoparticles did not appear to be toxic to the host cells.

Conclusions: Gold nanoparticles can act as an effective antimicrosporidial agent and hold promise to reduce disease in lizardfish aquaculture. Metal nanoparticles should be considered as an alternate choice for development of new antimicrosporidial drugs to combat disease problems in aquaculture.

Keywords: Gold nanoparticles, Microsporidia, *Heterosporis saurida*, Lizardfish, EK-1 cells

Background

Saurida undosquamis (Richardson, 1848) also known as Brushtooth lizardfish is fish species of the *Synodontidae* family. *S. undosquamis* is a Lessepsian migrant species distributed across the Indo-West Pacific including the Red Sea, Persian Gulf, Eastern Africa, Japan and Australia [1]. *S. undosquamis* invaded the Levant Basin of the Mediterranean Sea, from the Indo-West Pacific through the Suez Canal [2] and is considered one of the most successful colonizers of the Eastern Mediterranean, extending as far as the Aegean Sea [3]. The Mediterranean lizardfish population now has significant commercial value [4] in the eastern Mediterranean, where it is considered one of the most common species caught in the trawl fishery [5].

Diseases are a major obstruction to expansion of fresh water and marine aquaculture. Fish are susceptible to many pathogens, often with severe consequences [6].

Microsporidia are single-celled, obligate intracellular parasites that infect invertebrates and vertebrates. More than one thousand microsporidian species have been recognized as causing diseases in animals and humans [7]. Microsporidia are common in marine, fresh water and estuarine systems, and affect economically important fish species worldwide, including salmonids [8], flatfish [9], greater sand eels (*Hyperoplus lanceolatus*) [10] and ornamental fish, such as zebrafish (*Danio rerio*) [11] and killifish (Family Cyprinodontidae) [12]. Infections caused by microsporidia reduce the growth rate of fish and decrease production in aquaculture [13, 14]. Recently, *H. saurida* was isolated from lizardfish (Fig. 1) where it infects skeletal muscle, body cavity and mesenteric tissues and forms white, cyst-like structures, which contain numerous spores making the fish unsuitable for public consumption [15].

Only a small number of anti-parasitic drugs are permitted in aquaculture, as the cost of drug development is high and the market small. The few available treatments for microsporidiosis differ in their effectiveness, and as with many drug treatments, there is concern for

* Correspondence: Mansour.El-Matbouli@vetmeduni.ac.at
[1]Clinical Division of Fish Medicine, University of Veterinary Medicine, Veterinaerplatz 1, 1210 Vienna, Austria
Full list of author information is available at the end of the article

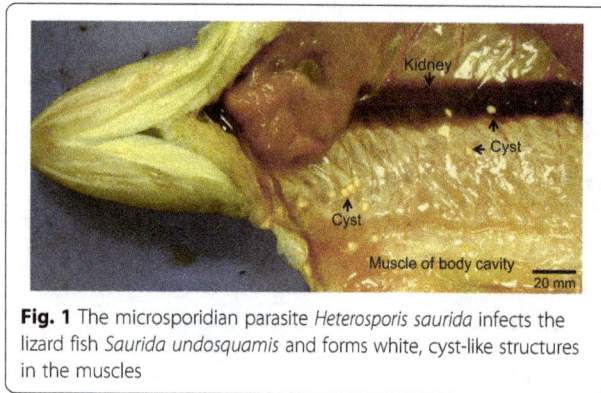

Fig. 1 The microsporidian parasite *Heterosporis saurida* infects the lizard fish *Saurida undosquamis* and forms white, cyst-like structures in the muscles

the pathogens developing resistance to one or multiple antibiotics [16]. A promising, alternative approach that has received recent attention is the use of metallic nanoparticles, which have distinct advantages over conventional antimicrobial agents [17, 18]. Nanometer-sized materials have unique, extraordinary and fascinating physical, chemical, and biological properties, particularly a large contact area with microorganisms because of their small size and higher surface-to-volume ratio; a property that expands their biological and chemical activity. Currently, nanoparticles with one dimension of 100 nm or less have received immense interest as an alternative means of combatting infectious agents in medicine. Metal based nanoparticles display broad spectrum antimicrobial activity against bacteria, fungi and viruses [19–24].

The most widespread antimicrobial compounds are silver and benzalkonium chloride [25, 26]. Unfortunately, in a comparable manner where scientists develop new efficient antimicrobial materials, there is no doubt that resistance to silver also is increasing [16]. Therefore, a number of metals, mainly copper, have been used as an antimicrobial agent. Gold has been little explored as an antimicrobial agent, although it has been used as a catalyst [27, 28].

Gold nanoparticles in particular, have a broad range of applications in nano-scale devices and technologies due to their chemical inertness and resistance to surface oxidation [29]. Gold nanoparticles have been investigated as an antimicrobial agent to inhibit the growth of common, waterborne, pathogens *Escherichia coli* and *Salmonella typhi*, which are developing resistance to common bactericides [30]. In aquaculture, several studies have been carried out to investigate gold nanoparticles as antimicrobial drugs [31–33].

In vivo efficiency trials for anti-parasitic drugs are expensive, time intensive, and need ethical permission, hence new and efficient systems to screen compounds while reducing animal experiments are required. One alternative, cost-effective approach is to screen compounds using relevant animal cell lines. In the case of *H.*

saurida, in vitro propagation has been demonstrated for both mammal (rabbit kidney; [34]) and fish (eel kidney EK-1; [35]) cell lines and an in vitro screening approach using the EK-1 cells to test antimicrosporidial agents against the parasite was also developed [36], however, our aim in the present study was to investigate the in vitro antimicrosporidial activity of gold nanoparticles as a potential agent against *H. saurida* infections.

Methods
Ethics statement
No ethical approval was necessary as this study did not involve laboratory animals; it comprised in vitro testing of cultured cell lines and microsporidian spores.

Propagation of *H. saurida* spores
Heterosporis saurida spores were grown in the eel fish kidney cell line (EK-1) using procedures previously described [35]. Briefly, *H. saurida* spores were collected from naturally infected lizard fish, *Saurida undosquamis* [15]. EK-1 cells were sub-cultured, seeded in 24-well plates in triplicate and supplemented with L-15 medium (Leibovitz) containing L-glutamine (Sigma-Aldrich), 10 % fetal bovine serum (FBS) (Sigma-Aldrich), 100 units/ml penicillin and 100 µg/ml streptomycin (Sigma-Aldrich, Vienna, Austria). Twenty four hours after seeding, 100 µl ($\sim10^7$ spores/ml) of spore suspension was added to each well. Twenty-four hour post-inoculation (p.i.), the medium was removed and the cells rinsed gently 3 times with fresh medium; the medium was replace twice per week.

Preparation and characterization of gold nanoparticles
We followed the protocol of Storhoff et al. [37] to synthesize gold nanoparticles (~13 nm diameter) by reduction of 10 mM tetrachloroauric acid ($HAuCl_4$) using sodium citrate (Sigma-Aldrich, Vienna, Austria). Briefly, an aqueous solution of $HAuCl_4.3H2O$ was boiled under reflux while being stirred. The color of the solution changed from yellow to deep red after rapid addition of 10 ml 1 % trisodium citrate. The color change signified formation of monodispersed spherical gold nanoparticles. The solution refluxed for an additional 15 min, then allowed to cool to room temperature. The solution was subsequently filtered through a 0.45 µm acetate filter and stored at 4 °C. A stock concentration of 1 mg/ml gold nanoparticles was used in the assays.

Morphology, size, and shape of synthesized gold nanoparticles were characterized using transmission electron microscopy (TEM). Samples were prepared by drop casting a 2.5 mL aliquot of the Au NPs suspension onto a 300 mesh carbon-coated copper grid. The gold suspension was dried at room temperature for 5 min and overload solution was removed from the grid using blotting paper. Particles were imaged using a Zeiss EM109. The size distribution of particles was estimated by images analysis of 100 nanoparticles located at different regions of the grid ($n = 3$). Images were taken of several samples ($n = 3$) to produce statistically meaningful results.

Measurement of anti-microsporidial activity of gold nanoparticles

Twenty-four well culture plates were loaded with EK-1 cells at a concentration of 1.5×10^5 cells/ml in L-15 medium containing 10 % FBS, and penicillin-streptomycin solution (Sigma-Aldrich, Vienna, Austria). The plates were incubated overnight at 26 °C to allow a cell monolayer to form. To reach a final ratio of 3:1 spores/cell, H. saurida spores were added in 1 ml volumes of medium at a concentration of 10^6 –10^7 spores/ml. Non-adherent spores were washed off after 24 h, and fresh medium with 0, 0.01, 0.1 and 1.0 μg/ml gold nanoparticles was added to wells, and incubated for 7 days. Media was replaced every three days. Cell monolayers were examined daily with an inverted microscope, and 10 cells in 10 fields were viewed per well using a 40X objective, for each treatment group (6 wells each treatment and control). Each concentration was tested in triplicate and the inhibition of H. saurida spore propagation was calculated as percent inhibition = 100 − [(mean number of H. saurida spores counted in treated cultures/mean number of H. saurida spores counted in non-treated cultures) × 100]. The differences between treated and non-treated H. saurida spores were analyzed using t-tests with Bonferroni α-correction. A p-value < 0.05 was regarded as significant for all statistical tests. Statistical analyses were carried out using SPSS version-20 software.

Visual observations and measurement of drug toxicity

EK-1 cells were plated in 96-well plates at approximately 1.5×10^4 cells per well. After 24 h, the medium was replaced with fresh medium containing different concentrations of gold nanoparticles as described above. Cellular viability of EK-1 cultures after introduction to the gold nanoparticles was examined as above. Any toxic effects were noted, such as cells becoming sub-confluent or altered in morphology compared with non-treated control cells. Plates were incubated at 26 °C for 1 week. The medium was then removed and the viability of cultures was assayed by incubating with MTT (3-[4,5-di-methylthiazol-2-yl]-2,5-diphenyl tetrazolium bromide, Sigma-Aldrich), following the method described by Mosmann [38]: 20 μl MTT (5 mg/ml in balanced salt solution) was added to each well and incubated for 2 h. After that, medium of each well was discarded, and 200 μl of MTT solubilization solution (Sigma-Aldrich) was added and the plates agitated with an orbital shaker. Triplicate absorbance values of each well were measured in a microplate reader at 570 nm against a reference wavelength of 690 nm. The percentage of cell viability was calculated as the optical density values of treated cells divided by the mean optical density of non-treated cells, multiplied by100.

Re-infection of EK-1 cells with H. saurida recovered after gold nanoparticles treatments

To determine if H. saurida spores were still infectious after treatment with gold nanoparticles, spores were recovered from each culture well on day 7, by addition of 100 μl of 10 % (w/v) sodium dodecyl sulfate. Released spores were centrifuged at 400 g for 15 min and washed 3 times with Tris-buffered saline containing Tween 20 (0.3 %). Spore pellets were re-suspended in medium and used to infect new cultures as previously described. A hemocytometer was used to count spores gold nanoparticles from treated and non-treated wells: 1 ml of spores suspension was adjusted to 1×10^4 spores/ml and then added to each well. Fresh medium without gold nanoparticles was added on day 3. Each culture well was observed under an inverted microscope and spores were counted 3 times (10 field/well).

Results

Gold nanoparticles

TEM revealed that the mean diameter of gold nanoparticles was 11.06–14.22 nm, and particles were spherical (Fig. 2). TEM also showed that the gold nanoparticles suspension was in a monodispersional state without obvious aggregations.

Measurement of anti-microsporidial activity of gold nanoparticles

Gold nanoparticles significantly reduce ($p < 0.001$) the number of H. saurida spores produced by infected cells, in a concentration-dependent manner (Fig. 3). The numbers of spores observed in 10 infected EK-1 cells in 10 fields of 6 wells were recorded and are listed in Table 1.

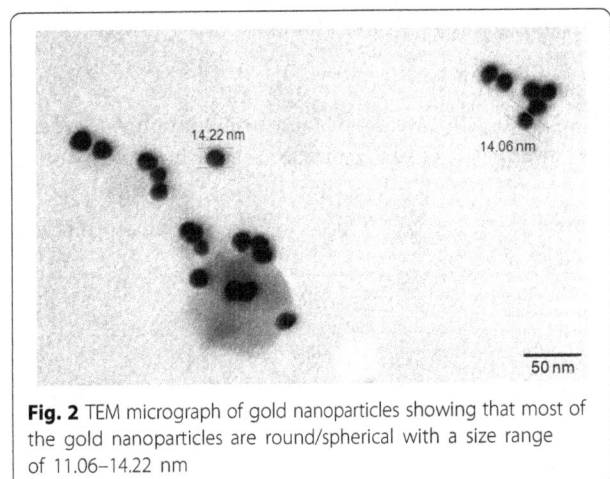

Fig. 2 TEM micrograph of gold nanoparticles showing that most of the gold nanoparticles are round/spherical with a size range of 11.06–14.22 nm

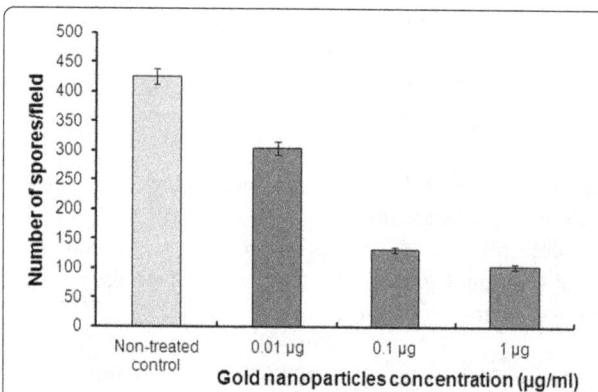

Fig. 3 Effect of gold nanoparticles against *Heterosporis saurida* in EK-1 cells. Cells were infected with the spores of *H. saurida* and incubated with different concentrations of gold nanoparticles. Data are mean (± SD) numbers of spores in 6 wells of infected EK-1 cells

Cultures with 0.01 µg/ml gold nanoparticles had fewer *H. saurida* spores than control cell cultures. Propagation of *H. saurida* spores was inhibited 68 and 75 % by 0.1 µg/ml and 1 µg/ml gold nanoparticles, respectively. Cellular and nuclear shapes appeared normal at all gold nanoparticle concentrations.

Drug toxicity measurements
Cell viability was monitored using MTT assay after incubation for 7 days with different concentrations of gold nanoparticles. Effects of gold nanoparticles tested concentrations were analyzed using MTT assay and results are shown in Table 1.

Re-infection of EK-1 cells with recovered *H. saurida* spores
Since it was not appropriate to verify if these spores were mature or infectious by microscopic observation, EK-1 cells were re-infected with recovered *H. saurida* spores after treatment.

Significantly fewer infectious microsporidia spores were recovered after treatments with gold nanoparticles in a concentration-dependent manner when compared with non-treated cultures (Table 1).

Discussion
Host- pathogen interactions are usually multivalent, and the interplay between microbes and host cells often

involves several copies of multiple receptors and ligands that bind in a coordinated way to allow the microbial agent to take the cell under control. Interfering with these recognition events, by effectively crowding out pathogen entry into the cells, is one of the most promising strategies being investigated for drug development [21]. Due to the emergence of diseases and increased mortalities in aquaculture, and the development of drug resistance by aquatic microbes, there is an ongoing effort to investigate alternative methods of prevention and control of diseases [24]. A growing attention in compounds with antimicrobial characteristics is rising due to their wide application potential in various fields including medicine [39, 40].

The present study was conducted to find out if gold nanoparticles demonstrate antimicrosporidial activity against the aquatic microsporidian *Heterosporis saurida* in vitro.

We synthesized the gold nanoparticles (13 nm diameter) by reduction of 10 mM tetrachloroauric acid (HAuCl4) with sodium citrate.

TEM shows that most of the gold nanoparticles are round and spherical in shape and in a monodispersional state without obvious aggregations that is due to the negatively charged coating layer of citrate ions, which leads to electrostatic repulsion and prevents aggregation of gold nanoparticles.

We screened different concentrations of the nanoparticles for activity against *H. saurida* in EK-1 cells. Cell cultures treated with even the lowest concentration (0.01 µg/ml) of gold nanoparticles produced fewer *H. saurida* spores than control cell cultures (Table 1). At a concentration of 0.1 µg/ml, production of spores was inhibited more than 65 %, and at 1.0 µg/ml, inhibition was more than 75 %. The inhibitory rates obtained in this study are close to those observed when other potential antimicrosporidial drugs were used [36].

We conducted MTT assays to determine if health of host cells was adversely affected, after incubation for 7 days with different concentrations of gold nanoparticles. Negligible cytotoxicity was observed up to concentrations of 0.01 µg/ml, and < 35 % toxicity was found at the highest concentrations tested (1 µg/ml). These results are consistent with the low cytotoxicity reported

Table 1 Effects of different concentrations of gold nanoparticles on proliferation of *Heterosporis saurida* and infectivity of the recovered spores in EK-1 cell cultures

Concentration of gold nanoparticles	Mean count of *H. saurida* spores	Mean percent inhibition on day 7	Cell viability (%)	Mean numbers of *H. saurida* spore (infected cells/10 fields)
0.01 g/ml	303 ± 12.3	28.4	89.6 ± 1.7	9
0.1 g/ml	133 ± 7.1	68.6	70.9 ± 2.2	5
1 g/ml	104 ± 6.7	75.5	69.8 ± 1.3	3
Non-treated control cells	423 ± 15.4	-	-	67

previously for gold nanoparticle conjugates [41]. It has been suggested that gold nanoparticles increase permeability of the cell wall that leads to leakage of cell contents and cell death. Furthermore, gold nanoparticles have been shown to bind to the DNA of microorganisms and inhibit the DNA transcription process [41, 42]. Recently, conjugates of gold nanoparticles were investigated and reported not to be generally cytotoxic and non-specific host cell membrane disruptors but affect the transcription of a number of micro-organisms genes including those involved in cell division [43]. Similarly, in this study gold nanoparticles have been shown not to be generally toxic because the viability of the EK-1 cells was not greatly affected as confirmed with MTT test. Gene expression studies would be required to clarify the molecular mechanistic effects of gold nanoparticles on *H. saurida*, though it has been suggested that the nanoparticles may alter expression of genes related to parasite cell division [43]. The mechanism of action may also involve an increase in permeability of the cell walls, leading to leakage of cell contents and death [41, 42].

Conclusions

This study shows that gold nanoparticles demonstrate a considerable antimicrosporidial activity against the fish microsporidian *H. saurida* in vitro. However, further investigations concerning mode of action and functionalization of gold nanoparticles to increase their antimicrosporidial activity, reduce possible in vivo accumulation related toxicity and enhance and promote their use in aquaculture are still needed.

Abbreviations
S. undosquamis: Saurida undosquamis; *H. saurida*: Heterosporis saurida; EK-1: eel kidney cell line.

Competing interests
The authors declare that they have no competing interests.

Authors' contributions
MS designed and accomplished the study and drafted the manuscript. GK helped with the propagation of the spores, MTT assay, figures preparations and revision of the manuscript. AA and SA dissected the fish and collected the spores. MEL supervised the study and helped revised the manuscript. All authors read and approved the final manuscript.

Acknowledgments
This work was funded in part by King Saud University, Riyadh, Saudi Arabia; the research group projects number ARP-32-19 and by the Austrian Science Fund (FWF) project no. P 27489-B22.

Author details
[1]Clinical Division of Fish Medicine, University of Veterinary Medicine, Veterinaerplatz 1, 1210 Vienna, Austria. [2]Zoology Department, College of Science, King Saud University, Riyadh, Saudi Arabia. [3]Zoology Department, Faculty of Science, Beni-Suef University, Beni-Suef, Egypt.

References
1. Froese R, Pauly D. Fishbase. World Wide Web electronic publication. 2015. http://www.fishbase.org. (version 10/2015).
2. Ben-Tuvia A. Red Sea fishes recently found in the Mediterranean. Copeia. 1966;2:254–75.
3. Bilecenoğlu M, Taşkavak E, Mater S, Kaya M. Checklist of the marine fishes of Turkey. Zootaxa. 2002;113:1–194.
4. Ben-Yami M, Glazer T. The invasion of *Saurida undosquamis* (Richardson) into the Levant Basin-an example of biological effect of interoceanic canals. Fish Bull. 1974;72(2):359–73.
5. Bingel F, Ozsoy E, Unluata U. A review of the state of the fisheries and the environment of the Northeastern Mediterranean (Northern Levantine Basin), Studies and Reviews, General Fisheries Council for the Mediterranenan, vol. 65. Rome: FAO; 1993. p. 74.
6. Kent ML, Speare DJ. Review of the sequential development of *Loma salmonae* (Microsporidia) based on experimental infections of rainbow trout (*Oncorhynchus mykiss*) and Chinook salmon (*O. tshawytscha*). Folia Parasitol. 2005;52(1–2):63–8.
7. Weiss LM. Microsporidia: emerging pathogenic protists. Acta Trop. 2001;78(2):89–102.
8. Kent ML. Marine netpen farming leads to infections with some unusual parasites. Int J Parasitol. 2000;30(3):321–6.
9. Matthews RA, Matthews BF. Cell and tissue reactions of turbot *Scophthalmus maximus* (L.) to *Tetramicra brevifilum* gen. n., sp. n. (Microspora). J Fish Dis. 1980;3(6):495–515.
10. Leiro J, Paramá A, Ortega M, Santamarina MT, Sanmartín ML. Redescription of *Glugea caullery*, a microsporidian parasite of the greater sand-eel, *Hyperoplus lanceolatus* (Le Sauvage), (Teleostei: Ammodytidae), as *Micro Gemma* caullery comb. nov. J Fish Dis. 1999;22(2):101–10.
11. de Kinkelin P. Occurrence of a microsporidian infection in zebra fish *Brachydanio rerio* (Hamilton-Buchanan). J Fish Dis. 1980;3(1):71–3.
12. Lom J, Noga E, Dykova I. Occurrence of a microsporean with characteristics of *Glugea anomala* in ornamental fish of the family Cyprinodontidae. Dis Aquat Org. 1995;21(3):239–42.
13. Constantine J. Estimating the cost of *Loma salmonae* to B.C. Aquaculture. British Columbia, Canada: Ministry of Agriculture and Food; 1999.
14. Canning EU. Phylum Microspora. In: Margulis L, Corliss JO, Melkonian M, Chapman DJ, editors. Handbook of protista. Boston, USA: Jones and Barlett Publishers; 1990. p. 53–72.
15. Al-Quraishy S, Abdel-Baki AS, Al-Qahtani H, Dkhil M, Casal G, Azevedo C. A new microsporidian parasite, *Heterosporis saurida* n. sp. (Microsporidia) infecting the lizardfish, *Saurida undosquamis* from the Arabian Gulf, Saudi Arabia: ultrastructure and phylogeny. Parasitology. 2012;139(4): 454–62.
16. Lallo MA, Vidoto da Costa LF, Manoel de Castro J. Effect of three drugs against *Encephalitozoon cuniculi* infection in immunosuppressed mice. Antimicrob Agents Chemother. 2013;57(7):3067–71.
17. Chaloupka K, Malam Y, Seifalian AM. Nanosilver as a new generation of nanoproduct in biomedical applications. Trends Biotechnol. 2010;28(11): 580–8.
18. Gunalan S, Sivaraj R, Rajendran V. Green synthesized ZnO nanoparticles against bacterial and fungal pathogens. Prog Nat Sci Mater Int. 2012;22(6):693–700.
19. Ren G, Hu D, Cheng EW, Vargas-Reus MA, Reip P, Allaker RP. Characterization of copper oxide nanoparticles for antimicrobial applications. Int J Antimicrob Agents. 2009;33(6):587–90.
20. Ali DM, Thajuddin N, Jeganathan K, Gunasekaran M. Plant extract mediated synthesis of silver and gold nanoparticles and its antibacterial activity against clinically isolated pathogens. Colloids Surf B. 2011;85(2):360–5.
21. Galdiero S, Falanga A, Vitiello M, Cantisani M, Marra V, Galdiero M. Silver nanoparticles as potential antiviral agents. Molecules. 2011;16(10):8894–918.
22. Nasrollahi A, Pourshamsian K, Mansourkiaee P. Antifungal activity of silver nanoparticles on some of fungi. Int J Nano Dim. 2011;1(3):233–9.
23. Seil JT, Webster TJ. Antimicrobial applications of nanotechnology: methods and literature. Int J Nanomed. 2012;7:2767–81.
24. Swain P, Nayak SK, Sasmal A, Behera T, Barik SK, Swain SK, et al. Antimicrobial activity of metal based nanoparticles against microbes associated with diseases in aquaculture. World J Microbiol Biotechnol. 2014; 30(9):2491–502.
25. Chopra I. The increasing use of silver-based products as antimicrobial agents: a useful development or a cause for concern? J Antimicr Chem. 2007;59(4):587–90.

26. Rees EN, Tebbs SE, Elliott TSJ. Role of antimicrobial-impregnated polymer and Teflon in the prevention of biliary stent blockage. J Hosp Inf. 1998;39(4):323–9.

27. Haruta M, Tsubota S, Kobayashi T, Kageyama H, Genet M, Delmon B. Low temperature oxidation of CO over gold supported on TiO_2, α-Fe_2O_3, and Co_3O_4. J Catal. 1993;144(1):175–92.

28. Huang J, Lima E, Akita T, Guzmán A, Qi C, Takei T, et al. Propene epoxidation with O_2 and H_2: Identification of the most active gold clusters. J Catal. 2011;278(1):8–15.

29. Sugunan A, Thanachayanont C, Dutta J, Hilborn JG. Heavy-metal ion sensors using chitosan-capped gold nanoparticles. Adv Mater. 2005;6:335–40.

30. Lima E, Guerra R, Lara V, Guzmán A. Gold nanoparticles as efficient antimicrobial agents for *Escherichia coli* and *Salmonella typhi*. Chem Cent J. 2013;7:11.

31. Soltani M, Ghodratnema M, Ahari H, Ebrahimzadeh Mousavi HA, Atee M, Dastmalchi F, et al. The inhibitory effect of silver nanoparticles on the bacterial fish pathogens, *Streptococcus iniae, Lactococcus garvieae, Yersinia ruckeri* and *Aeromonas hydrophila*. Int J Vet Res. 2009;3(2):137–42.

32. Vaseeharan B, Ramasamy P, Chen JC. Antibacterial activity of silver nanoparticles (AgNps) synthesized by tea leaf extracts against pathogenic *Vibrio harveyi* and its protective efficacy on juvenile *Feneropenaeus indicus*. Lett Appl Microbiol. 2010;50(4):352–6.

33. Ravikumar S, Gokulakrishnan R, Raj JA. Nanoparticles as a source for the treatment of fish diseases. Asian Pac J Trop Dis. 2012;2:S703–6.

34. Kumar G, Saleh M, Abdel-Baki AA, Al-Quraishy S, El-Matbouli M. In vitro cultivation model for *Heterosporis saurida* (Microsporidia) isolated from lizardfish, *Saurida undosquamis* (Richardson). J Fish Dis. 2014;37(5):443–9.

35. Saleh M, Kumar G, Abdel-Baki AA, El-Matbouli M, Al-Quraishy S. In vitro growth of the microsporidian *Heterosporis saurida* in the eel kidney EK-1 cell line. Dis Aquat Org. 2014;108(1):37–44.

36. Saleh M, Kumar G, Abdel-Baki AA, Dkhil M, El-Matbouli M, Al-Quraishy S. Development of a novel in vitro method for drug development for fish; application to test efficacy of antimicrosporidian compounds. Vet Rec. 2014;175(22):561.

37. Storhoff JJ, Elghanian R, Mucic RC, Mirkin CA, Letsinger RL. One-pot colorimetric differentiation of polynucleotides with single base imperfections using gold nanoparticle probes. J Am Chem Soc. 1998;120(9):1959–664.

38. Mosmann T. Rapid colorimetric assay for cellular growth and survival: application to proliferation and cytotoxicity assays. J Immunol Methods. 1983;65:55–63.

39. Hobman JL, Wilson JR, Brown NL. Microbial mercury reduction. In: Lovley DR, editor. Environmental metal-microbe interactions. Washington: ASM Press; 2000. p. 177–90.

40. Lewis K, Klibanov AM. Surpassing nature: rational design of sterile-surface materials. Trends Biotechnol. 2005;23(7):343–8.

41. Rai A, Prabhune A, Perry CC. Antibiotic mediated synthesis of gold nanoparticles with potent antimicrobial activity and their application in antimicrobial coatings. J Mater Chem. 2010;20(32):6789–98.

42. Prema P, Thangapandiyan S. In-vitro antibacterial activity of gold nanoparticles capped with polysaccharides stabilizing agents. Int J Pharm Pharm Sci. 2013;5:310–4.

43. Bresee J, Bond CM, Worthington RJ, Smith CA, Gifford JC, Simpson CA, et al. Nonoscale structure-activity relationships, mode of action, and biocompatibility of gold nanoparticles antibiotics. J Am Chem Soc. 2014; 136(4):5295–300.

A rare case of acute toxoplasmosis in a stray dog due to infection of *T. gondii* clonal type I: public health concern in urban settings with stray animals?

Sergio Migliore[1], Salvatore La Marca[1], Cristian Stabile[2], Vincenzo Di Marco Lo Presti[1] and Maria Vitale[1]*

Abstract

Background: Typing of *Toxoplasma gondii* strains is important in epidemiological surveys, to understand the distribution and virulence of different clones of the parasite among human and animal populations. Stray dogs can be consider sentinel animals for contaminated environments playing an important but probably under- evaluated role in the epidemiology of *T. gondii*. We reported a rare case of acute toxoplasmosis in a stray dog due to clonal type I infection. The clonal type I, sporadic in Europe, is frequently associated with severe toxoplasmosis in humans and the control of its circulation is particularly relevant for public health. The symptomatology suggested a potential infection with the high similar parasite *Neospora caninum* but differential diagnosis showed that only *T. gondii* was involved highlighting the importance of multiple diagnostic methods beyond the clinical signs.

Case presentation: A female stray dog approximately six-month of age presented muscular atrophy of the femoral region and hyperextension of hind limbs. Body condition score (BCS) was 20% below ideal weight, ribs had almost no fat and the sensor state was depressed. Haematological values were normal and the dog did not show any neurological abnormalities. Serological analysis showed a positive response for *T. gondii* immunoglobulin G (IgG) antibodies and exclude *N. caninum* infection.
To confirm *T. gondii* infection, a muscle biopsy was performed and genomic DNA was extracted. PCR analysis resulted positive to *T. gondii* and strain genotyping reveals clonal type I infection. The dog recovered after 4 weeks of treatment with clindamycin hydrochloride and aquatic physiotherapy.

Conclusions: Our study reports a rare and severe case of *T. gondii* clonal type I infection in a stray dog feeding in garbage containers. The data confirm the importance of an in vivo early diagnosis for toxoplasmosis in dog. Clinical signs are often related to specific *T. gondii* genotype and parasite genotyping is important in the epidemiological survey of toxoplasmosis in public health. The detection of parasitic DNA in the tissue could be an useful diagnostic method in facilitating early treatment of the disease, which is important for a timely clinical recovery.

Keywords: Dog toxoplasmosis, Differential diagnosis, Treatment, *T. gondii* typing, Epidemiological survey, Urban settings

* Correspondence: marvitus@yahoo.com
[1]Istituto Zooprofilattico Sperimentale of Sicily "A. Mirri", Via G. Marinuzzi 3, 90129 Palermo, Italy
Full list of author information is available at the end of the article

Background

Toxoplasmosis in dog, is recognized as an opportunistic disease which is characterized by neuromuscular, respiratory and gastrointestinal signs or by generalized infection [1]. Clinical canine toxoplasmosis rarely results from a primary infection [2] and congenital transmission by tachyzoites crossing the placenta from the infected mother to the foetus is also described [3]. In addition spontaneous abortion and foetal death have been observed in pregnant canines infected with oocysts or tachyzoites [4]. Toxoplasmosis is considered to be an important infectious disease in dogs with neurological signs but the similarity between symptomatic toxoplasmosis and neosporosis should be considered in the differential diagnosis [5].

Stray dogs in urban structures may play an underrated role in the *T. gondii* epidemiology also in humans, as they can easily act as mechanical carriers for oocyte parasites due to their frequent contact with contaminated environments [6]. They consume a variety of foods from garbage containers in the urban environment [7] and are highly likely to interact with synantropic animals such as stray cats by increasing the chance of spreading parasites [8]. The virulence of *T. gondii* is related to different genotypes that influence the progression and the severity of the disease in human and animals as well. Several studies in Europe and North America [9, 10] described that *T. gondii* presents a highly clonal population structure made up of three lineages: types I, II and III. The infection by types II and III lead to chronic persistence and production of tissue cysts in mice, whereas type I strain is extremely virulent, producing high levels of parasitemia, with increased risk of transplacentary transmission and severity of infection in developing foetuses [10]. Nevertheless, several studies of *T. gondii* isolates in human and animals in South America suggested a high genetic variability expressed by other genotypes [11–13].

Typing of *T. gondii* strains is important in epidemiological surveys, to know the distribution and virulence of different clones of the parasite among human and animal populations. Our study reports a severe clinical case of toxoplasmosis in a stray dog and showed that the detection of parasitic DNA in the tissue is a useful diagnostic method in facilitating early treatment of the disease, which is important for a prompt clinical recovery. These data confirm the importance of early diagnosis of toxoplasmosis in dog and how clinical signs are often related to specific genotypes.

Case presentation

A female stray dog approximately six-month of age was sighted nearby garbage containers with an evident paralysis of hind limbs by animalist volunteers in Santa Margherita Belice (37°41′34″N 13°01′16″E), in the province of Agrigento (south-west of Sicily, Italy). The dog was rescued and taken in a private veterinary clinic. The physical examination showed a muscular atrophy of the femoral region and hyperextension of hind limbs (Fig. 1). Body condition score (BCS) was 20% below ideal weight, ribs had almost no fat and the sensor state was depressed. Haematological values were normal and the dog did not show any neurological abnormalities. ELISA rapid tests (SNAP 4Dx® Plus; IDEEX) excluded tick-borne disease such as Lyme disease, ehrlichiosis and anaplasmosis diseases related to paralysis in dogs. A serological test for *N. caninum* (ID Screen® Neospora caninum indirect multi-species) resulted also negative but a positive response for *T. gondii* immunoglobulin G (IgG) antibodies was detected by agglutination test (ToxoScreen DA- Biomèrieux). Two dilutions 1:40 and 1:4000 to avoid prozone effect were assayed as described previously [14]. The dog was positive only to 1:40 dilution.

To confirm the suspect of *T. gondii* clinical infection, a muscle fibers biopsy was performed from superficial gluteus according to conventional method. Genomic DNA was extracted using E.Z.N.A Tissue DNA Kit (Omega bio-tek). PCR was performed to detect *N. caninum* or *T. gondii* DNA. Only an approximately 333 base pairs DNA fragment of *T. gondii* was amplified from the sample using a highly sensitive nested-PCR. The analyses were performed by a first PCR using NC 18S RNA sense primer (5′TGCGGAAGGATCATTCACACG 3′, Invitrogen) and NC25S RNA antisense primer

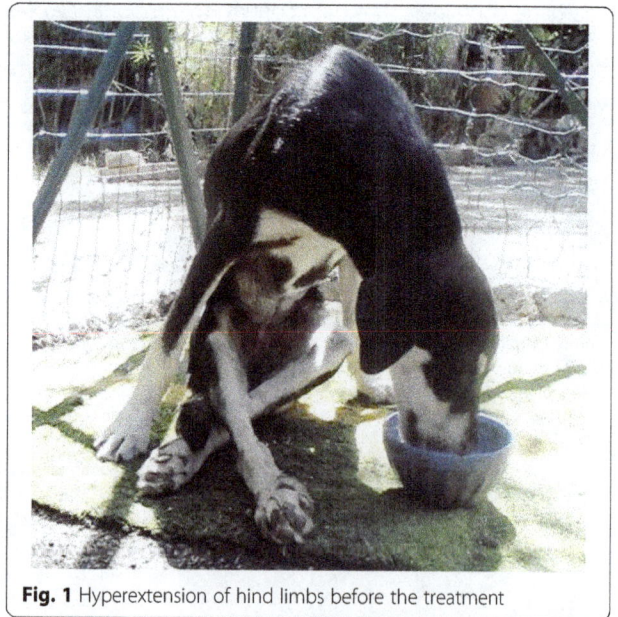

Fig. 1 Hyperextension of hind limbs before the treatment

Table 1 Genotyping results with 12 MS markers in a single multiplex PCR assay

Isolate (Genotype)	Microsatellite marker (size; base pairs)											
	TUB2 (287–291)	W35 (242–248)	TgM-A (203–211)	B18 (156–170)	B17 (334–366)	M33 (165–173)	IV.1 (272–282)	XI.1 (354–362)	M48 (209–243)	N82 (105–145)	N61 (79–123)	N83 (306–338)
sample	**291**	**247**	**209**	**160**	**343**	**169**	**274**	**358**	**209**	**121**	**87**	**308**
RH (I)	291	247	209	160	342	169	274	358	209	121	87	308
ME49 (II)	289	242	207	158	336	169	274	356	215	111	91	310
VEG (III)	289	242	205	160	336	165	278	356	213	111	89	312

The result was compared with 3 *Toxoplasma gondii* isolates corresponding to genotype I (RH), II (ME49) and III (VEG)
In bold the microsatellites results of the case study

(5'CCGTTACTAAGGGAATCATAGTT3', Invitrogen), followed by a nested PCR using Toxo ITS1sense primer (5'GATTTG– CATTCAAGAAGC TGATAGT AT3', Invitrogen) and Toxo ITS1 antisense primer (5'AGTTAGGAAGCA ATCTGAAAGCACATC, Invitrogen). as described in Vitale et al. [15].

The lineage type of *T. gondii* was determined by PCR-restriction fragment length polymorphism (RFLP) of the amplified SAG2 gene and by microsatellite (MS) markers in a multiplex PCR as described in Fuentes et al. [16] and Ajzenberg et al. [17] respectively. The amplified fragments of the SAG2 gene, 5'-end of 241 bp and 3'-end of 221 bp, were undigested with restriction enzymes *Sau*3AI (5'-end products) and with *Hha*I (3'-end products) clearly indicating genotype I.

Clonal type I infection was confirmed by MS analysis of the 12 alleles patterns (Table 1) estimated using GeneMapper analysis software (version 4.0; Applied Biosystem). Reference DNAs corresponding to the three main lineages (I, II and III) kindly donated by the European Reference Laboratory for Parasites in Rome were used for comparison and negative controls were run in each assay. To avoid cross contamination during molecular analysis all different steps (DNA extraction, PCR setting of all components,

Samples DNA and negative control, reference DNAs addition) were always performed in separate rooms.

The dog was treated according to the principles of good clinical practice and specific therapy for toxoplasmosis was initiated immediately after the diagnosis with Clindamycin hydrochloride (25 mg/kg orally twice daily for 4 weeks). In addition, classical and aquatic physiotherapy was performed to help solve the muscular atrophy. After the first week of treatment the dog started to move the hind limbs; after 2 weeks of treatment was able to stay in quadruped station (Fig. 2). In the third week of treatment the dog regained partial ambulation and after 4 weeks the ambulation returned to normal.

Discussion and conclusions

Our study reported a rare case of clinical toxoplasmosis in a stray dog due to clonal type I infection. The detection of parasitic DNA in the tissue can be a useful diagnostic method in vivo to facilitate early treatment of the disease, which is important for a timely clinical recovery.

Clonal type I is a particularly virulent strain in mice but has been associated with some severe cases of toxoplasmosis in humans [10, 16]. It is considered sporadic in Europe where a high prevalence of clonal type II with several subgroups has been observed in many cases [17–19]. The detection of this clonal type in Sicily in a stray dog suggests the opportunity for further studies in stray animal populations.

The control of its circulation is important for public health, especially in south Italy where a high population of stray cats and dogs is present in urban and periurban areas. Stray dogs, feeding at the same garbage containers where cats and rodents feed also, might have more chance to get contaminated with *T. gondii* oocysts and to spread them to larger areas of the cities.

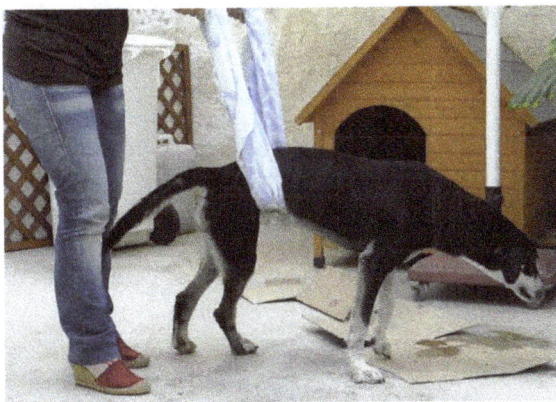

Fig. 2 Dog performance after two weeks of treatment. Fully recovery was obtained after four weeks

Abbreviations
BCS: Body condition score; MS: Microsatellite; RFLP: Restriction fragment length polymorphism

Acknowledgements
The authors thank Chiara Calasanzio and the "Amici di Olivia - ONLUS" association for their contribution. The European reference laboratory at

Istituto Superiore di Sanità in Rome is also acknowledged for the reference DNAs.

Funding
The work has been granted by Italian Ministry of Health RCSi 15/11 to M.V.

Authors' contributions
SM made the diagnosis, laboratory testing, data analysis and drafting of the article; SL participated in laboratory testing; CS collected the sample and was responsible for the clinical management; VDMLP participated in the coordination of the study; MV coordinated the study and participated in the drafting of the article. All authors have read and approved the final manuscript.

Consent for publication
Not applicable.

Competing interests
The authors declare that they have no competing interests.

Author details
[1]Istituto Zooprofilattico Sperimentale of Sicily "A. Mirri", Via G. Marinuzzi 3, 90129 Palermo, Italy. [2]Centro Veterinario "L'arca", Via V. Mazzini 112, 92013 Menfi, Italy.

References
1. Da Silva AV, Pezerico SB, Lima VY, D'arc Moretti L, Pinheiro JP, Tanaka EM, Ribeiro MG, Langoni H. Genotyping of Toxoplasma gondii strains isolated from dogs with neurological signs. Vet Parasitol. 2005;127:23–7.
2. Bresciani KDS, Costa AJ, Toniollo GH, Sabatini GA, Moraes FR, Paulillo AC, Ferraudo AS. Experimental toxoplasmosis in pregnant bitches. Vet Parasitol. 1999;86:143–5.
3. Wong SY, Remington JSC. Toxoplasmosis in pregnancy. Clin Infect Dis. 1994;18(6):853–61.
4. Dubey JP, Carpenter JL, Topper MJ, Uggla A. Fatal toxoplasmosis in dogs. J Am Anim Hosp Assoc. 1989;25:659–64.
5. Mineo TW, Silva DA, Costa GH, Von Ancken AC, Kasper LH, Souza MA, Cabral DD, Costa AJ, Mineo JR. Detection of IgG antibodies to Neospora caninum and Toxoplasma gondii in dogs examined in a veterinary hospital from Brazil. Vet Parasit. 2001;98:239–45.
6. Lindsay DS, Dubey JP, Butler JM, Blagburn BL. Mechanical transmission of Toxoplasma gondii oocysts by dogs. Vet Parasitol. 1997;73(1–2):27–33.
7. El Behairy AM, Choudhary S, Ferreira LR, Kwok OCH, Hilali M, Su C, Dubey JP. Genetic characterization of viable Toxoplasma gondii isolates from stray dogs from Giza, Egypt. Vet Parasit. 2013;1-3:25–9.
8. Otranto D, Cantacessi C, Pfeffer M, Dantas-Torres F, Brianti E, Deplazes P, Genchi C, Guberti V, Capelli G. The role of wild canids and felids in spreading parasites to dogs and cats in Europe: part I: protozoa and tick-borne agents. Vet Parasitol. 2015;213(1–2):12–23.
9. Dardé ML. Biodiversity in Toxoplasma gondii. Curr Top Microbiol Immunol. 1996;219:27–41.
10. Howe DK, Honore S, Derouin F, Sibley LD. Determination of genotypes T. Gondii strains isolated from patients with toxoplasmosis. J Clin Microbiol. 1997;35:1411–4.
11. Dubey JP, Cortés-Vecino JA, Vargas-Duarte JJ, Sundar N, Velmurugan GV, Bandini LM, Polo LJ, Zambrano L, Mora LE, Kwok OCH, Smith T, Su C. Prevalence of Toxoplasma gondii in dogs from Colombia, South America and genetic characterization of T. Gondii isolates. Vet Parasitol. 2007;145:45–50.
12. Pena HFJ, Gennari SM, Dubey JP, Su C. Population structure and mouse-virulence of Toxoplasma gondii in Brazil Int. J Parasitol. 2008;38:561–9.
13. Rajendran C, Su C, Dubey JP. Molecular genotyping of Toxoplasma gondii from central and South America revealed high diversity within and between populations. Infect Genet Evol. 2012;12(2):359–68.
14. Gebremedhin EZ, Tesfamaryam G, Yunus HA, Duguma R, Tilahun G, DI Marco V, Vitale M. Seroepidemiology of Toxoplasma gondii infection in free-range chickens (Gallus Domesticus) of Central Ethiopia. M Epidemiol Infect. 2014;24:1–10M.
15. Vitale M, Galluzzo P, Currò V, Gozdzik K, Schillaci D, Di Marco Lo Presti V. A high sensitive nested PCR for Toxoplasma gondii detection in animal and food samples. J Microb Biochem Technol. 2013;5:039–41.
16. Fuentes I, Rubio JM, Ramírez C, Alvar J. Genotypic characterization of Toxoplasma gondii strains associated with human toxoplasmosis in Spain: direct analysis from clinical samples. J Clin Microbiol. 2001;39(4):1566–70.
17. Ajzenberg D, Collinet F, Mercier A, Vignoles P, Dardé ML. Genotyping of Toxoplasma gondii isolates with 15 microsatellite markers in a single multiplex PCR assay. J Clin Microbiol. 2010;48:4641–5.
18. D. Ajzenberg, A.L. Bañuls, M. Tibayrenc, M.L. Dardé Microsatellite analysis of Toxoplasma gondii shows considerable polymorphism structured into two main clonal groups Int. J. Parasitol., 32 (2002), pp. 27–38.
19. Robert-Gangneux F, Dardé ML. Epidemiology of and diagnostic strategies for toxoplasmosis. Clin Microbiol Rev. 2012;25:264–96.

3

Emergence of *Brucella suis* in dogs in New South Wales, Australia: clinical findings and implications for zoonotic transmission

Siobhan M. Mor[1,2*], Anke K. Wiethoelter[1], Amanda Lee[3], Barbara Moloney[4], Daniel R. James[5] and Richard Malik[1]

Abstract

Background: Animal reservoirs of brucellosis constitute an ongoing threat to human health globally, with foodborne, occupational and recreational exposures creating opportunities for transmission. In Australia and the United States, hunting of feral pigs has been identified as the principal risk factor for human brucellosis due to *Brucella suis*. Following increased reports of canine *B. suis* infection, we undertook a review of case notification data and veterinary records to address knowledge gaps about transmission, clinical presentation, and zoonotic risks arising from infected dogs.

Results: Between 2011 and 2015, there was a 17-fold increase in the number of cases identified (74 in total) in New South Wales, Australia. Spatial distribution of cases largely overlapped with high feral pig densities in the north of the state. Ninety per cent of dogs had participated directly in pig hunting; feeding of raw feral pig meat and cohabitation with cases in the same household were other putative modes of transmission. Dogs with confirmed brucellosis presented with reproductive tract signs (33 %), back pain (13 %) or lameness (10 %); sub-clinical infection was also common (40 %). Opportunities for dog-to-human transmission in household and occupational environments were identified, highlighting potential public health risks associated with canine *B. suis* infection.

Conclusions: Brucellosis due to *B. suis* is an emerging disease of dogs in Australia. Veterinarians should consider this diagnosis in any dog that presents with reproductive tract signs, back pain or lameness, particularly if the dog has a history of feral pig exposure. Moreover, all people in close contact with these dogs such as hunters, household contacts and veterinary personnel should take precautions to prevent zoonotic transmission.

Keywords: Brucellosis, *Brucella suis*, Dog, Emergence, Zoonosis, Australia

Background

In a recent global review of diseases at the wildlife-livestock interface, brucellosis ranked amongst the top ten diseases [1]. Because the disease is readily transmitted between wildlife, domestic animals and humans, new and re-emerging foci represent an ongoing challenge worldwide with foodborne and occupational exposures to livestock and livestock products recognised as the main traditional risk factors in humans [2]. Increasingly, recreational activities such as hunting of feral animals and wildlife have emerged as an alternative risk factor [3]. Out of

* Correspondence: siobhan.mor@sydney.edu.au
[1]Faculty of Veterinary Science, The University of Sydney, Sydney 2006, NSW, Australia
[2]Tufts University School of Medicine, 145 Harrison Avenue, Boston 02111, MA, USA
Full list of author information is available at the end of the article

the four terrestrial zoonotic *Brucella* species – *B. melitensis*, *B. abortus*, *B. suis*, and *B. canis* – only *B. abortus* and *B. suis* have been frequently found in wildlife [4]. In particular, contact with bison (*Bison bison*), elk (*Cervus elaphus*) or African buffalo (*Syncerus caffer*) as well as reindeer (*Rangifer tarandus*) have been identified as important risk factors for human brucellosis due to *B. abortus* [3, 5, 6] and *B. suis* biovar 4 [7], respectively.

Australia is currently free of many of the human pathogenic *Brucella* species; *B. melitensis* and *B. canis* are exotic and *B. abortus* was eradicated from cattle and buffalo by 1989 [8]. However, *B. suis* biovar 1 is endemic in feral pigs (*Sus scrofa*), and was thought to be limited to east Queensland (QLD) [9–12] until recently when seropositive feral pigs were identified in northern New South Wales (NSW) [13]. Hunting and dressing of carcasses of feral pigs has been associated with human *B.*

suis biovar 1 infections in Australia [14, 15] and the United States (US) [16].

Feral pigs are one of the most successful invasive species worldwide due to their adaptable, highly reproductive and opportunistic omnivore nature [17]. Due to the severely negative impacts on crop and livestock farming as well as wildlife predation and habitat degradation, they are regarded as a threat to biodiversity in Australia. Consequently, land owners in the state of NSW are required by law to institute control measures (e.g. hunting, trapping or poisoning) on their properties [18]. Hunting is also permitted on public land and state forests [19]. An estimated 100–200,000 hunters kill up to 500,000 feral pigs per year in Australia [20] and dogs are widely used to bail, locate and hold feral pigs [21].

Since 2011, a growing number of *B. suis* infections have been reported in dogs in NSW. Prior to 2011, the only published evidence for canine infection in Australia was a single laboratory report citing isolation of *B. suis* from a canine testis in QLD in 1968 [12]. However, sporadic case reports from other countries confirm that dogs can be infected [22–33]. Since *B. suis* biovar 1 is second only to *B. melitensis* in terms of pathogenicity for humans [34], concerns about the potential for dog-to-human transmission in NSW initially led to the recommendation that affected dogs be euthanized [35]. However, knowledge of the natural history of infection, clinical presentation and zoonotic implications of canine *B. suis* infection is meagre and the policy is under review. There is a need for better scientific evidence to underpin sound, risk-based policy responses.

To address these gaps, we documented the epidemiology and clinical findings of canine *B. suis* cases diagnosed between 2011 and 2015. Whether infected dogs pose an ongoing threat to their owners and household contacts and/or other dogs is of principal interest to policy makers. Thus, we examined exposure histories of affected dogs with a view to expanding current understanding of modes of acquisition in dogs. We also reviewed veterinary records to identify opportunities for occupational and household exposure.

Methods

Data on cases notified between 1 January 2011 and 31 December 2015 were obtained from NSW Department of Primary Industries (DPI), which incorporates the State Veterinary Diagnostic Laboratory (SVDL). SVDL is the only veterinary laboratory that performs serological testing for brucellosis in NSW. As a notifiable disease, other laboratories which diagnose cases through other means (e.g. culture) are required to report cases to DPI. To ensure that no cases had been unreported, DPI staff contacted private laboratories to request information on cases they had diagnosed.

Suspect cases were initially screened at SVDL using the sensitive Rose-Bengal agglutination test (RBT). Dogs with RBT agglutination scores of 1+ (low positive) to 3+ (high positive) were subjected to confirmation using the more specific complement fixation test (CFT). A positive case was defined as a dog with positive culture, or positive RBT and reciprocal CFT titre ≥16. Since neither of these serological tests is perfect, dogs with positive RBT, but anti-complimentary CFT or reciprocal CFT titre <16 and history (pig hunting, eating raw feral pig meat, contact with a positive case) and/or indicative clinical signs were considered inconclusive cases. Data accompanying the laboratory records included: date of blood collection, name and location of referring veterinarian, serology results, signalment (gender, breed, age), and history as provided in the laboratory submission form or obtained during follow-up of cases by DPI. In addition, data on the total number of dogs tested were obtained from DPI. Dogs that underwent repeat testing were only counted once. Following preliminary analysis, veterinarians attending cases were contacted and invited to share the full records of affected dogs. Owner details were removed from records to ensure confidentiality. A unique identifier was retained enabling dogs with the same owner to be linked.

To assess temporal trends, the number of dogs tested and positive/inconclusive cases identified annually were plotted in R (v3.1.3, R Foundation, Vienna, Austria) taking into consideration repeat testing of individual animals. Spatial distribution of cases aggregated by town was mapped in ArcMAP (v10; ESRI, Redlands, CA). Data on feral pig density was obtained from DPI surveys conducted in 2009 [36]. To examine transmission pathways at household level, network analysis was performed using the igraph package in R [37]. A cluster was defined as a household that included ≥1 dog that tested positive/inconclusive for *B. suis*.

Demographic and clinical information were extracted from veterinary records, tabulated in Excel and summarized as counts and percentages. Fisher's exact test was used to investigate associations between clinical presentation and signalment. As body temperature was not reliably documented in the majority of cases, we elected not to report on this measurement. We note, however, that fever was not invariably present in dogs for which temperature was recorded. Where absence of other clinical signs was not specifically mentioned in the case notes, these were presumed not to be present. Subclinical cases were defined as cases that did not have any clinical signs consistent with brucellosis but which were reactive on RBT/CFT.

Results

Between 2011 and 2015, 437 unique dogs were tested for brucellosis at SVDL, of which 72 (16.5 %) were seroreactive (46 positive, 26 inconclusive cases). One additional case was notified to DPI but was excluded since the dog resided in QLD. A further case was excluded because it was identified as part of a research study and the dog was not subjected to evaluation sufficient to determine exposure history or clinical status. During follow-up with private laboratories, a further two cases (both positive) were identified. Thus, we present the clinical findings from 74 dogs, diagnosed by either SVDL or private laboratories. Veterinary records and/or additional information were provided by the referring veterinarian for 50 of these 74 cases (67.6 %). Since information on possible incontact animals was not available for the cases diagnosed by private laboratories, assessment of household clustering and potential exposure pathways was limited to the 72 cases diagnosed at SVDL.

Epidemiology and transmission

Figures 1 and 2 show the temporal trend and geographic distribution of cases, respectively. The proportion of positive/inconclusive dogs increased from around 9 % in 2012/13 to 17–22 % in 2014/15. Cases were largely spatialised to northern NSW, where feral pig density is highest.

Forty one discrete clusters were reported to SVDL (Fig. 3). Records revealed linkages across clusters. For example, dogs from different households were sometimes taken on the same hunting trips. Typically, index cases presented with clinical findings consistent with brucellosis or following injuries sustained during pig hunting. Clinical suspicion led to testing of these index cases, confirmation of which led to further testing of incontact animals and detection of sub-clinical cases in the same household. Only three index cases presented sub-clinically; in all cases there was a history of pig hunting and/or feeding of raw feral pig meat. The two earliest clusters in NSW had links to QLD. The first (October 2011) involved a dog that had been pig hunting in QLD. The second (June 2012) involved a dog mated to a female 'pig dog' from QLD 5 weeks earlier. The latter dog was used for pig hunting but had not been hunting in QLD for 4 years.

Potential exposure histories were available for 57/72 cases diagnosed by SVDL (38/41 household clusters). Pig hunting was practiced by 36/38 households and was the most plausible source of infection in 51/57 cases (89.4 %). However, within pig hunting households, not all seroreactive dogs had participated in this activity (Fig. 3: M1, fed raw feral pig meat; O1, no known contact with feral pigs).

Serology was performed on offspring of seroreactive dogs in two pig hunting households. In one household the female (Fig. 3: P1) and male (P2) canine parents tested seropositive and inconclusive, respectively, while the 5-month old offspring tested seronegative. Review of veterinary records revealed that 2 pups from the same litter had been aborted prematurely; the remaining five pups were delivered by caesarean. In the other household, the female (P3) tested seropositive when her offspring were 12 months old; only one of the two offspring (full siblings) was seropositive on subsequent testing. Another dog in this household (M2) was inseminated by a dog that later tested positive (M1), although the former was found to be seronegative on subsequent testing.

Pig hunting status was not known for the three remaining household clusters. In two of these clusters, index cases had a history of being fed raw feral pig meat (Fig. 3: M3, M4) and were the only seropositive cases detected in these households. The remaining dog (O2) had no known contact with feral pigs or infected dogs and was not fed raw feral pig meat according to the current owner, although this dog was adopted from a pound and exposure history prior to this was unobtainable.

Clinical presentation and outcome in dogs

Tables 1 and 2 show the signalment and clinical presentation of dogs, respectively. The median age of affected dogs was 2 years (range 5 months to 12 years). There were no clear relationships between age and clinical presentation, with dogs aged ≤24 months just as likely to present with certain clinical signs as those aged >24 months ($p > 0.05$ for all signs). De-sexed dogs were more likely than reproductively intact animals to present with back pain (50 % versus 10.3 %; $p = 0.074$) and lameness (50 % versus 7.4 %, $p = 0.045$), while females were more likely than males to be sub-clinically affected (53.6 % versus 31.8 %, $p = 0.087$). No other significant associations existed between gender, reproductive status and specific signs. Dogs with clinical

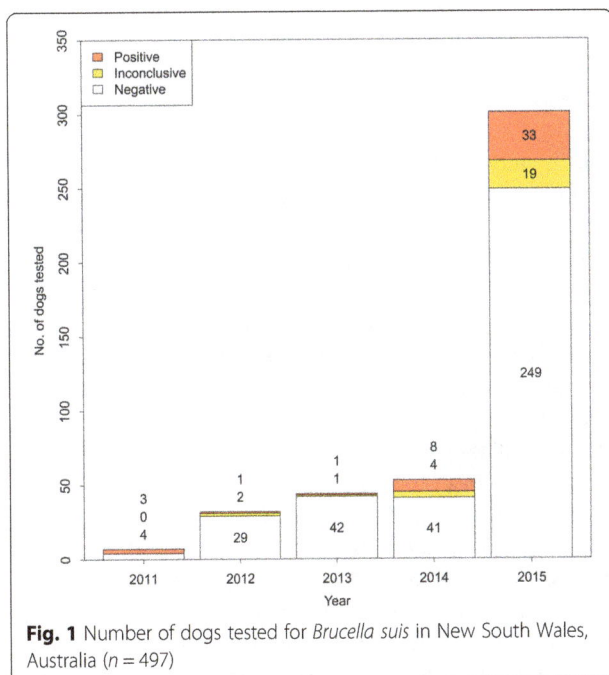

Fig. 1 Number of dogs tested for Brucella suis in New South Wales, Australia ($n = 497$)

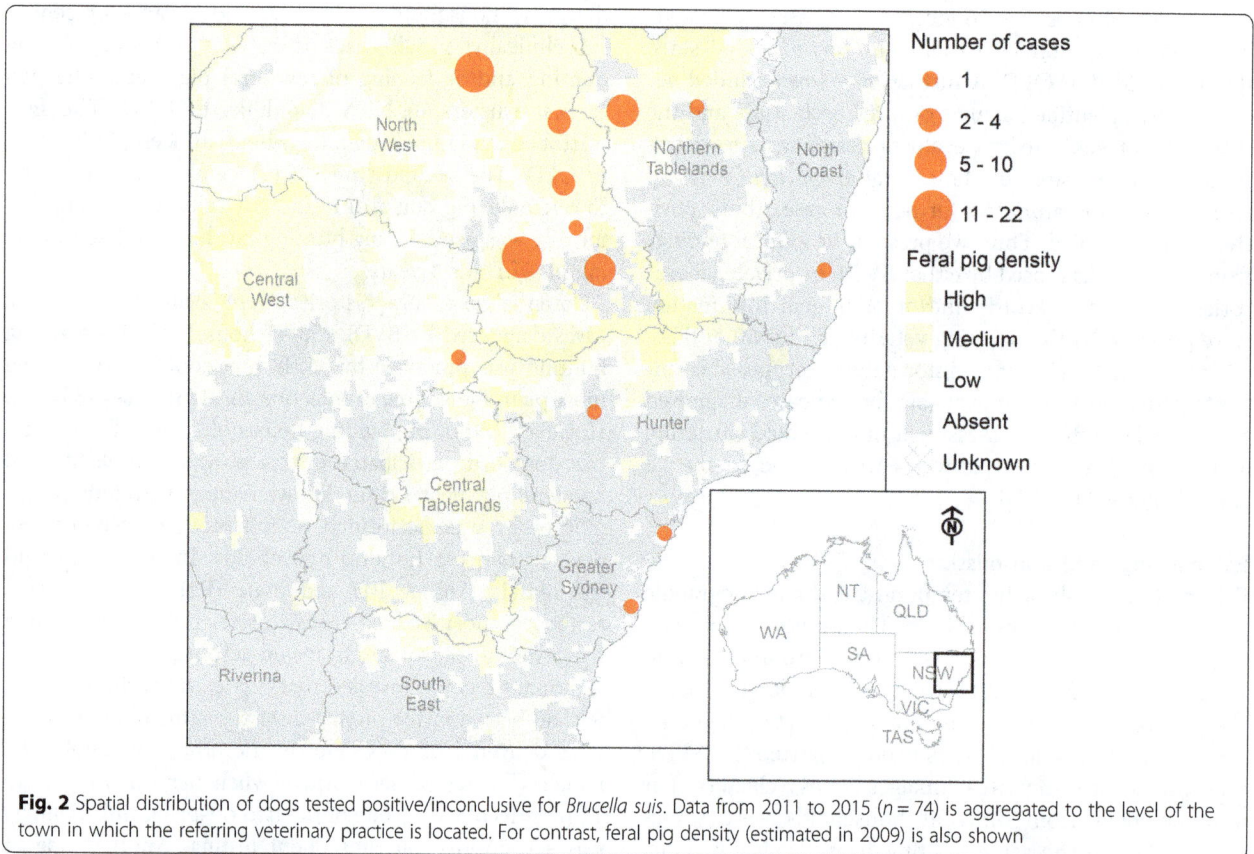

Fig. 2 Spatial distribution of dogs tested positive/inconclusive for *Brucella suis*. Data from 2011 to 2015 (*n* = 74) is aggregated to the level of the town in which the referring veterinary practice is located. For contrast, feral pig density (estimated in 2009) is also shown

signs were just as likely as dogs without clinical signs to have an inconclusive sero-status (35 % versus 37.5 %, *p* = 1.0).

Signs consistent with reproductive tract involvement were the most common presenting problem and occurred across a range of ages (1–9 years). Among 21 dogs with orchitis/epididymitis, presentation was unilateral in 12 cases and bilateral in eight (one unspecified). Serology conducted on one female at the time of abortion was negative; retesting 8 months later however showed an inconclusive result.

Nine dogs presented with back pain, four of which also presented with intermittent lameness, while one presented with concurrent reproductive tract signs. Back pain was mostly localized to the thoracolumbar junction (five out of six cases). Two dogs were diagnosed with discospondylitis with localized empyema adjacent to affected vertebrae. While there was no bacterial growth following culture of cerebrospinal fluid, *B. suis* was cultured from soft tissue material collected during decompressive hemilaminectomy in both animals.

Three dogs presented with lameness without back pain. In one case (Bull-Mastiff, 22 months), the dog presented with a history of shifting lameness and swollen joints followed by an acute episode of dyspnoea. A large, oedematous mass cranial to the larynx was palpable and considered to be impeding airflow. Generalised lymphadenomegaly was also evident and unilateral orchitis/epididymitis and pyrexia developed one week later. The dog was castrated and euthanised following culture of *B. suis* biovar 1 from the affected testis. A second dog (Kelpie X, 33 months) presented with painful, dorsally-swollen left carpus. *B. suis* biovar 1 was cultured from joint fluid collected from the inter-carpal joint.

Public health considerations

In two separate clusters, veterinary records indicated that the dogs' owner had been diagnosed with brucellosis prior to presentation of the dog. Both households practiced pig hunting. Other potentially risky practices identified from veterinary records included assistance with whelping and on-sale of live-born offspring prior to diagnosis in the parent dogs. A woman in at least two households was reported as being pregnant at the time of canine diagnosis.

Opportunities for potential occupational exposure were noted in records of several cases. Four dogs were de-sexed during the episode of illness as part of clinical management of reproductive tract signs, while two underwent spinal surgery. Infection status of these dogs was unknown at the time of the procedure, and thus the surgical teams are presumed to have taken no special

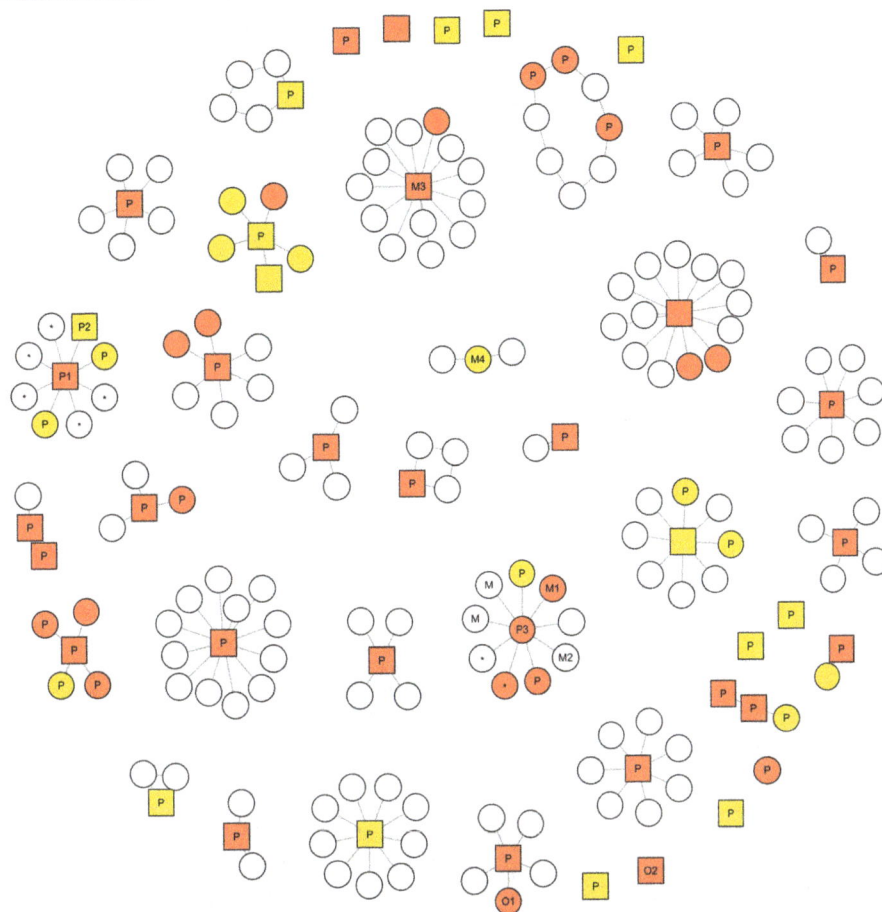

Fig. 3 Network analysis of canine *Brucella suis* cases in New South Wales, Australia. Positive (*red*), inconclusive (*orange*) and negative (*white*) dogs clustered within the same household. Index cases and in-contact dogs appear as hub and spoke, while dogs presenting simultaneously appear as other formations. Dogs with and without clinical signs are depicted as squares and circles, respectively. Relevant exposure histories are shown where known (P = pig hunting, M = fed raw feral pig meat, * = offspring of seropositive dog(s), O = other exposure history). See main text for further description of individual animals (P1, P2, P3, M1, M2, M3, M4, O1 and O2)

precautionary measures to minimise the risk of infection. Likewise, bacterial culture was performed by unsuspecting laboratory staff involved in the diagnosis of two cases.

Discussion

This article comprises the largest and most detailed compilation of canine *B. suis* cases reported to date. Previous cases have been recorded in Bulgaria [31], Brazil [25, 28, 29], Germany [27], Hungary [26], India [23] and the US [22, 24, 30, 32]. Many of these were documented in the mid-20th century when commercial piggeries constituted the main reservoir of *B. suis* biovar 1. With eradication having been achieved in many of these countries, infection dynamics have shifted considerably, as have exposure risks [16].

We observed a 17-fold increase in the number of canine cases detected in NSW between 2011 and 2015. A similar trend has been documented in Georgia, US in association with recreational pig hunting activities [22]. The extent to which this increase reflects true emergence versus enhanced detection of previously unrecognized foci of infection is unclear. Certainly awareness for the disease is growing in NSW, as evidenced by the increasing number of dogs presented for testing. However, the incursion of seropositive feral pigs in NSW lends biological plausibility to a novel source of infection, a finding supported by the high degree of spatial overlap between feral pigs and canine cases reported here. We suspect *B. suis* was introduced following deliberate transportation of feral pigs across state borders by recreational hunters, a practice which is illegal but, anecdotally, widely practiced [20]. Natural migration of infected feral pigs across the NSW-QLD border is also likely [13]. Movements of up to 12 km per day as well as swimming across rivers and off coastlines have been observed in feral pigs and seem to be largely driven by external factors such as human

Table 1 Signalment of dogs diagnosed with *Brucella suis* in New South Wales, Australia (*n* = 74)

Characteristic	Positive (*n* = 48) No. (%)	Inconclusive (*n* = 26) No. (%)
Age		
≤24 months	16 (33)	6 (23)
>24 months	26 (54)	18 (69)
Unknown	6 (13)	2 (8)
Gender		
Male intact	26 (54)	16 (62)
Male de-sexed	1 (2)	1 (4)
Female intact	17 (35)	9 (35)
Female de-sexed	2 (4)	0
Unknown	2 (4)	0
Breed		
Boxer/Boxer X[a]	5 (10)	0
Bull Arab/Bull Arab X	11 (23)	5 (19)
Bull Mastiff/Bull Mastiff X	9 (19)	6 (23)
Cattle dog/Collie/Kelpie	5 (10)	3 (12)
Wolfhound/Wolfhound X	2 (4)	4 (15)
Pig dog, unspecified breed	6 (13)	5 (19)
Other[b]	8 (17)	3 (12)
Unknown	2 (4)	0

Cases from 2011 to 2015 (*n* = 74) are presented
[a]X - cross-breed
[b]Other includes: Great Dane/Great Dane X (*n* = 3), Bull Terrier/Bull Terrier X (2), Catahoula (1), Dachshund (1), Jack Russell Terrier (1), Staffordshire Terrier (1), Staghound (1), and cross-bred, breeds unspecified (1)

Table 2 Clinical presentation of dogs diagnosed with *Brucella suis* in New South Wales, Australia (*n* = 74)

Clinical presentation	Positive (*n* = 48) No. (%)	Inconclusive (*n* = 26) No. (%)
Sub-clinical infection[a]	19 (40)	12 (46)
Male	8 (30)	6 (35)
Female	9 (47)	6 (67)
Reproductive tract signs[b]	14 (33)	11 (44)
Orchitis/epididymitis[c]	12 (46)	9 (56)
History of abortion[c]	2 (12)	2 (22)
Lethargy/'off-colour'	13 (27)	8 (31)
Discospondylitis/ back pain	6 (13)	3 (12)
Intact	4 (9)	3 (12)
De-sexed	2 (67)	0
Lameness	5 (10)	2 (8)
Intact	3 (7)	2 (8)
De-sexed	2 (67)	0
Other[d]	7 (15)	4 (15)

Cases from 2011 to 2015 (*n* = 74) are presented. Denominators are adjusted for gender and reproductive status, where applicable
[a]Gender of two sub-clinically affected dogs was unknown (see Table 1)
[b]Reproductively intact animals only (see Table 1)
[c]Other includes: superficial abscess (*n* = 4), haematuria (2), prostatitis (2), vomiting (2), weight loss (2), lymphoadenomegaly (2), suppurative endometritis (1)

disturbance, weather conditions, food and habitat availability [38].

Given co-occurrence of exposures in the same households and potential for casual contact between dogs (e.g. through sharing feed bowls), it is difficult to draw definitive conclusions about transmission. Direct involvement in pig hunting was the most plausible mode of transmission for the majority (90 %) of dogs, while feeding of raw feral pig meat resulted in infection of dogs not involved directly with hunting. Evidence for vertical transmission was limited in cases reported here, although we presume it occurs by extrapolation from other *Brucella* spp. [39]. Pig-to-dog transmission of *B. suis* through hunting or co-habitation with domestic pigs has been reported [22, 28]. Precisely how dogs acquire the infection from pigs is not known. Given the nature of pig hunting – which involves a high frequency of injuries to both animals and humans – we suspect transfer likely occurs through blood-borne contact and/or direct inoculation by contamination of wounds, transmission via mucous membranes or via ingestion of pig offal or meat. Ingestion of aborted foetal material has also been proposed [27]. A number of dogs in this study presented for

treatment of sub-cutaneous abscesses most likely sustained as a result of pig hunting. Cutaneous lesions due to *B. suis* have been described in humans [40] and may be consistent with traumatic inoculation at these sites.

Little is published on the risk of foodborne transmission of *B. suis* biovar 1 via meat, although the first canine case was linked to this practice [33]. Further, Hellmann and Sprenger [27] postulated that raw pet food obtained from Eastern European countries was the likely source of infection for dogs in Germany. The likelihood that *B. suis* may be transmitted via feral pig meat has implications for human and animal health. At one time Australia supplied as much as 30 % of wild boar meat consumed globally, with a smaller quantity being sold domestically and by-products/substandard carcasses used as pet food [41]. Proper cooking and/or canning will destroy *Brucella* spp., thus the main risk comes from handling and consumption of undercooked meat [42]. Raw pet food diets are becoming popular in Australia and elsewhere, and concerns have been raised following detection of a number of zoonotic foodborne hazards in raw pet food [43, 44]. We are not aware of any studies that have specifically tested commercial raw food diets for *B. suis* in Australia or elsewhere.

It is generally assumed that hunters acquire brucellosis following direct contact with blood and other fluids and/or aerosols during field slaughter of feral pigs [14, 42]. Risk reduction strategies have therefore focused on preventing transmission at slaughter, including promoting use of personal protective clothing, such as mesh gloves to prevent abrasions and cuts to the hands [45]. The extent to which infected dogs present an ongoing risk to humans in the household is unknown but plausible in the view of the authors. A single 1967 case report found that a woman in Massachusetts most likely acquired *B. suis* following unprotected disposal of aborted dog foetuses [30]. The dog, which was confirmed at necropsy to be infected, had been allowed to roam freely and likely acquired the infection from a swine farm nearby. Other case reports have implicated dogs as the source of human infection with *B. abortus* [46], *B. canis* [47, 48], and *B. melitensis* [49, 50], establishing that pathogen excretion and/or contact sufficient to lead to human infection can occur.

In reviewing veterinary records, opportunities for human exposure through contact with body fluids within a household environment (e.g. aborted foetuses, placenta) as well as occupational exposure of veterinary staff via routine (e.g. diagnostic specimen collection and processing, castration and ovariohysterectomy) and advanced procedures (e.g. spinal surgery) were identified. High speed burr was used in the latter case, increasing risk of aerosolisation. Veterinary staff should be encouraged to adopt strict precautions, including use of masks, gloves and eye shields when handling dogs with a history of pig hunting. Further, following presumptive diagnosis by serology, preliminary antimicrobial therapy may make subsequent surgery less hazardous by reducing viability of organisms in vivo. We also recommend that specimens collected from pig hunting dogs be clearly identified as such, so that laboratory staff can perform subsequent manipulations under safe conditions even if specimens are not specifically tested for brucellosis. Finally, we advise that pregnant women (in the household and in the workplace) should avoid contact with hunting dogs.

Dogs with brucellosis presented with one of three syndromes consistent with involvement of the reproductive tract, axial skeleton or appendicular skeleton, although combinations were possible also. Reproductive tract involvement is recognized as a clinical feature of brucellosis in a number of animal species, including dogs [25, 27, 29, 33]. Discospondylitis due to *B. suis* has also been previously described in one dog [24] and spondylitis is a well-known complication of *B. suis* infections in humans [51]. The detailed clinical findings and successful treatment of one discospondylitis case reported here (Fig. 3: O2) as well as two orchitis cases is described elsewhere (James et al. 2016, *in review*). We found that dogs that had been de-sexed were more likely to present with back pain and/or lameness than reproductively intact animals, suggesting that *B. suis* may display tropism for bones or joints when the preferred site (reproductive tract) is not present.

A considerable number of dogs without clinical signs were reactive on RBT/CFT and were presumed to be sub-clinically infected. These cases present a particular challenge in terms of detection and clinical management. Sub-clinical infection has been reported in both naturally occurring [26] and experimental infections in dogs [52]. The finding that females were more likely to be sub-clinically infected may reflect a bias towards detection in males, with owners more likely to recognize and investigate enlarged testes. Alternatively, veterinary records may have failed to adequately document a history of abortion in healthy female dogs that present later for testing. Given the high frequency of sub-clinical infection, regular testing of pig hunting dogs and in-contact animals, particularly prior to invasive surgeries or breeding, is advised.

This study has a number of limitations. Clinical and exposure histories were limited for some dogs, making conclusions about source of infection and onset of illness difficult in these cases. Further, the location and timing of hunting trips was not disclosed. Such information would be useful in guiding surveillance and control activities in the feral pig population, as well as updating knowledge on incubation period in dogs. Diagnosis remains a particular challenge with a number of dogs deemed to have inconclusive serological results. To our knowledge, necropsy was not performed on any dog after euthanasia nor was sequential serology performed on animals that were not euthanised (with exception of the case described by James et al., *in review*). Culture is the gold standard for diagnosing brucellosis but was not pursued in the majority of cases. The sensitivity and specificity of the serological tests used has not been determined, nor is it known whether seropositive cases are actively infected or rather previously exposed but with elimination of all foci of disease. This distinction has major implications for evaluating public health risks associated with canine infection and, for this reason, molecular-based methods are being pursued by DPI.

Conclusions

In conclusion, brucellosis is an emerging disease of dogs in NSW with the principal risk being involvement in feral pig hunting. Veterinarians should consider this diagnosis in any dog that presents with reproductive tract signs, back pain or lameness, particularly if the dog has a history of feral pig exposure. The extent to which infected dogs present an ongoing risk to humans and/or other dogs in the household is unknown but plausible. Therefore all people in close contact with infected dogs such as hunters, household contacts and veterinary personnel should take precautions to prevent zoonotic transmission. More research into the natural history of infection and treatment is needed to formulate more evidenced-based advice on clinical management of infected dogs.

Acknowledgments

The authors wish to thank Kelli Johnson and Sally Spence (NSW DPI) for assistance with the canine data and Peter West (NSW DPI) for sharing data on feral pigs from NSW DPI pest surveys. Richard Malik's position is supported by the Valentine Charlton Bequest to the Centre for Veterinary Education.

Funding

None.

Authors' contribution

SM coordinated the case series, planned the study design, conducted the data analysis and drafted the manuscript; AW contributed to the study design, reviewed the literature and drafted the manuscript; AL, BM, DJ and RM provided case data, contributed to the study design and revised the manuscript. All authors read and approved the final manuscript.

Authors' information

SM is a public health epidemiologist and veterinarian-researcher based at The University of Sydney. Her interests include emerging zoonoses, and informing evidence-based practices to controlling the same.

Competing interests

The authors declare that they have no competing interests.

Consent for publication

Not applicable.

Author details

[1]Faculty of Veterinary Science, The University of Sydney, Sydney 2006, NSW, Australia. [2]Tufts University School of Medicine, 145 Harrison Avenue, Boston 02111, MA, USA. [3]New South Wales Department of Primary Industries, Woodbridge Road, Menangle 2568, NSW, Australia. [4]New South Wales Department of Primary Industries, 161 Kite Street, Orange 2800, NSW, Australia. [5]Small Animal Specialist Hospital, 1 Richardson Place, North Ryde 2113, NSW, Australia.

References

1. Wiethoelter AK, Beltran-Alcrudo D, Kock R, Mor SM. Global trends in infectious diseases at the wildlife-livestock interface. Proc Natl Acad Sci U S A. 2015;112(31):9662–7.
2. Seleem MN, Boyle SM, Sriranganathan N. Brucellosis: a re-emerging zoonosis. Vet Microbiol. 2010;140(3-4):392–8.
3. Godfroid J, Cloeckaert A, Liautard JP, Kohler S, Fretin D, Walravens K, Garin-Bastuji B, Letesson JJ. From the discovery of the Malta fever's agent to the discovery of a marine mammal reservoir, brucellosis has continuously been a re-emerging zoonosis. Vet Res. 2005;36(3):313–26.
4. Godfroid J, Garin-Bastuji B, Saegerman C, Blasco JM. Brucellosis in terrestrial wildlife. Rev - Off Int Epizoot. 2013;32(1):27–42.
5. Alexander KA, Blackburn JK, Vandewalle ME, Pesapane R, Baipoledi EK, Elzer PH. Buffalo, bush meat, and the zoonotic threat of brucellosis in Botswana. PLoS One. 2012;7(3):e32842.
6. Rhyan JC, Nol P, Quance C, Gertonson A, Belfrage J, Harris I, Straka K, Robbe-Austerman S. Transmission of brucellosis from elk to cattle and bison, Greater Yellowstone area, U.S.A., 2002-2012. Emerging Infect Dis. 2013;19(12):1992–5.
7. Hueffer K, Parkinson AJ, Gerlach R, Berner J. Zoonotic infections in Alaska: disease prevalence, potential impact of climate change and recommended actions for earlier disease detection, research, prevention and control. Int J Circumpolar Health. 2013;72:19562.
8. Animal Health Australia. Animal Health in Australia 2014. Canberra: Animal Health Australia; 2015.
9. Mason RJ, Fleming PJ. Serological survey for Brucella antibodies in feral pigs from eastern Australia. Aust Vet J. 1999;77(5):331–2.
10. Crichton R, Medveczky NE. The identity, distribution and epizootiological significance of Brucella isolates in Australia, 1981 to 1985. Aust Vet J. 1987; 64(2):48–52.
11. Norton TH, Thomas AD. Brucella suis in feral pigs. Aust Vet J. 1976;52(6):293–4.
12. Aldrick SJ. Typing of Brucella strains from Australia and Papua-New Guinea received by the regional WHO Brucellosis Centre. Aust Vet J. 1968;44:130–3.
13. Ridoutt C, Lee A, Moloney B, Massey P, Charman N, Jordan D. Detection of brucellosis and leptospirosis in feral pigs in New South Wales. Aust Vet J. 2014;92(9):343–7.
14. Eales KM, Norton RE, Ketheesan N. Brucellosis in northern Australia. Am J Trop Med Hyg. 2010;83(4):876–8.
15. Irwin MJ, Massey PD, Walker B, Durrheim DN. Feral pig hunting: a risk factor for human brucellosis in north-west NSW? N S W Public Health Bull. 2009; 20(11-12):192–4.
16. CDC. Brucella suis infection associated with feral swine hunting - three states, 2007-2008. MMRW. 2009;58(22):618–21.
17. Bevins SN, Pedersen K, Lutman MW, Gidlewski T, Deliberto TJ. Consequences associated with the recent range expansion of nonnative feral swine. Bioscience. 2014;64(4):291–9.
18. NSW Government. Rural Lands Protection (Feral pigs) Pest Control Order. 2011.
19. NSW Government. Game and Feral Animal Control Regulation. 2012.
20. Tisdell CA. Wild pigs: environmental pest or economic resource? 1st ed. Sydney: Pergamon Press; 1982.
21. Sparkes J, Ballard G, Fleming PJS. Cooperative hunting between humans and domestic dogs in eastern and northern Australia. Wildl Res. 2016;43(1):20.
22. Ramamoorthy S, Woldemeskel M, Ligett A, Snider R, Cobb R, Rajeev S. Brucella suis infection in dogs, Georgia, USA. Emerg Infect Dis. 2011;17(12):2386–7.
23. Thanappa Pillai M, Nedunchelliyan S, Raghavan N. Brucellosis in a dog caused by Brucella suis biovar 1 in Madras. Cherion. 1990;19(2):97–8.
24. Barr SC, Eilts BE, Roy AF, Miller R. Brucella suis biotype 1 infection in a dog. J Am Vet Med Assoc. 1986;189(6):686–7.
25. Correa WM, Correa CNM, Iamaguti P. Canine brucellosis by Brucella suis-1, atypical. Arq Bras Med Vet Zoot. 1984;36(4):397–405.
26. Koermendy B, Nagy G. The supposed involvement of dogs carrying Brucella suis in the spread of swine brucellosis. Acta Vet Acad Sci Hung. 1982;30(1-3):3–7.
27. Hellmann E, Sprenger HU. Brucella suis infection in dogs. Berl Muench Tieraerztl Wochenschr. 1978;91(19):385–7.
28. de Miranda JCB, Sei VLB, Sandoval LA, Teruya JM. Isolation of Brucella suis in an infected pig herd, with involvement of dog and man. Biol. 1978;44(9): 205–10.
29. Gomes OG, Portugal MASC, Giorgi W, Franca EN. Brucella suis biotype 1 infection in a dog. Arq Inst Biol (Sao Paulo). 1972;39(4):251–5.
30. Nicoletti PL, Quinn BR, Minor PW. Canine to human transmission of brucellosis. N Y State J Med. 1967;67:2886–7.
31. Pavlov P, Krastev V, Matev M, Milanov M, Tatarov B, Tschilev D. Recherches sur les reservoirs de Brucella chez le porc vivant en liberte. Bull Off Int Epizoot. 1960;53:1511–26.
32. Nolan AF. A sporadic case of brucellosis in the dog. Cornell Vet. 1940;30:542–5.
33. Planz JF, Huddleson IF. Brucella infection in a dog. J Am Vet Med Assoc. 1931;79:251–2.
34. Woldemeskel M. Zoonosis due to Bruella suis with special reference to infection in dogs (Carnivores): A brief review. Open J Vet Med. 2013;03(03): 213–21.
35. Brucellosis (Brucella suis) in dogs. http://www.dpi.nsw.gov.au/__data/assets/ pdf_file/0007/577411/information-sheet-brucellosis-in-dogs.pdf. Accessed 15 July 2016.
36. Feral pig density. http://www.dpi.nsw.gov.au/agriculture/pests-weeds/ vertebrate-pests/distribution-maps-for-vertebrate-pests. Accessed 11 Mar 2016.
37. Csardi G, Nepusz T. The igraph software package for complex network research. InterJournal. 2006;Complex Systems:1695.
38. Morelle K, Podgórski T, Prévot C, Keuling O, Lehaire F, Lejeune P. Towards understanding wild boar Sus scrofa movement: a synthetic movement ecology approach. Mamm Rev. 2014;45:15–29.

39. Diaz AE. Epidemiology of brucellosis in domestic animals caused by *Brucella melitensis*, *Brucella suis*, and *Brucella abortus*. Rev - Off Int Epizoot. 2013;32(1): 53–60.

40. Christianson HB, Pankey GA, Applewhite ML. Ulcers of skin due to *Brucella suis*. Report of a case. Arch Dermatol. 1968;98(2):175–6.

41. Ramsay BJ. Commercial use of wild animals in Australia. 1st ed. Canberra: Australian Government Publishing Service; 1994.

42. Gibbs EPJ. The public health risks associated with wild and feral swine. Rev - Off Int Epizoot. 1997;16(2):594–8.

43. Nemser SM, Doran T, Grabenstein M, McConnell T, McGrath T, Pamboukian R, Smith AC, Achen M, Danzeisen G, Kim S, et al. Investigation of *Listeria*, *Salmonella*, and toxigenic *Escherichia coli* in various pet foods. Foodborne Pathog Dis. 2014;11(9):706–9.

44. Mehlenbacher S, Churchill J, Olsen KE, Bender JB. Availability, brands, labelling and *Salmonella* contamination of raw pet food in the Minneapolis/ St. Paul area. Zoonoses Public Health. 2012;59(7):513–20.

45. Massey P, Polkinghorne B, Durrheim D, Lower T, Speare R. Blood, guts and knife cuts: reducing the risk of swine brucellosis in feral pig hunters in north- west New South Wales, Australia. Rural Remote Health. 2011;11(4):1793.

46. Feldman WH, Mann FC, Olson CJ. The spontaneous occurrence of *Brucella* agglutinins in dogs. J Infect Dis. 1935;56(1):55–63.

47. Dentinger CM, Jacob K, Lee LV, Mendez HA, Chotikanatis K, McDonough PL, Chico DM, De BK, Tiller RV, Traxler RM, et al. Human *Brucella canis* infection and subsequent laboratory exposures associated with a puppy, New York City, 2012. Zoonoses Public Health. 2015;62(5):407–14.

48. Lucero NE, Corazza R, Almuzara MN, Reynes E, Escobar GI, Boeri E, Ayala SM. Human *Brucella canis* outbreak linked to infection in dogs. Epidemiol Infect. 2010;138(2):280–5.

49. Ostertag HG, Mayer H. Verbreitung der Schafbrucellose bei Herdenhunden. Rindertuberkulose und Brucellose. 1958;7:57–70.

50. Dargein P. Relation d'une épidémie de mélitococcie. Bull Mem Soc Med Hop Paris. 1922;46:1373–7.

51. Kelly PJ, Martin WJ, Schirger A, Weed LA. Brucellosis of the bones and joints. J Am Med Assoc. 1960;174(4):347–53.

52. Feldman WH, Bollmann JL, Olson CJ. Experimental brucellosis in dogs. J Infect Dis. 1935;56:321–32.

4

First clinical case report of *Cytauxzoon* sp. infection in a domestic cat in France

Jean-Pierre Legroux[1], Lénaïg Halos[2]*, Magalie René-Martellet[3,4], Marielle Servonnet[2], Jean-Luc Pingret[5], Gilles Bourdoiseau[3,4], Gad Baneth[6] and Luc Chabanne[3,4]

Abstract

Background: Feline cytauxzoonosis is an emerging infection caused by tick-transmitted apicomplexan parasites of the genus *Cytauxzoon*. The association of clinical disease with *Cytauxzoon* infection appears to be limited to *C. felis* infections in the Americas. Sporadic infections of wild and domestic felids with *Cytauxzoon* sp. were recently described in European countries but clinical reports of the infection are rare and incomplete. This case report brings new interesting information on cytauxzoonosis expression in Europe.

Case presentation: A 9-years-old castrated European shorthair cat living in rural area of north-eastern France (Saint Sauveur, Bourgogne-Franche-Comté region), without any travel history was presented for consultation due to hyperthermia, anorexia, depression and prolonged fever that didn't respond to antibiotic therapy. The cat had outdoor access with a history of vagrancy and was adequately vaccinated (core vaccines and FeLV vaccine). During biological investigations, intraerythrocytic inclusions were observed on blood smear and were further investigated by PCR analysis and sequencing. Molecular analyses confirmed *Cytauxzoon* sp. infection. The cat was treated with a subcutaneous injection of imidocarb dipropionate (3.5 mg/kg). One week after treatment, the cat improved clinically, although parasitic inclusions within erythrocytes persisted, and only a mild lymphocytosis was found. Two weeks after treatment, the cat appeared in excellent health, appetite was normal and parasitemia was negative. However, one month after treatment the cat relapsed with hyperthermia, anorexia, and depression. Blood smears and PCR were once again positive. Subsequently, the cat received an additional dose of imidocarb dipropionate (3.5 mg/kg SC) and recovered rapidly without other clinical signs. Two weeks after the second imidocarb injection, the cat was hit by a car and died.

Conclusion: This case provides the first clinical description of infection by *Cytauxzoon* sp. in a domestic cat in France. These findings support the fact that cytauxzoonosis should be considered in the differential diagnosis of acute febrile illness which does not respond to antibiotic in cats with outdoor access especially in areas where populations of wild felids are present.

Keywords: Case report, *Cytauxzoon* sp., Cat, Feline piroplasmosis, Acute febrile illness, Persistent parasitemia

Background

Feline cytauxzoonosis is an emerging infectious disease with an expanding geographic distribution caused by tick-borne apicomplexan parasites of the genus *Cytauxzoon*. Cytauxzoonosis was first identified in 1973 as the cause of mortality in domestic cats in Missouri, USA [1].

Cytauxzoon or *Cytauxzoon*-like parasites have been reported in various domestic and wild felids throughout the World [2, 3]. *Cytauxzoon felis* is considered as the main agent of the disease in domestic cats, mostly described in USA. *Dermacentor variabilis* and *Amblyomma americanum* have been shown to be the tick vectors of this pathogen [4, 5]. *C. felis* is responsible for a severe, often fatal disease associating clinical signs such as anemia, depression, anorexia, vomiting, icterus, splenomegaly, hepatomegaly and high fever [6].

However, with rare exceptions, the recognition of clinical disease caused by parasites of the genus *Cytauxzoon* appears limited to *C. felis* infections in the Americas.

* Correspondence: Lenaig.HALOS@Merial.com
[2]Merial, Lyon, France
Full list of author information is available at the end of the article

Sporadic infections of wild and domestic felids with a new and genetically distinct species described as "*Cytauxzoon* sp." were reported in European countries such as Spain [7–11], France [11], Italy [12–14], Portugal [15], and Romania [16], but reports presenting clinical expression of the infection are rare and incomplete. *Cytauxzoon* sp. in Europe seems less virulent than *C. felis* and it was suggested that disease associated with it could develop preferentially in case of concurrent disease or immunodeficiency [12]. Hemolytic anemia, lethargy, fever, anorexia, weight loss, diarrhea and vomiting were occasionally described in association with *Cytauxzoon* sp. infection [12, 13, 15]. A high rate of asymptomatic carriage of *Cytauxzoon* sp. in domestic cats was reported in a study conducted in Northern Italy [12]. In France, a previous study reported the case of a cat found co-infected with *Hepatozoon canis* and *Cytauxzoon* sp. The agents were molecularly characterized but no information on the epidemiology, clinical history, clinical course of infection and therapy was available [11]. Consequently, knowledge on the epidemiology, risk factors and clinical course of infection of felids with *Cytauxzoon* sp. in European countries and in particular in France is still unclear and needs further investigation. This study provides the first clinical description of infection by *Cytauxzoon* sp. in a domestic cat in France.

Case presentation
Clinical history
A 9-years-old neutered male European shorthair cat weighting 6 kg and living in a rural area (Saint Sauveur, France: 47°48′N, 6°23′E), without any travel history was presented to consultation for lethargy, anorexia, hemorrhagic diarrhea, and abdominal pain. The cat had permanent outdoor access and was vaccinated against feline panleukopenia, viral rhinotracheitis, calicivirus and feline leukemia virus.

Two weeks before consultation, the cat came back from 4 days vagrancy with hyperthermia (41 °C), lethargy, anorexia, dehydration and weight loss. The cat didn't recover within the following 15 days despite antibiotic therapy of amoxicillin and clavulanic acid at 10 mg and 2.5 mg/kg respectively (Clavaseptin, Vetoquinol) administered orally every 12 h for 10 days.

Clinical findings and investigation (Table 1)
Clinical examination showed hyperthermia (40.5 °C), abdominal pain and subcutaneous hematomas on the abdomen. Sepsis resulting from a possible fight during vagrancy was suspected and subcutaneous injections of marbofloxacin (Marbocyl, Vetoquinol, 2 mg/kg) and carprofen (Rimadyl, Zoetis, 4 mg/kg) were performed followed by marbofloxacin (Marbocyl, Vetoquinol) 2 mg/

Table 1 Timeline table of the information of the case report

Day (D)	Findings		Treatment
	Clinical observation	Clinical investigation	
D-14	Clinical history: hyperthermia (41 °C), lethargy, anorexia, dehydration and weight loss after 4 days vagrancy		amoxicillin (10 mg/kg) + clavulanic acid (2.5 mg/kg) orally every 12 h for 10 days.
D0	hyperthermia (40.5 °C), abdominal pain and subcutaneous hematomas on the abdomen		marbofloxacin (2 mg/kg) and carprofen (4 mg/kg) marbofloxacin (2 mg/kg PO once daily for 10 days
D7 to D29		neutrophilic leukocytosis at the complete blood counts (CBC), biochemical, serological and molecular analyses for different infectious disease: all negative Abdominal, pulmonary and oral X-ray: normal except a marked splenomegaly oropharyngeal swab for the detection of calicivirus and feline herpes virus were conducted	meloxicam 0.05 mg/kg PO once daily for 5 days
D29	no clinical improvement vomiting, stomatitis, abdomen pain, hyperthermia, anorexia, severe depression	Stained blood smear of peripheral blood: small inclusions within erythrocytes PCR identification of *Cytauxzoon* sp.	imidocarb dipropionate 3.5 mg/kg/ subcutaneous injection).
Day 37	Clinical improvement	Inclusions present in the blood smear	
Day 46	Excellent general conditions	No more inclusions in the blood smear	
Day 63	Relapse: hyperthermia, anorexia depression and stomatitis	Inclusions present in the blood smear PCR positive for *Cytauxzoon* sp.	imidocarb dipropionate 3.5 mg/kg/ subcutaneous injection).
Day 69	Clinical recovery	hypergammaglobulinemia with hyperproteinemia (91 g/L; reference range: 57 – 94 g/L) with an hematocrit at the lower limit of the reference range (28 L/L; reference range: 28 – 45). Absence of inclusion in the blood smear	
Day 76	Death by car accident		

kg PO once daily for 10 days and meloxicam (Metacam, Boehringer Ingelheim) at 0.05 mg/kg PO once daily for 5 days for pain and fever relief.

The cat was rechecked 29 days later. The owner reported no clinical improvement despite proper administration of the treatment and subsequent vomiting, stomatitis, cranial right abdomen pain, hyperthermia, anorexia and severe depression were noticed. The cat was hospitalized and received symptomatic treatment against vomiting (maropitant, Cerenia, Zoetis, SC injection, 1 mg/kg) as well as a corticosteroid (dexamethasone tebutate, Dexamedium, MSD, SC injection, 0.1 mg/kg) and antibiotics (amoxicillin, Duphamox LA, Zoetis, SC injection, 15 mg/kg every other day for 1 week, followed by cefovecine, Convenia, Zoetis, SC injection, 8 mg/kg).

Blood samplings were performed on days 7, 18, 21 and 29 for complete blood counts (CBC), and/or biochemical, serological and molecular analyses of common infectious diseases. Abdominal, pulmonary and oral X-ray with oropharyngeal swab for the detection of calicivirus and feline herpes virus were conducted.

Differential diagnosis

The rapid immune-migration test for feline leukemia virus and feline immunodeficiency virus diagnosis (Witness®, Synbiotics corp.), Coombs test and PCR for the detection of feline hemotropic mycoplasms (*Mycoplasma haemofelis* and *Candidatus Mycoplasma haemominutum*) were all negatives. PCR detection of calicivirus and feline herpes virus on the oropharyngeal swab were also negative and the X-rays were interpreted as normal with the exception of a marked splenomegaly.

The CBC performed on day 7 (Table 2) showed red blood cells count within normal limits, an increased white blood cells count (WBC: 25.3×10^9/L; reference range: 5 – 11) with neutrophilic leucocytosis (neutrophils: 17.7×10^9/L, confirmed on blood smear with relatively frequent Döhle inclusion bodies; reference range: 3 – 11), and eosinophilia (eosinophils: 1.8×10^9/L; reference range: 0 – 0.6).

Serum biochemistry indicated an hypertriglyceridemia (7.14 mmol/L; reference range: 0.13 – 1.61) whereas all other biochemical parameters tested including urea, creatinine, glucose, ALT, ALKP, and lipase were within normal limits.

The stained blood smear of peripheral blood examined on day 29 revealed small inclusions within erythrocytes (Fig. 1) with uniform distribution on the smear (one red blood cell inclusion for two fields at high magnification: ×1000). The inclusions had an annular shape and were 0.5-0.8 μm in diameter suggesting the possibility of infection with and unidentified small piroplasmid parasite. A marked agglutination of erythrocytes was also noted on slide. No schizont-infected myeloid cells were detected. The blood smears done previously (on day 7, 18 and 21) were not available to be re-assessed.

Final diagnosis

DNA was extracted from whole blood collected in EDTA on day 29 and was simultaneously analyzed by PCRs on the 18S rRNA gene of the Piroplasmida in three different laboratories (Scanelis laboratory, Toulouse, France; Laboratory of Parasitology and Parasitic diseases, Vetagro Sup, Marcy-l'Etoile, France; and Koret School of Veterinary Medicine laboratory at the Hebrew University) following the conditions summarized in Table 3 [17, 18]. PCR was positive in all laboratories and the amplified DNA was sequenced. The three overlapping sequences of 18S rDNA

Table 2 Summary of blood cell counts at the time of diagnosis and at the last recheck before the cat's death with maximum and minimum values observed during the 78 days of follow-up

Parameter (unit)	Reference interval	Initial analysis (day 7)	Last analysis (day 69)	Minimum and maximum value during follow-up
RBC[a] (10^{12}/L)	5 – 10	8.00	8.73	6.75 – 8.73
Hemoglobin (g/L)	90 – 150	122	115	102 – 115
Hematocrit (L/L)	28 – 45	36.0	28	28 – 37.1
MCV[b] (fL)	40 – 55	45	32	32 – 47
MCHC[c] (g/L)	310 – 350	339	410	280 – 345
WBC[d] (10^9/L)	5 – 11	25.3	15.0	11 – 12.8
Neutrophils (10^9/L)	3 – 11	17.7	7.6	5.4 – 9.25
Eosinophils (10^9/L)	0 – 0.6	1.8	0.95	0.15 – 0.5
Monocytes (10^9/L)	0 – 0.5	0.500	0.55	0.15–1.85
Lymphocytes (10^9/L)	1 – 6	5.3	5.9	3–6.5
Platelets (10^9/L)	150 – 550	165	305	305 – 441

[a] *RBC* red blood cells count
[b] *MCV* mean corpuscular volume
[c] *MCHC* mean corpuscular hemoglobin concentration
[d] *WBC* white blood cells count

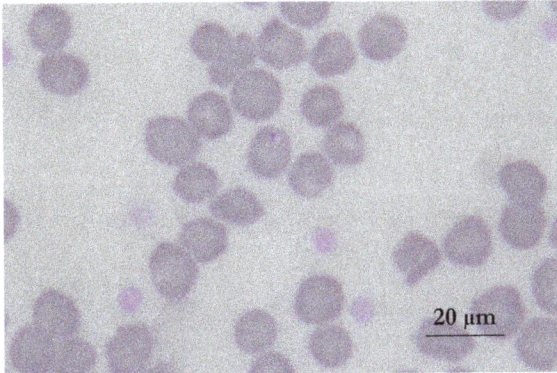

Fig. 1 Stained blood smear showing *Cytauxzoon* sp. parasite in cat erythrocyte

fragments obtained from each laboratory were 100% homologous to each other in the common fragments. A consensus sequence of 944 bp was deposited in Genbank under accession number KX881967. Comparison of this consensus sequence to sequences deposited in GenBank° using the basin local alignment search tool (BLAST) (https://blast.ncbi.nlm.nih.gov/Blast.cgi) as well as phylogenetic analyses (Fig. 2) affiliated the organism found in the cat's blood to *Cytauxzoon* sp. with 99% identity with sequences of *Cytauxzoon* sp. previously detected from domestic cats in France (EU622908) and Spain (AY309956) and from wild lynxes in Spain (EF094468 to EF094473). It also had a 99% identity with *Cytauxzoon manul* from Mongolian wild cats (AY485690 and AY485691).

Treatment, outcome and follow-up

On day 29, the cat was treated with a subcutaneous injection of imidocarb dipropionate (Carbesia, MSD, 3.5 mg/kg).

One week after treatment (day 37), the cat improved clinically, however, intraerythrocytic inclusions were still present, and a mild lymphocytosis was noticed on the blood smear.

Two weeks after treatment (day 46), the cat appeared in excellent health, appetite was normal and parasitemia was negative by blood smear microscopic examination.

However, one month after treatment (day 63) the cat relapsed and was presented with a new episode of hyperthermia, anorexia depression and stomatitis. CBC was within the normal values, but intraerythrocytic inclusions were again present on the blood smears and PCR was positive. The cat received an additional injection of imidocarb dipropionate (3.5 mg/kg SC) and recovered rapidly without other clinical signs. An extended CBC and a serum protein analysis performed 7 days later (on day 69) indicated an hypergammaglobulinemia with hyperproteinemia (91 g/L; reference range: 57 – 94 g/L) with an hematocrit at the lower limit of the reference range (28 L/L; reference range: 28 – 45). Oropharyngeal examination was normal.

Unfortunately, two weeks after the second imidocarb injection (day 76), the cat was hit by a car and died. This didn't allow further clinical investigations.

Post-mortem examination

No specific macroscopic lesions related to the cat's disease were found on gross pathology. *Post-mortem*

Table 3 List of the primers used for the amplification of 3 overlapping fragments of 18S rDNA of piroplasms

Primer names	Primers sequences	Product size bp	PCR conditions	Reference
Nested PCR: BTF1(external) BTR1 (external)	GGCTCATTACAACAGTTATAG CCCAAAGACTTTGATTTCTCTC	930 bp	94 °C 3 min, 58 °C 1 min 72 °C 2 min 45 cycles: 94 °C 30s, 58 °C 20s 72 °C 30s 72 °C 7 min	[17]
BTF2 (internal) BTR2 (internal)	CCGTGCTAATTGTAGGGCTAATAC GGACTACGACGGTATCTGATCG	836 bp	Same conditions for the secondary round with an annealing temperature of 62 °C	
Paraseq1F_scanelis 18seq1R_scanelis	TGGCTCATTAMAACAGTTATAGTTTA AGACAAATCRCTCCACCAAC	1188	94 °C 3 min 45 cycles: 94 °C 20 s 56 °C 30 s 72 °C 45 s 72 °C 7 min	Unpublished
Piro-A Piro-B	AAT ACC CAA TCC TGACAC AGG G TTA AAT ACG AAT GCC CCC AAC	408 bp	94 °C 1 min 39 cycles 94 °C 45 s, 62 °C 45 s, 72 °C 45 s. 72 °C 7 min	[18]

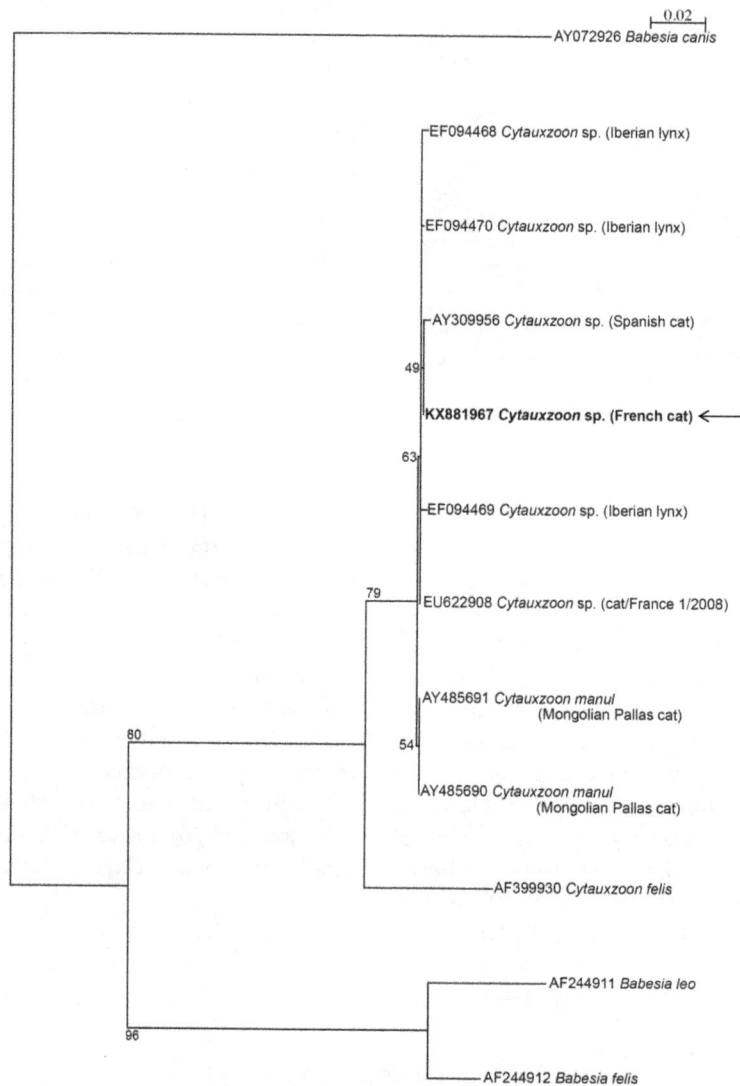

Fig. 2 Phylogenetic analysis based on 944-bp of 18S rDNA sequences of *Babesia* and *Cytauxzoon* species infecting wild and domestic Felids. Consensus sequence from the infected cat described in the present case report is indicated by an arrow. Identity and Genbank® accession numbers are indicated for each sample. The phylogenetic tree was constructed using the Hasegawa, Kishino and Yano maximum likelihood method, with bootstrap analysis with 1000 replicates. The tree was rooted using *Babesia canis* as an outgroup. Subsequent analyses using the Kimura's two-parameter (K2P) distance and the parsimony methods in the same conditions confirmed the topology of the tree

samples from the liver, spleen, kidney, iliac lymph node, lung and bone marrow as well as smears from the lung, spleen and marrow were collected and sent to the laboratory of Histology, VetAgro Sup, Marcy l'Etoile, France, for cytology and histology. *Cytauxzoon* schizonts were not encountered in the macrophages of any tissue. Layers from lungs showed suspicious inclusions in macrophages that could not be more precisely characterized. The histopathological findings observed included hyperplasia of the pancreas and of the spleen as well as an extended renal cortical inflammatory lesion. Changes in the lungs tissues related to the car crash were also noticed.

Discussion

The present case is the first report of a relapsing fever responsive to treatment with imidocarb dipropionate associated with *Cytauxzoon* sp. infection in a cat in France. It describes the course of the infection and brings new information about clinical expression of suspected cytauxzoonosis in the domestic cat in Europe.

The clinical signs reported here correspond to the signs previously described during infection with *Cytauxzoon* sp. (and usually described in case of piroplasms infection in other species). The facts that (i) no other cause (infectious in particular) could be evidenced, that (ii) intra-erythrocytic inclusions were systematically detected in acute phases of the disease and that (iii) clinical improvement was noticed after treatment with imidocarb dipropionate, highly comfort the role of Cytauxzoon sp. in the clinical signs observed. However it is not possible to ascertain that no other concurrent disease was present. Experimental infection should be conduct in the future to assess the clinical expression of European Cytauxzoon sp. infection.

Based upon results from the sequencing and the phylogenetic analyses performed on the 18S ribosomal RNA genes, Cytauxzoon sp. detected in this clinical case presented a high homology (99%) with Cytauxzoon sp. and Cytauxzoon manul previously detected in wild and domestic felids from Europe and Mongolia [7, 9, 11, 19]. In contrast, the sequence revealed an identity of only 95% with C. felis sequences deposited in GenBank®. The parasites described from Europe as Cytauxzoon sp. are closely related and may belong to the same species. They are distinct from Cytauxzoon felis, the agent of feline cytauxzoonosis in the New World.

Epidemiological and clinical data on Cytauxzoon sp. infection in domestic and wild felids in Europe have rarely been reported and originate from Spain, Italy, France, Portugal and Romania [7, 9–13, 15, 16].

In the domestic cat, single occasional molecular detections of Cytauxzoon sp. have been described in France [11] and Spain [11] with no associated clinical finding. More recently, widespread Cytauxzoon sp. infection (up to 23% prevalence by PCR) have been documented in a population of domestic cats living in Trieste in North-Eastern Italy [12]. Infection was sub-clinical in the majority of infected cats, however, clinical signs were described in 3 cats. Additional clinical cases have been reported in 2 young cats from Central Italy [13] and in a domestic cat from Portugal [15]. The clinical signs and history reported for Italian cats [12, 13], included gastro-intestinal disorders (vomiting, diarrhea), weight loss, hyperthermia (>40 °C), stomatitis, ulcerative dermatitis, and lethargy. Persistent parasitemia was also described [12]. A similar clinical pattern was observed in the present case characterized by nonspecific signs of acute febrile illness including lethargy and hyperthermia without a marked impact on the CBC and serum biochemical parameters. Stomatitis and persistent parasitemia despite clinical improvement were also described. This pattern appears to differ in severity compared to what is described in the US. Cytauxzoonosis due to C. felis is characterized by an acute febrile illness with profound fever (although hypothermia may be identified in moribund cats), depression and vocalization (so-called death yowl). Laboratory abnormalities at the time of presentation are more marked and include frequent thrombocytopenia and neutropenia as well as non-regenerative anemia,

leukopenia, hyperbilirubinemia and bilirubinuria, mild elevations in liver enzymes, hyperglycemia and hypoalbuminemia [2, 3]. Interestingly, the Portuguese case was evocative of the American disease. The cat displayed a panel of signs compatible with a severe hemolytic disease including anemia, leukocytosis, thrombocytopenia and azotemia [15]. However, genetic analyses clustered the Portuguese sequence with European Cytauxzoon sp. [15].

Supportive and critical treatment is a mainstay of therapy for American cytauxzoonosis [2, 3, 20]. Clinical recovery is not rapid with most patients getting worse during the first 24-48 h followed by a gradual improvement over the next several days. A randomized clinical trial demonstrated survival rates of 60% with a combination of atovaquone and azithromycin compared to 27% with imidocarb dipropionate [21]. In the Italian studies, treatments were based on different combinations of antiprotozoal drugs with antibiotics and steroids. One cat received a combination of imidocarb dipropionate and enrofloxacin 15 days apart followed by doxycycline, azithromycin and atovaquone without clinical improvement and was eventually euthanized. A second was treated with azithromycin, enrofloxacin and prednisone and survived, while a third cat received a single administration of azithromycin and imidocarb dipropionate and was euthanized in the absence of improvement [12]. The two other cats [13] were initially treated with doxycycline, followed by imidocarb dipropionate injections (5 mg/kg, IM injection, for two times 2 weeks apart). The 2 cats improved during a follow-up period of 175 days and 130 days respectively, and the treatment seemed to eliminate Cytauxzoon sp. infection. The Portuguese cat received daily administration of azithromycin (10 mg/kg) alone, and the animal died despite supportive care [15].

In our case, it is difficult to assert the clinical improvement as the cat accidentally died after a relapse and a second treatment with imidocarb dipropionate at a monthly interval.

Interestingly, detection of schizont-infected white blood cells on the initial blood smear wasn't noticed in any of the European cases, including the present one. In the US, the identification of schizont-infected myeloid cells confirms acute cytauxzoonosis due to C. felis. The absence of detection of schizonts may be related to a difference in the schizogony of the species present in Europe. This would need further investigation. No schizont-infected cells were either identified at necropsy.

Infection with Cytauxzoon sp. is usually associated with an outdoor life style. This is probably consistent with the suspected tick-borne transmission mode of this infection. The vector species of cytauxzoonosis in Europe is not identified yet. Interestingly, as for the Italian study of Carli et al. in 2012 [12], the cat in our report originated from an area close to the region where the presence of Eurasian lynx (*Lynx lynx*) was documented and where wild cats (*Felis silvestris*) are also present. *Cytauxzoon* sp. was also detected in Iberian lynxes (*Lynx pardinus*) from southern Spain [9, 10] suggesting a circulation of this parasite in wild and domestic felid populations of given areas. Additional studies are needed to understand the biology of the European species of *Cytauxzoon* and their distribution in European countries.

Conclusion

This case provides the first clinical description of disease associated with *Cytauxzoon* sp. in a domestic cat in France. While further investigations are needed to understand the relationship of the European strains of *Cytauxzoon* with the observed symptoms, these findings support the fact that cytauxzoonosis should be considered in the differential diagnosis of acute fever not responsive to antibiotic treatment in cats with outdoor access, especially in areas where populations of wild felids are present.

Funding
Not applicable.

Authors' contributions
JPL handled the case; MS was involved in the initial follow up of the case; JLP, Gad.B and MRM performed the molecular analyses; GB was involved in the diagnosis and draft of the article; MRM, LC and LH drafted the first version of the manuscript which was then substantially revised by all authors. All authors read and approved the final manuscript.

Competing interests
The authors declare that they have no competing interests.

Consent for publication
Consent was obtained from the owner of the animal for publication of this case report and any accompanying images.

Author details
[1]Clinique vétérinaire La Toison d'Or, Dijon, France. [2]Merial, Lyon, France. [3]University of Lyon, VetAgro Sup – Veterinary Campus of Lyon, Marcy l'Etoile, France. [4]EPIA (Epidémiologie animale Unit), INRA, Saint Genès Champanelle, France. [5]Scanelis, Colomiers, France. [6]Koret School of Veterinary Medicine, Hebrew University, Rehovot, Israel.

References
1. Wagner JE. A fatal cytauxzoonosis-like disease in cats. J Am Vet Med Assoc. 1976;168(7):585–8.
2. Cohn LA, Birkenheuer AJ. Cytauxzoonosis. In: Greene CE, editor. Infectious diseases of the dog and cat. 4th ed. St Louis: Elsevier Saunders; 2012. p. 764–71.
3. Lloret A, Addie DD, Boucraut-Baralon C, Egberink H, Frymus T, Gruffydd-Jones T, Hartmann K, Horzinek MC, Hosie MJ, Lutz H, Marsilio F, Pennisi MG, Radford AD, Thiry E, Truyen U, Möstl K, European Advisory Board on Cat Diseases. Cytauxzoonosis in cats. ABCD guidelines on prevention and management. J Feline Med Surg. 2015;17(7):637–41.
4. Blouin EF, Kocan AA, Glenn BL, Kocan KM, Hair JA. Transmission of *Cytauxzoon felis* kier, 1979 from bobcats, *Felis rufus* (Schreber), to domestic cats by *Dermacentor variabilis* (say). J Wildl Dis. 1984;20(3):241–2.
5. Reichard MV, Edwards AC, Meinkoth JH, Snider TA, Meinkoth KR, Heinz RE, Little SE. Confirmation of *Amblyomma americanum* (Acari: Ixodidae) as a vector for *Cytauxzoon felis* (Piroplasmorida: Theileriidae) to domestic cats. J Med Entomol. 2010;47(5):890–6.
6. Birkenheuer AJ, Le JA, Valenzisi AM, Tucker MD, Levy MG, Breitschwerdt EB. Cytauxzoon felis infection in cats in the mid-Atlantic states: 34 cases (1998-2004). J Am Vet Med Assoc. 2006;228(4):568–71.
7. Criado-Fornelio A, Gónzalez-del-Río MA, Buling-Saraña A, Barba-Carretero JC. The "expanding universe" of piroplasms. Vet Parasitol. 2004;119(4):337–45.
8. Luaces I, Aguirre E, García-Montijano M, Velarde J, Tesouro MA, Sánchez C, Galka M, Fernández P, Sainz A. First report of an intraerythrocytic small piroplasm in wild Iberian lynx (*Lynx pardinus*). J Wildl Dis. 2005;41(4):810–5.
9. Millán J, Naranjo V, Rodríguez A, de la Lastra JM, Mangold AJ, de la Fuente J. Prevalence of infection and 18S rRNA gene sequences of Cytauxzoon species in Iberian lynx (*Lynx pardinus*) in Spain. Parasitology. 2007;134(7):995–1001.
10. Millán J, Candela MG, Palomares F, Cubero MJ, Rodríguez A, Barral M, de la Fuente J, Almería S, León-Vizcaíno L. Disease threats to the endangered Iberian lynx (*Lynx pardinus*). Vet J. 2009;182(1):114–24.
11. Criado-Fornelio A, Buling A, Pingret JL, Etievant M, Boucraut-Baralon C, Alongi A, Agnone A, Torina A. Hemoprotozoa of domestic animals in France: prevalence and molecular characterization. Vet Parasitol. 2009;159(1):73–6.
12. Carli E, Trotta M, Chinelli R, Drigo M, Sinigoi L, Tosolini P, Furlanello T, Millotti A, Caldin M, Solano-Gallego L. *Cytauxzoon* sp. infection in the first endemic focus described in domestic cats in Europe. Vet Parasitol. 2012; 183(3-4):343–52.
13. Carli E, Trotta M, Bianchi E, Furlanello T, Caldin M, Pietrobelli M, Solano-Gallego L. *Cytauxzoon* sp. infection in two free ranging young cats: clinicopathological findings, therapy and follow up. Turkiye Parazitol Derg. 2014;38(3):185–9.
14. Veronesi F, Ravagnan S, Cerquetella M, Carli E, Olivieri E, Santoro A, Pesaro S, Berardi S, Rossi G, Ragni B, Beraldo P, Capelli G. First detection of *Cytauxzoon* spp. infection in European wildcats (*Felis silvestris silvestris*) of Italy. Ticks Tick Borne Dis. 2016;7(5):853–8.
15. Alho AM, Silva J, Fonseca MJ, Santos F, Nunes C, de Carvalho LM, Rodrigues M, Cardoso L. First report of *Cytauxzoon* sp. infection in a domestic cat from Portugal. Parasit Vectors. 2016;9(1):220.
16. Gallusová M, Jirsová D, Mihalca AD, Gherman CM, D'Amico G, Qablan MA, Modrý D. *Cytauxzoon* infections in wild felids from Carpathian-Danubian-Pontic space: further evidence for a different *Cytauxzoon* species in European felids. J Parasitol. 2016 Jun;102(3):377–80.
17. Jefferies R, Ryan UM, Irwin PJ. PCR-RFLP for the detection and differentiation of the canine piroplasm species and its use with filter paper-based technologies. Vet Parasitol. 2007;144:20–7.
18. Olmeda AS, Armstrong PM, Rosenthal BM, Valladares B, del Castillo A, de Armas F, Miguelez M, Gonzalez A, Rodriguez JA, Spielman A, Telford SR. A subtropical case of human babesiosis. Acta Trop. 1997;67:229–34.
19. Reichard MV, Van Den Bussche RA, Meinkoth JH, Hoover JP, Kocan AA. A new species of *Cytauxzoon* from Pallas' cats caught in Mongolia and comments on the systematics and taxonomy of piroplasmids. J Parasitol. 2005;91(2):420–6.
20. Sherrill MK, Cohn LA. Cytauxzoonosis: diagnosis and treatment of an emerging disease. J Feline Med Surg. 2015;17(11):940–8.
21. Cohn LA, Birkenheuer AJ, Brunker JD, Ratcliff ER, Craig AW. Efficacy of atovaquone and azithromycin or imidocarb dipropionate in cats with acute cytauxzoonosis. J Vet Intern Med. 2011;25(1):55–60.

5

Knowledge, attitudes, and practices regarding cystic echinococcosis and sheep herding in Peru: a mixed-methods approach

Veronika Merino[1*], Christopher M. Westgard[2], Angela M. Bayer[3,4] and Patricia J. García[4]

Abstract

Background: The parasitic disease, cystic echinococcosis (CE), is prevalent in low-income, livestock-raising communities and 2000 new people will be diagnosed this year in South America alone. The disease usually passes from livestock to dogs to humans, making it a zoonotic disease and part of the One Health Initiative. Control of CE has been infamously difficult; no endemic areas of South America have succeeded in maintaining sustainable eradication of the parasite.

For the current study, we aimed to gain a better understanding of the knowledge, attitudes, and practices of rural sheep farmers and other community leaders regarding their sheep herding practices and perspectives about a control program for CE. We also hope to identify potential barriers and opportunities that could occur in a control program.

The authors conducted Knowledge, Attitude and Practices (KAP) surveys and semi-structured interviews in rural communities in the highlands of Peru. The KAP surveys were administered to 51 local shepherds, and the semi-structured interviews were administered to 40 individuals, including shepherds, community leaders, and health care providers.

Results: We found that the shepherds already deworm their sheep at a median of 2 times per year ($N = 49$, range 2–4) and have a mean willingness-to-pay of U.S. $ 0.60 for dog dewormer medication ($N = 20$, range = 0.00- $2.00 USD). We were not able to learn the deworming agent or agents that were being used, for neither sheep nor dogs. Additionally, 90% of shepherds slaughter their own sheep ($N = 49$). We also learned that the main barriers to an effective control program include: lack of education about the cause and control options for CE, accessibility to the distant communities and sparse grazing pastures, and a lack of economic incentive.

Conclusions: Findings suggest it may be feasible to develop an effective CE control program which can be used to create an improved protocol to control CE in the region.

Keywords: Echinococcosis, *Echinococcus granulosus*, Zoonoses, Surveys, Peru

Background

Cystic echinococcosis (CE) is one of the most prevalent zoonotic diseases in South America [1]. It is caused by an infection of the larvae of the parasite *Echinococcus granulosus*. Humans can become infected by ingesting the eggs excreted by a dog or any other canid (definite hosts); however, humans cannot transmit the disease (accidental host). The eggs ingested by humans and/or intermediate hosts (livestock, such as sheep, cattle, horses, etc.) reach the gastrointestinal tract where they hatch, freeing oncospheres that are transported through lymphatic and cardiovascular circulation to various organs, usually the liver or lungs, where they will lodge and slowly form cysts, causing CE [2, 3].

CE is considered by the World Health Organization (WHO) to be a neglected disease [4], and it remains a persistent problem in areas of low socio-economic status and livestock production. The present study was set in the Central and Southern Andes of Peru, regions where sheep-herding communities are found. While some of these communities also raise bovines and South American camelids, and CE can be present in these species as well, the study focused in sheep-herding

* Correspondence: veronika.merino@upch.pe
[1]Kuskaya: An Interdisciplinary Training Program for Innovation in Global Health, School of Public Health, Universidad Peruana Cayetano Heredia, Av. Honorio Delgado 431 San Martin de Porres, Lima, Peru
Full list of author information is available at the end of the article

communities given that the prevalence of the disease has been reported to be higher in sheep raising regions.

This disease causes a substantial burden in highly endemic areas of South America, including Peru [5]. The WHO Informal Working Group on Cystic Echinococcosis Surveillance, Prevention and Control [6] estimates that CE results in 1 to 3 million Disability-Adjusted Life Years (DALYs) per year. The disease increases vulnerability for the poorest populations due to medical costs and loss of human and livestock productivity [7, 8]. Some studies have shown that CE can result in a 10% decrease in productivity of infected animals, lowering quality of meat, production of fiber and milk, and number of surviving offspring [9].

For effective control of *E. granulosus,* it is necessary to stop the parasite's development at different stages of its life cycle [10]. There are several control strategies that have been studied and have proven to be successful in different scenarios [10, 11]; some of the control strategies that have been studied are: dog deworming, sheep deworming and sheep vaccination [12–16]. Mathematical modelling has shown that the most effective intervention was a combination of vaccinating sheep and dog deworming treatment [10].

There have been several attempts at controlling CE in endemic countries around the world; however, most endemic areas, like Latin America, have not achieved sustainable control. Potential barriers have been discussed in various control studies, including unsustainable financial and political support, inaccessible roads and communities, poor evaluation efforts, lack of education and supplies in the control authority, and ineffective infrastructure to administer frequent dog deworming [1, 13]. Most of these studies include administrative difficulties as one of the main barriers, but lack in-depth information regarding the perspectives and daily practices of intervention recipients.

Therefore, the aim of the present study is to explore: the knowledge, attitudes and practices of shepherds regarding CE; the shepherds' willingness-to-pay for certain key control strategies; and the perspectives of community leaders, health center representatives, and local municipality employees regarding CE. With a better understanding of the perspectives of diverse stakeholders we hope to identify and target barriers to the implementation of an effective control program.

Methods
Study design
This was a descriptive, cross-sectional, mixed methods study. The qualitative semi-structured interviews provide a cross reference to responses given in the KAP survey. Triangulation between the qualitative and quantitative

data helped generate a comparative analysis, increase the credibility of results and limit misinterpretations [17].

Study area
The study was conducted from November to December 2014, in the central and southern highlands of Peru, in the provinces of Junin, Huancavelica, Puno, and Cusco. Villages from 14 districts with sheep husbandry practices were sampled. The villages are located at high altitudes, normally varying between 3200 to 4100 m above sea level. Transportation to these villages takes from 1 to 6 h by car from the capital of each department. The villages within each region were chosen using purposive sampling to ensure that different areas of the region were represented in our sample population.

Preliminary work
The research team conducted a stakeholder analysis to identify the actors at the national level (in Lima) that have knowledge regarding CE and its control. The authors received assistance from representatives from the Pan American Health Organization (PAHO) and Universidad Peruana Cayetano Heredia (UPCH) to coordinate with other political and academic experts. Representatives from the Ministry of Health, Ministry of Agriculture, and Ministry of Housing, Construction and Sanitation – Programa Nacional TAMBO (PNT) [18] assisted in introducing the research team to contacts within the study communities and facilitating logistical information. The PNT provides, in isolated high poverty areas of Peru, buildings designed to host representatives of National, Regional and Local institutions to facilitate the access to this often-neglected population and ensure they can be reached and covered by different services and programs. These buildings include dormitories; media-equipped offices and meeting/conference rooms; and a storage room stocked with emergency equipment and supplies.

Data collection and analysis methods
Quantitative methodology
The quantitative component was carried out with community members within sheep raising communities. The research team utilized purposive sampling within the communities by traveling through the streets or pastures searching for individuals that owned sheep and/or owned dogs and approaching them to inquire about participation in the study.

All participating community members completed a Knowledge, Attitudes and Practices (KAP) survey. The KAP survey was administered, with the interviewer reading the questions in Spanish, without presenting the response options so that participants could provide the answers they deemed most appropriate. If the participant provided an answer that was not listed as an option, the new answer was included in the questionnaire under 'Other'. The KAP survey was divided into three sections and included questions regarding the shepherds' knowledge and experience with CE in animals and humans; demographics of their animals; and medication and slaughter practices for their animals. The KAP survey included 47 questions and took approximately 20 to 30 min to complete.

A randomly selected sub-group of participating shepherds was asked to complete a willingness-to-pay survey, which was presented following the KAP survey and a short description of the disease and of each of the three control strategies considered in the study. The shepherds were asked how much they would be willing to pay for the medication for each control strategy. The three control strategies presented were: (1) Praziquantel to deworm dogs every 45 days, (2) Oxfendazole to deworm sheep every three months, and (3) EG95 vaccine to vaccinate sheep three times in their first year of life. The shepherds were asked how much they would pay per dose. The interviewer started by asking if they would pay 20 Soles (U.S. $6.35), which is a very high price, considering the average shepherd's economy (U.S. $ 100 per month, as stated in the interviews). If the shepherd declined that price, the interviewer proceeded to present lower and lower prices until the shepherd agreed on the price he would be willing to pay. Often the latter process was not necessary since after declining the high price, the shepherds would state the price they were willing to pay.

The data from the KAP surveys were entered in a database in Microsoft Excel® and reviewed for errors by another member of the research team. Data was analyzed using EpiInfo version 3.5.4 (Epidata Association; Odense, Denmark). First, descriptive data analysis was run, which included calculating frequency of responses, mean, and median. Then, univariate logistic regression models were applied to analyze correlations between the community members' experience with CE, and the shepherds' practices that would contribute to effective CE prevention. The authors wanted to see if previous exposure to information regarding CE had contributed to a positive change in practices. Prevalence ratios (PR) and their corresponding 95% Confidence Intervals, along with p values from the 2-tailed Fisher's exact test, are provided for each regression.

Qualitative methodology

The qualitative component was carried out with community members including: shepherds; community leaders, health center representatives; and personnel from local municipalities. The qualitative component also utilized purposive sampling to seek out relevant participants. For non-shepherds, a few key actors were identified in the villages and in department capitals and they were asked to provide introductions to others that could offer relevant information. A semi-structured guide was used to interview participants in greater depth about their perspectives regarding the barriers to CE control programs in their communities. The interview began by asking participants what they and others in their community think about CE control programs, including difficulties they may face for each control program alternative. The interviews also engaged participants about the three potential control strategies (dog deworming, sheep deworming, and sheep vaccination) to learn about their associated barriers. The conversation was audio recorded with prior written consent, and later transcribed.

For the qualitative data analysis, the study team identified a set of sub-themes from the responses to generate an initial codebook. These codes were applied to two transcripts (one from shepherds, one from non-shepherds) to standardize the coding process. The resulting modified codebook and transcripts were entered into Dedoose (SocioCultural Research Consultants; Manhattan Beach, CA). Next, the team coded the remaining transcripts. Finally, they explored similarities and differences in perspectives of participants within and across participants.

Results
Quantitative
Cystic echinococcosis -relevant knowledge, Attitudes and practices among shepherds

Fifty-one (51) participants, individuals that either owned sheep and/or owned dogs, completed the KAP survey (the results of the KAP survey can be found in Additional file 1). The demographic information of the KAP participants, as well as information regarding their sheep and dogs and their practices with these animals, is displayed in Table 1. Of the interview participants (51), 49 owned sheep, with a median of 24 sheep per shepherd. Only 12% of shepherds have veterinary supervision of their sheep and 90% slaughter their own sheep. 41 out of 51 participants (80%) owned dogs, with a median of 2 dogs per shepherd.

We found that 98% of the shepherds currently deworm their sheep, 60% of them to treat *Fasciola hepatica* (common liver fluke), while the rest deworm against diverse intestinal parasites and ectoparasites, at a median of 2 times per year, and at a median price of $0.38 per dose of dewormer. About 69% of the shepherds that deworm their sheep administer the medicine themselves or with a community member and 31% use a vet/technician. Regarding sheep vaccination, we learned that the shepherds referred to

Table 1 Characteristics of Knowledge, Attitudes and Practices (KAP) survey shepherd participants and information regarding their ownership of sheep and dogs and their practices with these animals, Peru, 2014

	Number (%)	Median (Range)
CHARACTERISTICS OF KAP SURVEY PARTICIPANTS, N = 51		
Gender	-	-
Male	30 (59)	-
Female	21 (41)	-
Age	-	45.5 (20–75)
CHARACTERISTICS OF SHEEP OWNED BY PARTICIPANTS		
Number of sheep owned	-	24 (2–417)
Sheep receive veterinarian supervision	6 (12)	-
Participants slaughter own livestock	44 (90)	-
Location of slaughter	-	-
Only in backyard	48 (98)	-
Backyard and Slaughterhouse	4 (10)	-
Backyard and Common area	1 (2)	-
Use of meat from sheep	-	-
Personal consumption	48 (98)	-
Sell meat in market	34 (69)	-
Does not use it (Sell sheep alive)	20 (41)	-
Age of sheep at slaughter or sale (years)	-	1.5 (0.5–5)
Maximum age of sheep (years)	-	10
CHARACTERISTICS OF DOGS OWNED BY PARTICIPANTS		
Owns a dog	41 (80)	-
Number of dogs owned	-	2 (1–6)

vaccines as anything injectable. Therefore, we were not able to differentiate between the use of vaccines and other injections like antibiotics or vitamins. 53% of shepherds provide injections at a median of 2 times per year and at a median price of $0.32 per injection. Less than half (39%) of shepherds that provide injectable medicine to their livestock administer the injections themselves, and 16% use a vet/technician. We also learned that most of the shepherds have seen cysts in their sheep's viscera (89%). The shepherds indicated that they often bury (73%) or burn (35%) the viscera, if it is infected with cysts.

Of the participants who declared to own dogs, 73% currently deworm them, and at a median of 2 times per year. We were not able to learn the deworming agent or agents that were being used. More than half of the dog-owners feed sheep viscera to their dogs (56%). 83% of them indicated that they feed the viscera cooked (58%), and 15% of dog owners said that they do not feed them viscera if it has cysts.

Of all the shepherds surveyed, only 33% indicated they had heard of CE. When asked how the disease is transmitted to humans, only 4% correctly mentioned that it is transmitted through infected dog feces. 15% incorrectly responded that the disease is contracted by eating infected meat or viscera. After the participants learned about CE and its health consequences in humans, 35% of them stated that they knew someone that had contracted the disease (35%); of those infected people, 94% needed surgery.

Willingness-to-pay for cystic echinococcosis control strategies among shepherds

The Willingness-to-pay survey was administered to 22 individuals. The following number of participants responded to the three willingness-to-pay questions regarding three potential control strategies: dog dewormer ($n = 19$), sheep dewormer ($n = 17$), sheep vaccine ($n = 20$). The number of shepherds that answered each question of the *Willingness-To-Pay* survey varied because some were not able or did not agree to answer one or two of them. The results display the average the shepherd is willing to pay for one dose of the required medication to control the spread of CE in U.S. Dollars (3.15 Peruvian Soles = 1 USD; at the time of the study). The responses for how much they would be willing to pay were higher than the responses in the KAP survey regarding how much they currently pay for dewormer and vaccines for their sheep (U.S. $ 0.56 vs U.S. $ 0.38, and U.S. $ 0.70 vs U.S. $ 0.32, respectively). The averages for willingness-to-pay for all three medications are substantially lower in Puno than the other two provinces (See Table 2).

Association between cystic echinococcosis knowledge and experiences and cystic echinococcosis-relevant practices among shepherds

The relationships between knowledge of CE were regressed against the shepherds' practices that would have an influence reducing CE. The results are displayed in Table 3. The only significant correlation is between

Table 2 Willingness-To-Pay for CE control strategies among Shepherds, Peru, 2014

AVERAGE WILLINGNESS-TO-PAY	CUSCO (U.S.$/dose)	PUNO (U.S.$/dose)	JUNIN (U.S.$/dose)	AVERAGE (U.S.$/dose)
Dog Dewormer	0.71	0.18	1.04	0.60
Sheep Dewormer	0.71	0.15	0.61	0.56
Sheep Vaccine	0.84	0.14	1.01	0.71

Table 3 Results for Univariate Logistic Regression

	Deworms sheep ≥2 times per year	Deworms dogs ≥3 times per year	Feeds infected viscera to dogs
	Prevalence Ratios (95% CI). p-value		
Participated in CE[a] control program	0.58 (0.23–1.45), $p = 0.24$	0.49 (0.21–1.16). $p = 0.02$[b]	0.94 (0.13–6.87), $p = 1.00$
Heard of CE[a]	0.82 (0.49–1.38), $p = 0.54$	0.92 (0.70–1.38), $p = 1.00$	0.83 (0.17–4.01), $p = 1.00$
Knew someone with CE[a]	1.18 (0.75–1.85), $p = 0.55$	0.76 (0.52–1.12), $p = 0.22$	0.30 (0.04–2.33), $p = 0.37$

[a]*CE* Cystic echinococcosis
[b]significant at confidence of 95%

having previously participated in a control program for CE and deworming their dogs 3 or more times per year ($p = 0.02$). The other correlations between knowledge of CE and CE-related practices were not significant.

Qualitative

Semi-structured interviews were held with 40 participants. The population included 19 shepherds; 10 community leaders, who also owned sheep; 5 health care providers from local Health Centers, including doctors, medical technicians and a nurse; and 6 Ministry of Housing, Construction and Sanitation – TAMBO National Program representatives. The quotes used to present these results can be found in Additional file 2.

Knowledge related to cystic echinococcosis

We found that most of the interviewees, including health care providers, did not have a clear notion of what CE is, nor how it is transmitted. Some interviewees thought that CE was transmitted through contact with cat hair, while others were convinced that CE was caused by the ingestion of meat from infected animals. Although some of them were aware that dogs are involved in the transmission of CE, they did not fully understand that livestock and humans are infected by ingesting *E. granulosus* excreted by dogs.

In regards of presence of CE in their community, some of the interviewees confirmed that they were familiar with some positive cases within their community. Some of these known cases were patients that had gone through surgery after symptoms became severe, and some other patients had passed away.

Barriers for a cystic echinococcosis control program

When shepherds and community leaders were asked about their perspective on a control program for CE, we obtained answers that reflected some of the most important barriers for a successful program, including: understanding the benefits of the program, their willingness to participate in a program, and difficulties accessing the population. Rural populations will only participate in a new program if they can see and experience immediate benefits. When they were asked about participating, some replied that currently one of the greatest incentive to participate in health programs and/

or campaigns, like vaccination for children, is the presence of 'Programa Juntos´, a Peruvian Government cash transfer program to aid poor populations, financed by the Ministry of Social Inclusion and Development that places conditions for funding, such as maintaining children good school attendance, children vaccines up to date, etc.

There are some areas where pilot programs have been present, and have exposed the community to information about CE. However, several communities were omitted from pilot programs and other social initiatives due to their inaccessibility. Some of these villages do not have roads and it could take up to 10 h on foot to reach them. Interviewees from such populations stated that they feel like they have been neglected.

We found that for a significant number of shepherds, lack of knowledge and awareness about CE is an important barrier. For this population, education and training are immensely important, and are key factors to an effective and sustainable control program. They believe that continuous training and informative campaigns for shepherds would aid the fight against CE and other zoonotic diseases in livestock. Some community members consider that education must be conducted using strategies specifically designed for the target population. These strategies need to reflect their culture, be accessible and engaging. They recognize that raising livestock is their main source of income and that keeping their animals free of disease will translate into better economy.

Another interesting finding was that shepherds and other community members suggested having people from the community actively involved, and that they would prefer a member of their own community, rather than an "outsider" to act as a promoter, distributing preventive medicine. Some of the reasons they presented include the fact that they would be more familiar with their livestock, costumes and routine, and would be more responsible and involved with his or her community's interests.

Perspectives on cystic echinococcosis control strategies

The implementation of dog deworming is a challenging procedure because sheep dogs are working dogs, and behave very differently than domestic dogs in urban areas.

Shepherds acknowledge that sheep dogs are more difficult to handle and to medicate on a regular basis. In addition, local government representatives consider this option less viable, since they perceive that communities do not have *"a set routine, not even for themselves. They don't go or take their kids to the health center. It is less likely that they would do it for their animals."*

When asked about sheep vaccination interventions, interviewees presented different reactions. Some believe that sheep vaccination could be valuable, but were concerned about the difficulties in successfully tracing all the sheep from all the shepherds. Other shepherds were in complete agreement of implementing a vaccination intervention, since it would prevent the disease in animals, and therefore in humans as well. Additionally, people had different perspectives about the effect of the vaccination on the quality and flavor of the meat. Some shepherds recognized the potential benefit of producing better quality meat from disease-free animals; on the other hand, others were worried about the possibility of the vaccine altering the flavor of the meat, following their experience with their potato crops after artificial fertilizers were introduced.

Shepherds and community leaders were also inquired about deworming of sheep. Their responses show that deworming could be a potential strategy if the medication is long-lasting and low-cost, but challenges would include perceptions about investing in sheep that will soon be slaughtered. Shepherds also showed concern about the drug's withdrawal period, its efficacy, and frequency of dosage.

Willingness to pay for cystic echinococcosis control strategies

Some shepherds indicated that if the medicine were provided for free by a program, they would have less confidence in the control program. They mentioned that if the drugs were distributed for free, they would be afraid that the medication would not be safe for their animals, that it might be expired or even toxic. A community leader said: *"Most of the people will want to make sure that the medicine they are getting is real, and of good quality, or at least the same quality as the medicine they regularly buy themselves. If they can make sure of that, they will accept it."* Additionally, paying for treatment might increase compliance, since it is less likely that shepherds will not use something they already have paid for.

While shepherds stated that they will be willing to pay for intervention strategies, some ministries representatives, such as a PNT representative reported that in impoverished areas, having to pay could be a potential barrier: *"In Huancavelica, in the isolated areas, like the estancias, people only make a living from the sale of their livestock. In a month, they possibly sell one or two sheep, obtaining a monthly income of 200 to 300 Soles [U.S. $ 63 – U.S. $95]. If they need to invest an amount close to 10% of their monthly income, it is very unlikely that they will agree to it."*

Discussion

Our findings highlight the difficulties faced by a control initiative in poor, hard to reach regions, but also identify several opportunities. Even though CE can develop in most livestock, the study focused on sheep, because the highest prevalence of CE in humans is found in populations that raise sheep [19]. The study found that shepherds know very little regarding CE and that they deworm their sheep and dogs already to control intestinal parasites, but the frequency and the drugs they are currently using are not necessary effective against *E. granulosus*. However, they are willing to improve their deworming practices if they receive education about the benefits. The lack of awareness and understanding of the disease, and the low profit margins shepherds earn from their livestock could be some of the reason why control has been so ineffective. The intervention strategies to control CE that have been effective in wealthy countries have not been effective at achieving long-term control of the disease in low income countries [11]. In Peru, between 2002 and 2013, there were 33,838 human CE cases reported. The province of Pasco has the highest prevalence of CE, reporting 108 cases per 100,000 persons, followed by Huancavelica (43/100,000) [20]. These two regions are the hardest to reach; the poorest and several of the comments in these regions noted the lack of government assistance they receive.

In fact, the barriers to an effective control program in the highlands of Peru are likely greater than any other region in South America. The communities are in high-altitude, difficult to reach regions of the Andes, shepherds are some of the poorest populations in Peru, and the education system is often very low-quality in remote regions. Also, the inability of programs to effectively control CE could be attributed to the fact that chronic diseases with low fatality rates that are limited to poor rural areas are particularly "unattractive" to researchers and funders who depend on relatively immediate results. CE shares this situation with other communicable diseases, such as neurocysticercosis and Buruli disease [21]. Effective control is hindered because surveillance is difficult in animals and humans, infection is asymptomatic in dogs, clinical signs in livestock are not easily perceived by shepherds and the disease can take 5–10 years to be symptomatic in humans [4].

Many of our findings are contradictory to beliefs held by some policy makers in the country's capital of Lima. During the preliminary phase of the study we held meetings with policymakers, some of whom perceived that people in rural areas will not accept CE-related intervention programs. Our results show that most of the people we interviewed would be willing to adopt a new program if they are provided with sufficient education about benefits and risks. Also, as previously mentioned, they are already deworming (although not in the right frequency and/or dosage recomemended to control Echinococcosis) and report being willing to pay for deworming medicine. People in the areas we visited, along with previous studies, consider education to be the key to any sustainable program [2]. Shepherds showed great interest in the topic of CE once they recognized the potential risks for their families' health and the negative effect on their income.

Many policy makers and experts were not aware that shepherds already deworm their livestock and dogs. Since 73% of dog owners already deworm their dogs, and 98% of shepherds already deworm their sheep to control intestinal parasites, a control program would only need to explain and encourage increased frequency and dosage for their sheep and assure the correct drugs to treat Echinococcosis are used, while complementing the control of other parasites. Currently shepherds deworm their sheep before and after rain season (December to March), therefore any new deworming protocol should expand on the same deworming schedule [11].

The price for preventative medication was one of the main barriers we heard from shepherds and community leaders for adopting CE prevention strategies. Although, they are willing to pay for interventions, they are reluctant to increase the expenses needed to raise their sheep, specifically new medications that are unknown to them and are unsure of the efficacy. The study's *willingness-to-pay* analysis found that the median willingness-to-pay amount for preventive medication was well below the market price of the drugs in some provinces and for certain control strategies, such as dog dewormer in Junin and Cusco. In poorer provinces, like Puno, the willingness-to-pay amount was significantly less than the market price for all control medication options. This aligns with the fact that Puno is the most impoverished of the three departments [22]. In poorer provinces like this, there would need to be substantial financial support. In regions with higher willingness-to-pay for control strategies, it should be relatively easily to implement a program, with appropriate education and logistical support.

Creating the required behavior change by shepherds to halt the spread of CE is another issue to address [15]. If the shepherds stopped feeding their dogs the sheep viscera, the spread of CE would come to a halt. A previous study in Peru showed that 83% of shepherds feed their

dogs infected viscera [23]. Although 73% of shepherds indicated that they bury the infected viscera in our study, it is highly unlikely this occurs, due to social desirability; and when it does occur it is likely that they are not burying the viscera deep enough to prevent the dogs from digging it up and eating it. The effort that it would take to bury viscera deeper than a dog would dig, in the rocky ground of the Andes, is tremendous. Performing this act, every time a shepherd slaughters a sheep, is unreasonable. However, the shepherds still indicate that they do so. Also, because we found that 90% of shepherds slaughter their own sheep, we cannot rely on slaughterhouses to handle the disposal of the infected viscera. Behavior change must occur at the household level. Therefore, a better disposal strategy for sheep viscera must be developed.

35% of shepherds answered that they knew someone that had suffered from CE, and only 6% of the shepherds identified the correct form of disease transmission. Many of the shepherds were aware that CE is present in their communities, but did not know how it got there. Most of them think that it is due to ingesting infected sheep viscera. Most think that to prevent CE, they should offer sheep viscera to their dogs instead of to their families, inadvertently completing the biological cycle of *E. granulosus*.

Another important barrier for a control program is the difficult access to communities [10]. Usually, shepherding communities are in districts far from the province capital, and the shepherds spend many weeks at a time away in higher lands where better pastures can be found. These areas are between 1 and 10 h away on foot from their communities, and are hardly accessible by motor vehicles. This creates a burden for the shepherds to obtain preventive medicine from their communities.

Some shepherds said they are not willing to administer new medicine to their animals if they do not see any immediate benefit. Neither the dogs nor the sheep show evident clinical signs when infected with *E. granulosus*, so it is difficult to encourage compliance from owners to deworm their animals, especially if they are asked to do so frequently. Also, deworming dogs is very challenging. Handling sheepdogs is much more difficult than handling pet dogs, and it is difficult to monitor and ensure that dogs are getting the medicine they need in the frequency and dose required.

One of the limitations of the present study is related to data collection. It involved only 51 participants for the quantitative interviews and 40 participants for the qualitative interviews. For the study population to be more representative, it would have benefitted from a larger number of participants for the KAP surveys. The research team was not able to survey more shepherds due to limited accessibility and great distance to most sheep grazing fields and the fact that rural sheep-raising communities are highly dispersed. Another important limitation in this study is the potential bias on the willingness-to-pay values, due to that they were mostly based on responses from shepherds that already deworm their animals.

Conclusion

The findings of this study illustrate that any effective and sustainable efforts to control CE require addressing the barriers perceived by the shepherds and to identify opportunities. The main barriers identified by this study include: lack of education about the cause and control options for CE; accessibility to the distant communities and sparse grazing pastures; complications in coordinating the administration of preventative medicine; and lack of economic incentives for CE control.

The opportunities found in this study are: most shepherds already deworm their sheep at a median of 2 times per year, slaughter their sheep at 1.5 years old or younger, and deworm their dogs at least twice a year; willingness to pay, at least a small amount, for interventions; and the acceptance of community workers to distribute preventive medicine and health messages. The findings can be used to create an improved, expanded protocol to control CE in the region.

As proposed in previous studies, education on Echinococcosis and its economic and public health impact on humans and animals, will support the behavior change needed to halt transmission of the parasite [24].

Abbreviations

CE: Cystic echinococcosis; DALYs: Disability-Adjusted Life Years; KAP: Knowledge Attitudes and Practices; PNT: Programa Nacional TAMBO; PR: Prevalence ratios (PR); WHO: World Health Organization

Acknowledgements

We wish to thank the representatives of the Pan American Health Organization (PAHO), the Ministry of Health, the Ministry of Agriculture, and the Programa Nacional TAMBO (PNT) of the Ministry of Housing, Construction and Sanitation for their collaboration during the preliminary phase of the study, and the introductions to stakeholders at the regional and local levels.

Funding

This article was supported by the NIH Research Training Grant 5D43TW009375–02 awarded to Kuskaya: An Interdisciplinary Training Program for Innovation in Global Health from the Fogarty International Center, United States National Institutes of Health.

Authors' contributions

VM, CW conceived the study. VM, CW, AB, PG participated in its design. VM, CW developed the data collection instruments, performed the data analysis and drafted the manuscript. All authors read and approved the final manuscript.

Consent for publication

Not applicable.

Competing interests

The authors declare that they have no competing interests.

Author details

[1]Kuskaya: An Interdisciplinary Training Program for Innovation in Global Health, School of Public Health, Universidad Peruana Cayetano Heredia, Av. Honorio Delgado 431 San Martin de Porres, Lima, Peru. [2]Kuskaya: An Interdisciplinary Training Program for Innovation in Global Health, School of Public Health, University of Washington, Seattle, USA. [3]Division of Infectious Diseases, David Geffen School of Medicine, University of California, Los Angeles, California, Los Angeles, USA. [4]Unit of Epidemiology, STD and HIV, School of Public Health and Administration, Universidad Peruana Cayetano Heredia, Lima, Peru.

References

1. Larrieu E, Zanini F. Critical analysis of cystic echinococcosis control programs and praziquantel use in South America, 1974-2010. Rev Panam Salud Pública. 2012;31:81–7.
2. Eckert J, Gemmell M, Meslin F, Pawlowski Z. WHO/OIE manual on Echinococcosis in humans and animals: a public health problem of global concern. World Organ Anim Health Off Int Epizoot World Health Organ. 2001;
3. Moro P, Schantz PM. Echinococcosis: a review. Int J Infect Dis. 2009;13:125–33.
4. Daumerie D, Savioli L: Working to Overcome the Global Impact of Neglected Tropical Diseases: First WHO Report on Neglected Tropical Diseases. David William Thomasson Cromptopn and Patricia Peters; 2010.
5. Torgerson PR, Budke CM. Echinococcosis – an international public health challenge. Res Vet Sci. 2003;74:191–202.
6. Report of the WHO Informal Working Group on cystic and alveolar echinococcosis surveillance, prevention and control, with the participation of the Food and Agriculture Organization of the United Nations and the World Organisation for Animal Health [http://apps.who.int/iris/handle/10665/44785].
7. Moro PL, Budke CM, Schantz PM, Vasquez J, Santivañez SJ, Villavicencio J. Economic impact of cystic echinococcosis in peru. PLoS Negl Trop Dis. 2011;5:e1179.
8. Torgerson PR: Economic effects of echinococcosis. Acta Trop 2003, 85:113–118. [New Dimensions in Hydatidology in the New Millenium].
9. Battelli G. Echinococcosis: costs, losses and social consequences of a neglected zoonosis. Vet Res Commun. 2009;33(Suppl 1):47–52.
10. Craig PS, McManus DP, Lightowlers MW, Chabalgoity JA, Garcia HH, Gavidia CM, et al. Prevention and control of cystic echinococcosis. Lancet Infect Dis. 2007;7:385–94.
11. Heath D, Yang W, Li T, Xiao Y, Chen X, Huang Y, Yang Y, Wang Q, Qiu J: Control of hydatidosis. Parasitol Int 2006, 55, Supplement:S247–S252. [Taeniasis/Cysticercosis and Echinococcosis with Focus on Asia and the Pacific].
12. Cabrera PA, Lloyd S, Haran G, Pineyro L, Parietti S, Gemmell MA, et al. Control of Echinococcus granulosus in Uruguay: evaluation of different treatment regimes for dogs. Vet Parasitol. 2002;103:333–40.
13. Plumb D.C. Veterinary Drug Handbook. Ames (Iowa): Wiley-Blackwell; 2011. p.2792-2799.
14. Gavidia CM, Gonzalez AE, Barron EA, Ninaquispe B, Llamosas M, Verastegui MR, et al. Evaluation of Oxfendazole, Praziquantel and Albendazole against cystic Echinococcosis: a randomized clinical trial in naturally infected sheep. PLoS Negl Trop Dis. 2010;4:e616.
15. Heath DD, Jensen O, Lightowlers MW: Progress in control of hydatidosis using vaccination—a review of formulation and delivery of the vaccine and recommendations for practical use in control programmes. Acta Trop 2003, 85:133–143. [New Dimensions in Hydatidology in the New Millenium].
16. Larrieu E, Mujica G, Gauci CG, Vizcaychipi K, Seleiman M, Herrero E, et al. Pilot field trial of the EG95 vaccine against ovine cystic Echinococcosis in Rio Negro, Argentina: second study of impact. PLoS Negl Trop Dis. 2015;9:e0004134.

Knowledge, attitudes, and practices regarding cystic echinococcosis and sheep herding...

35

17. Riviere-Cinnamond A, Eregae M: Community-Based Animal Health Workers in Pastoralist Areas of Kenya: A Study on Selection Processes, Impact and Sustainability. 2003.
18. Programa Nacional de Tambos [http://apu.vivienda.gob.pe/tambook/inicio].
19. Center for Disease Control. Cystic Echinococcosis (CE) FAQs. [https://www.cdc.gov/parasites/echinococcosis/index.html].
20. Oficina General de Estadística en Informática - Sistema HIS. Health Ministry of Peru: 2012.
21. Brunetti E, Garcia HH, Junghanss T. On behalf of the members of the international CE workshop in lima P 2009: cystic Echinococcosis: chronic, complex, and still neglected. PLoS Negl Trop Dis. 2011;5:e1146.
22. Robles M, Ramirez R: Mapa de Pobreza Provincial y Distrital 2009. 2010.
23. Moro PL, Cavero CA, Tambini M, Briceño Y, Jiménez R, Cabrera L. Prácticas, conocimientos y actitudes sobre la Hidatidosis Humana en poblaciones procedentes de zonas endémicas. Rev Gastroenterol Perú. 2008;28:43–9.
24. Moro PL, Lopera L, Bonifacio N, Gonzales A, Gilman RH, Moro MH. Risk factors for canine echinococcosis in an endemic area of Peru. Vet Parasitol. 2005;130:99–104.

6

High genotypic diversity among methicillin-resistant *Staphylococcus pseudintermedius* isolated from canine infections in Denmark

Peter Damborg[1*], Arshnee Moodley[1], Bent Aalbæk[1], Gianpiero Ventrella[2], Teresa Pires dos Santos[1] and Luca Guardabassi[1,3]

Abstract

Background: Methicillin-resistant *Staphylococcus pseudintermedius* (MRSP) has emerged globally in companion animals in the last decade. In Europe, the multidrug-resistant sequence type (ST)71 is widespread, but recently other clones have appeared. The objective of this study was to examine genotypic diversity and antimicrobial resistance of clinical MRSP isolates obtained from dogs, including dogs sampled on multiple occasions, in Denmark over a six-year period. For that purpose a total of 46 clinical MRSP isolates obtained from 36 dogs between 2009 and 2014 were subjected to antimicrobial susceptibility testing, multilocus-sequence typing (MLST) and SCC*mec* typing.

Results: Twenty-three sequence types were identified with ST71, mostly associated with SCC*mec* II-III, as the most common occurring in 13 dogs. Among the remaining 33 isolates, 19 belonged to clonal complex (CC)258 comprising ST258-SCC*mec* IV and its single- and double-locus variants. These were susceptible to 4–7 of the 22 antibiotics tested, whereas CC71 isolates were susceptible to only 2–5 antibiotics. Clone-specific differences were especially pronounced for fluoroquinolones and aminoglycosides with most CC71 isolates being resistant and almost all CC258 isolates being susceptible. Sixteen of the 19 CC258 isolates had oxacillin MICs of 0.5 g/L, whereas MICs for CC71 isolates were consistently above 4 g/L. Four of five dogs representing multiple isolates had distinct STs on different sampling events.

Conclusions: The overall genotypic diversity of MRSP is high in Denmark indicating multiple acquisitions of SCC*mec* into distinct clones, and mutational evolution, which appears to be particularly rapid for certain ancestral clones such as ST258. ST71-SCC*mec* II-III is the most common MRSP lineage and is typically multidrug-resistant. CC258-SCC*mec* IV isolates, which emerged in Denmark since 2012, display susceptibility to a wider range of antimicrobials. The isolation of distinct STs in individual dogs over time suggests repeated exposure or short-term genetic evolution of MRSP clones within patients.

Keywords: MRSP, Dog, Antibiotic resistance, Multilocus sequence typing, ST71, ST258

Background

Staphylococcus pseudintermedius is an opportunistic pathogen in dogs causing mainly integumentary infections [1]. In the last decade, methicillin-resistant *S. pseudintermedius* (MRSP) has emerged globally. MRSP is resistant to all beta-lactams, and multidrug-resistance occurs frequently, especially among multilocus sequence type (ST)71 and ST68, which predominate in dogs across Europe and North America, respectively [2]. Recently, other clones such as ST258 and closely related variants have been detected with relatively high frequency in Norway [3, 4] and the Netherlands [5], and sporadically in other EU countries [6–9]. Apart from often being resistant to fewer antimicrobial classes, these clones appear to be less virulent than ST71 as suggested by a lower tendency to produce biofilm [3] and less adherence to canine corneocytes [10]. The aim of this study was to assess the genotypic diversity and antimicrobial susceptibility of canine clinical MRSP isolates in Denmark over a 5-year period, with

* Correspondence: pedam@sund.ku.dk
[1]Department of Veterinary Disease Biology, Faculty of Health and Medical Sciences, University of Copenhagen, Stigbøjlen 4, 1870 Frederiksberg C, Denmark
Full list of author information is available at the end of the article

emphasis on temporal shifts in the general dog population and in individual dogs sampled on multiple occasions.

Methods

A total of 46 clinical MRSP isolates obtained from integumentary infections ($n = 37$), mucosal sites ($n = 4$) or other sites ($n = 5$) were collected at the University of Copenhagen veterinary diagnostic laboratory Sund Vet Diagnostik from 36 dogs between 2009 and 2014. All isolates were verified as MRSP by *nuc* and *mecA* PCR [11, 12]. Isolates were tested for antimicrobial susceptibility using Sensititre COMPAN1F broth microdilution plates (Thermo Fisher Scientific, Hvidovre, Denmark) according to the Clinical Laboratory Standards Institute [13]. Separately for doxycycline, susceptibility was tested by disk diffusion according to the breakpoints established by Maaland et al. [14]. Isolates were also subjected to Staphylococcal Cassette

Chromosome (SCC) *mec* typing [11] and multilocus sequence typing (MLST) [15]. STs were compared to the existing *S. pseudintermedius* database using the eBURST V3 software [16]. We used an arbitrary definition of clonal complexes (CCs) that included major group/subgroup founders (with more than 3 single-locus links) from the MLST database and respective single- and double locus variants (SLVs and DLVs).

Results and discussion

A total of 23 STs were detected among the 36 dogs (Table 1), including two STs (ST258 and ST273) occurring repeatedly in individual dogs at different sampling times (Table 2). This high overall genotypic diversity is notable and resembles what was recently observed in Norway and the Netherlands [4, 5]. With regards to number of dogs infected, ST71 predominated and was detected in 13 dogs, whereas the second most common

Table 1 Characteristics of the 46 MRSP isolates included in the study

Clonal Com-plex	MLST type	No. of isolates	No. of dogs	SCCmec type	No. (type) of antibiotics susceptible to[a]
CC45	ST45	3	3	NT[b]	2-3 (AMI, CHL, GEN, RIF, SXT)
	ST288[c]	1	1	V	3 (AMI, CHL, RIF)
CC68	ST271[c]	1	1	V	4 (AMI, CHL, GEN, RIF)
CC71	ST71	13	13	II–III ($n = 11$) NT ($n = 2$)	2–5 (AMI, CHL, DOX, GEN, RIF, SXT)
	ST270[c]	1	1	II–III	3 (CHL, RIF, SXT)
	ST272[d]	1	1	II–III	2 (CHL, RIF)
CC258	ST118[d]	1	1	IV	7 (AMI, CHL, ENR, GEN, MAR, RIF, SXT)
	ST258	7	2	IV	4–6 (AMI, CHL, ENR, GEN, MAR, RIF)
	ST261[c]	1	1	IV	5 (AMI, CHL, GEN, MAR, RIF)
	ST265[d]	1	1	IV	4 (CHL, ENR, MAR, RIF)
	ST267[d]	1	1	IV	6 (AMI, CHL, ENR, GEN, MAR, RIF)
	ST273[c]	2	1	IV	6 (AMI, CHL, ENR, GEN, MAR, RIF)
	ST277[c]	1	1	IV	6 (AMI, ENR, GEN, MAR, RIF)
	ST290[d]	2	2	IV, NT	6 (AMI, CHL, ENR, GEN, MAR, RIF)
	ST301[d]	1	1	IV	4 (CLI, ERY, MAR, RIF)
	ST414[d]	1	1	IV	5 (AMI, CHL, GEN, RIF, SXT)
	ST430[d]	1	1	IV	7 (AMI, CHL, ENR, GEN, MAR, RIF, SXT)
NA[e]	ST431	1	1	V	7 (AMI, CHL, CLI, DOX, ERY, GEN, RIF)
	ST268	1	1	IV	7 (AMI, CHL, ENR, GEN, MAR, RIF, SXT)
	ST269	2	2	IV	6–7 (AMI, CHL, ENR, GEN, MAR, RIF, SXT)
	ST284	1	1	V	3 (AMI, RIF, SXT)
	ST286	1	1	IV	6 (AMI, CHL, ENR, GEN, MAR, RIF)
	ST295	1	1	NT	7 (AMI, DOX, ENR, GEN, MAR, RIF, SXT)

AMI amikacin, *CHL* chloramphenicol, *CLI* clindamycin, *DOX* doxycycline, *ENR* enrofloxacin, *ERY* erythromycin, *GEN* gentamicin, *MAR* marbofloxacin, *RIF* rifampicin, *SXT* sulphamethoxazole and trimethoprim

[a]Out of the 22 antibiotics in the COMPAN1F broth microdilution panel. Underlined antibiotics are those for which some isolates within an ST were susceptible and others resistant

[b]NT, not typeable with the method of Kondo et al. [11]

[c]SLV of the founder of the clonal complex

[d]DLV of the founder of the clonal complex

[e]NA, not applicable as the STs are singletons

Table 2 MRSP clones over time in dogs that were MRSP positive on at least two sampling occasions

Dog ID	Date of isolation (month/year)	MLST type	Relatedness of clones
A	12/09	ST268	6 of 7 alleles in common (SLVs)
	08/10	ST269	
B	12/12	ST45	1 of 7 alleles in common
	01/13	ST71	
C	07/12	ST258	–
	10/12	ST258	
D	10/12	ST71	2 of 7 alleles in common
	11/12	ST295	
E	01/12	ST258	6 of 7 alleles in common (SLVs)
	03/12	ST273	
	06/12	ST273	
	07/12	ST258	
	11/12	ST258	
	12/12	ST258	
	02/13	ST258	

type (ST45) occurred in 3 dogs (Table 1). The frequent detection of ST71 was not surprising given its widespread appearance, and the occurrence of two closely related variants (ST270 and ST272) corroborates a recent Japanese study showing that the ST71 lineage is not as clonal as previously believed [17]. ST45 is the predominant MRSP clone in distant countries such as Australia, Thailand and Israel [18–20], but it is also relatively common in Europe. In fact, similar to our findings, it was the second most frequent MRSP clone after ST71 in both the Netherlands and in Finland [5, 21]. The eleven STs belonging to CC258 were detected in 13 dogs (Table 1). The presence of all these closely related variants of ST258 could indicate that this clone has existed and evolved for a longer time in Denmark than ST71. However, the vast majority (95 %) of ST258 isolates and variants from this study were obtained after 2012. A more plausible explanation may therefore be that the ST258 clone has a higher evolutionary rate than ST71, or that some unknown factor has favoured its recent dissemination. Interestingly, a partial and gradual replacement of CC71 with CC258 MRSP isolates was also noted in the Netherlands recently [5].

SCCmec typing confirmed the well-known association between ST71 and the SCCmec II-III element [2], except in two isolates where no SCC element could be identified (Table 1). SCCmec type IV was associated with 14 MLST types. Even though many of these types are closely related within CC258, the occurrence also in distantly related types (ST268, ST269, and ST286) suggests enhanced mobility or a low fitness cost of this element

as seen in methicillin-resistant *Staphylococcus aureus* (MRSA) [22]. SCCmec was non-typeable in the three ST45 isolates. This may reflect presence of the pseudo-SCCmec element ($\Psi SCCmec_{57395}$) that was recently discovered in this clone by Perreten et al. [18].

Antibiotic susceptibility testing revealed the multidrug-resistant nature of MRSP with only limited susceptibility to veterinary licensed antibiotics. This was particularly pronounced for certain clones (Table 1), for example ST71 with three isolates being susceptible only to chloramphenicol and rifampicin. Isolates belonging to CC258 were generally susceptible to more antibiotic classes compared to CC71 isolates (Table 1), thus supporting the findings by Kjellman et al. [4] and Duim et al. [5]. One of the major differences was that all 15 CC71 isolates were resistant to fluoroquinolones compared to only 1 of 19 CC258 isolates (Table 1). A similar picture was observed for aminoglycosides, since 10 of 15 CC71 isolates and 2 of 19 CC258 isolates were gentamicin resistant. Interestingly, the opposite trend was evident for doxycycline, with only 8 of 15 CC71 isolates and all 19 CC258 isolates displaying resistance. Rifampicin resistance was rarely detected (1/46 isolates), thus illustrating the potential use of this drug in systemic therapy against MRSP. However, rifampicin is registered for use in humans only and should be used with caution given its potential side effects such as hepatotoxicity. Furthermore, it should not be used as monotherapy but in combination with other antibiotics, since mutations conferring resistance readily develop during rifampicin therapy [23]. A closer look at the susceptibility data showed that 16 of the 19 CC258 isolates had oxacillin MICs of 0.5 g/L, whereas MICs for CC71 isolates were consistently above 4 g/L. This could have important implications, as commercial agar plates used by some laboratories for selective isolation of MRSP were originally designed for detection of MRSA, which have a higher oxacillin breakpoint than MRSP [13] and may not allow growth of strains with low-level oxacillin resistance. In order to check this we streaked all 46 isolates on Brilliance MRSA 2 agar plates (Thermo Fisher Scientific) followed by overnight incubation at 37 °C. Only one CC258 isolate failed to grow on this medium, whereas various levels of growth were detected among remaining isolates, irrespective of their oxacillin MIC (data not shown). This indicates that at least this commercial medium has a high sensitivity for detection of MRSP, although growth may not always be as pronounced as for MRSA.

Two of the five dogs representing multiple isolates had genetically unrelated MRSP clones isolated on different sampling occasions (Dogs B and D, Table 2). Two previous longitudinal studies detected MRSP from carrier sites such as the nose and perineum for several months following MRSP infections in dogs [24, 25]. In these studies the same clone was always recovered over time in individual dogs. This difference to our study is difficult to explain, although we analysed clinical isolates and not isolates from carrier sites. Dogs B and D may have been exposed to MRSP on multiple occasions, either in their normal environment or, perhaps more likely, at the veterinary clinics they visited during infection. In Dogs A and E (Table 2), the MRSP isolates were closely related (SLVs), suggesting that these dogs might have been infected by a single clone, which later evolved within the host. In all these dogs (A, B, D, and E), infection or colonization with multiple MRSP clones at the same time is possible, since Paul et al. [26] showed high heterogeneity amongst *S. pseudintermedius* isolates originating from different body sites of the same dog. Presence of multiple clones would have gone unnoticed in this study and in many other veterinary diagnostic laboratories, which usually select only one colony representing each morphological type for susceptibility testing.

Two cases of likely dog-dog transmission were observed based on the epidemiological information we retrieved. One case concerned the two ST71 isolates with an unknown SCC*mec*. These isolates had the same susceptibility profile and originated from two unrelated dogs attending the same hospital with a 2-week interval, suggesting transmission via the hospital environment. Another case comprised two dogs living in the same family. These dogs visited a veterinary hospital two weeks apart with skin infections caused by MRSP ST71 and ST270, respectively. These STs are SLVs, and the isolates shared the same antibiotic susceptibility profile. In this case transmission between the dogs, either before or after short-term evolution of ST71, is a likely scenario, although independent acquisition of these strains cannot be ruled out.

Conclusions

In conclusion, Danish clinical MRSP isolates are genotypically diverse indicating multiple acquisitions of SCC*mec* by distinct genetic backgrounds and rapid evolution of certain clones such as ST258. ST71-SCC*mec* II-III is the most common MRSP clone but the recent emergence of the less resistant ST258-SCC*mec* IV and related variants, signals a shift in the MRSP clonal population, which is similar to the gradual shift observed in the Netherlands recently. Further studies are needed to clarify lineage-specific virulence properties, and to assess whether the recent emergence of ST258 and related types in Europe has potential impact on veterinary care. Our results support previous evidence that MRSP can be a nosocomial pathogen [27]. Veterinary practitioners should therefore focus on hygiene measures and promote prudent antibiotic use to prevent spread of MRSP between patients.

Abbreviations
CC, clonal complex; DLV, double-locus variant; MIC, minimum inhibitory concentration; MLST, multilocus sequence typing; MRSA, methicillin-resistant *Staphylococcus aureus*; MRSP, methicillin-resistant *Staphylococcus pseudintermedius*; SCC*mec*, Staphylococcal Cassette Chromosome *mec*; SLV, single-locus variant; ST, sequence type

Acknowledgements
Thanks to Ljudmila Troianova and Jan Pedersen for technical assistance, and to Danish veterinary clinics for sending diagnostic specimens. This study was supported by internal funding.

Authors' contributions
LG and PD conceived the study and planned the experiment. Sample processing and laboratory analysis were done by AM, BA, PD, and LG. Data analysis was done by AM, PD, TP and LG. All authors contributed to the final version of the manuscript. All authors read and approved the final manuscript.

Competing interests
The authors declare that they have no competing interests.

Consent for publication
Not applicable.

Author details
[1]Department of Veterinary Disease Biology, Faculty of Health and Medical Sciences, University of Copenhagen, Stigbøjlen 4, 1870 Frederiksberg C, Denmark. [2]Department of Veterinary Medicine, Università degli Studi di Bari, Strada P.le per Casamassima Km 3, Valenzano-Bari 70010, Italy. [3]Department of Biomedical Sciences, Ross University School of Veterinary Medicine, Basseterre, West Indies, St Kitts and Nevis.

References
1. Bannoehr J, Guardabassi L. Staphylococcus pseudintermedius in the dog: taxonomy, diagnostics, ecology, epidemiology and pathogenicity. Vet Dermatol. 2012;23:253–66.
2. Perreten V, Kadlec K, Schwarz S, Grönlund Andersson U, Finn M, Greko C, et al. Clonal spread of methicillin-resistant Staphylococcus pseudintermedius in Europe and North America: an international multicentre study. J Antimicrob Chemother. 2010;65:1145–54.
3. Osland AM, Vestby LK, Fanuelsen H, Slettemeås JS, Sunde M. Clonal diversity and biofilm-forming ability of methicillin-resistant Staphylococcus pseudintermedius. J Antimicrob Chemother. 2012;67:841–8.
4. Kjellman EE, Slettemeås JS, Small H, Sunde M. Methicillin-resistant Staphylococcus pseudintermedius (MRSP) from healthy dogs in Norway - occurrence, genotypes and comparison to clinical MRSP. Microbiologyopen. 2015;4:857–66.
5. Duim B, Verstappen KM, Broens EM, Laarhoven LM, van Duijkeren E, Hordijk J, et al. Changes in the population of methicillin-resistant Staphylococcus pseudintermedius and dissemination of antimicrobial-resistant phenotypes in the Netherlands. J Clin Microbiol. 2016;54:283–8.
6. Haenni M, Alves De Moraes N, Châtre P, Médaille C, Moodley M, Madec JY. Characterisation of clinical canine meticillin-resistant and meticillin-susceptible Staphylococcus pseudintermedius in France. J Global Antimicrob Res. 2014;2:119–23.
7. Swedres-Svarm 2014. Consumption of antibiotics and occurrence of antibiotic resistance in Sweden. Solna/Uppsala, Sweden.
8. Rota A, Corrò M, Drigo I, Bortolami A, Börjesson S. Isolation of coagulase-positive staphylococci from bitches' colostrum and milk and genetic typing of methicillin-resistant Staphylococcus pseudintermedius strains. BMC Vet Res. 2015;11:160.

9.   PubMLST database. http://pubmlst.org. Accessed 28 June 2016.

10. Latronico F, Moodley A, Nielsen SS, Guardabassi L. Enhanced adherence of methicillin-resistant *Staphylococcus pseudintermedius* sequence type 71 to canine and human corneocytes. Vet Res. 2014;45:70.

11. Kondo Y, Ito T, Ma XX, Watanabe S, Kreiswirth BN, Etienne J, et al. Combination of multiplex PCRs for staphylococcal cassette chromosome *mec* type assignment: rapid identification system for *mec*, *ccr*, and major differences in junkyard regions. Antimicrob Agents Chemother. 2007;51:264–74.

12. Sasaki T, Tsubakishita S, Tanaka Y, Sakusabe A, Ohtsuka M, Hirotaki S, et al. Multiplex-PCR method for species identification of coagulase-positive staphylococci. J Clin Microbiol. 2010;48:765–9.

13. Clinical Laboratory Standards Institute (CLSI). Performance standards for antimicrobial disk and dilution susceptibility tests for bacteria isolated from animals; second informational supplement. CLSI document VET01S2. Wayne, Pennsylvania, USA: CLSI, Wayne; 2013.

14. Maaland MG, Papich MG, Turnidge J, Guardabassi L. Pharmacodynamics of doxycycline and tetracycline against *Staphylococcus pseudintermedius*: proposal of canine-specific breakpoints for doxycycline. J Clin Microbiol. 2013;51:3547–54.

15. Solyman SM, Black CC, Duim B, Perreten V, van Duijkeren E, Wagenaar JA, et al. Multilocus sequence typing for characterization of *Staphylococcus pseudintermedius*. J Clin Microbiol. 2013;51:306–10.

16. Eburst V3 software. http://Eburst.mlst.net. Accessed 28 June 2016.

17. Ishihara K, Koizumi A, Saito M, Muramatsu Y, Tamura Y. Detection of methicillin-resistant *Staphylococcus pseudintermedius* ST169 and novel ST354 SCC*mec* II-III isolates related to the worldwide ST71 clone. Epidemiol Infect. 2015 [in press].

18. Perreten V, Chanchaithong P, Prapasarakul N, Rossano A, Blum SE, Elad D, et al. Novel pseudo-staphylococcal cassette chromosome *mec* element (ψSCC*mec*57395) in methicillin-resistant *Staphylococcus pseudintermedius* CC45. Antimicrob Agents Chemother. 2013;57:5509–15.

19. Siak M, Burrows AK, Coombs GW, Khazandi M, Abraham S, Norris JM, et al. Characterization of meticillin-resistant and meticillin-susceptible isolates of *Staphylococcus pseudintermedius* from cases of canine pyoderma in Australia. J Med Microbiol. 2014;63:1228–33.

20. Kadlec K, Weiß S, Wendlandt S, Schwarz S, Tonpitak W. Characterization of canine and feline methicillin-resistant *Staphylococcus pseudintermedius* (MRSP) from Thailand. Vet Microbiol. 2016 (in press).

21. Grönthal T, Ollilainen M, Eklund M, Piiparinen H, Gindonis V, Junnila J, et al. Epidemiology of methicillin resistant *Staphylococcus pseudintermedius* in guide dogs in Finland. Acta Vet Scand. 2015;57:37.

22. Lee SM, Ender M, Adhikari R, Smith JM, Berger-Bächi B, Cook GM. Fitness cost of staphylococcal cassette chromosome *mec* in methicillin-resistant *Staphylococcus aureus* by way of continuous culture. Antimicrob Agents Chemother. 2007;51:1497–9.

23. Kadlec K, van Duijkeren E, Wagenaar JA, Schwarz S. Molecular basis of rifampicin resistance in methicillin-resistant *Staphylococcus pseudintermedius* isolates from dogs. J Antimicrob Chemother. 2011;66:1236–42.

24. Laarhoven LM, de Heus P, van Luijn J, Duim B, Wagenaar JA, van Duijkeren E. Longitudinal study on methicillin-resistant *Staphylococcus pseudintermedius* in households. PLoS One. 2011;6:e27788.

25. Windahl U, Reimegård E, Holst BS, Egenvall A, Fernström L, Fredriksson M, et al. Carriage of methicillin-resistant *Staphylococcus pseudintermedius* in dogs - a longitudinal study. BMC Vet Res. 2012;8:34.

26. Paul NC, Bärgman SC, Moodley A, Nielsen SS, Guardabassi L. *Staphylococcus pseudintermedius* colonization patterns and strain diversity in healthy dogs: a cross-sectional and longitudinal study. Vet Microbiol. 2012;160:420–7.

27. Lehner G, Linek M, Bond R, Lloyd DH, Prenger-Berninghoff E, Thom N, et al. Case–control risk factor study of methicillin-resistant *Staphylococcus pseudintermedius* (MRSP) infection in dogs and cats in Germany. Vet Microbiol. 2014;168:154–60.

7

Toxoplasma gondii and *Neospora caninum* in farm-reared ostriches (*Struthio camelus*) in China

Yongjie Feng[1], Yaoyao Lu[1], Yinghua Wang[2], Longxian Zhang[1] and Yurong Yang[1*] ⓘ

Abstract

Background: The parasites *Toxoplasma gondii* (*T. gondii*) and *Neospora caninum* (*N. caninum*) are globally distributed; they infect warm-blooded animals, including many avian species. The aim of this study was to evaluate the presence of these parasites in ostriches from central China. In total, 402 ostrich (*Struthio camelus*) samples (293 hearts, 77 brains, and 32 serum) from slaughterhouses of the Henan Province and Hebei Province were collected. The heart juice (*n* = 283) and serum samples (*n* = 32) were tested for antibodies to *T. gondii* using the modified agglutination test (MAT). Hematoxylin and eosin (H&E) staining, immunohistochemical (IHC) staining, and the polymerase chain reaction were used to examine the cysts and DNA of *T. gondii* and *N. caninum* parasites, respectively.

Results: Antibodies to *T. gondii* were detected in 6.4% (20/315) (cut-off, 25). No cysts or DNA of *T. gondii* or *N. caninum* were observed in any of the 293 hearts and 77 brains.

Conclusion: The results showed a low prevalence of *T. gondii* antibody in ostriches, compared to that in the other animals. *N. caninum* occurs at low to negligible frequencies in ostriches from China. This is the first report on screening ostriches in China for *T. gondii* antibodies.

Keywords: Antibody, Cysts, DNA, Epidemiology, Modified agglutination test

Background

Toxoplasma gondii is an obligate cyst-forming parasite known to infect many species of warm-blooded animals, including ostrich [1, 2]. Infection with *T. gondii* is usually asymptomatic, but it can cause severe illness in both humans and animals with weakened immune systems, and in the case of pregnancy [3]. *Neospora caninum* is a parasite similar to *T. gondii* in many respects as it causes abortion in cattle and paralysis in dogs [4, 5].

The breeding of ostriches for eggs, feathers, skin and meat is growing in China and its meat, in particular, is low in fat and highly palatable. The prevalence of *T. gondii* in free-range chickens is a good indicator of the presence of oocysts in the environment [6], and ostrich is much like free-range chickens that feed directly from the ground. It was speculated that *T. gondii* and *N. caninum* infection in ostriches may assess the presence of oocysts in the local soil and environment. Furthermore, the consumption of undercooked ostrich meat containing *T. gondii* cysts might be a source of infection to consumers. Although the prevalence of *T. gondii* in ostriches has been reported in various countries [7–13], no research studies on *T. gondii* infection in ostriches from China have been conducted to date. Recently, the first report of isolation of *T. gondii* from ostriches was published [2]. The aim of this study was to determine the presence of *T. gondii* and *N. caninum* in farm-raised ostriches from China and attempt to isolate *T. gondii*.

Methods
Sample collection
A total of 402 ostrich (*Struthio camelus*) samples (283 fresh hearts, 77 fresh brains, 32 fresh sera, and 10 formalin-fixed hearts) from slaughterhouses in two provinces (Henan Province: 165 hearts, 77 brains, 32 sera and 10 formalin-fixed hearts samples; Hebei

* Correspondence: yangyu7712@sina.com
[1]Laboratory of Veterinary Pathology, College of Animal Science and Veterinary Medicine, Henan Agricultural University, Zhengzhou 450002, People's Republic of China
Full list of author information is available at the end of the article

Province: 118 hearts) were collected between 2012 and 2015 (Table 1). All ostriches was above 10 months old, however the sex was unknown. The provinces of Henan (31.38° to 36.37°N and 110.35° to 116.65°E) and Hebei (36.08° to 42.67° N and 113.45° to 119.83°E) are located in central China. Unfrozen and fresh samples were transported to the Laboratory of Veterinary Pathology, Henan Agricultural University in cooler boxes. The ostriches were bred in paddocks and fed from the ground with greens and nutritious additives. Heart juice from 283 hearts was collected and centrifuged (1000 g, 5 min) and then assayed for antibodies against *T. gondii*. A total of 315 samples (283 heart juice and 32 sera) were screened for *T. gondii* antibodies. The samples were kept in a refrigerator with a temperature range of 2 °C to 4 °C until analysis (within 1 week).

Screening of ostriches body fluids for *T. gondii* antibodies

Using the modified agglutination test [14] at a dilution of 1:25, 1:50, 1:100 and 1:200, 315 body fluid samples (283 heart juice and 32 sera) were screened for *T. gondii* antibodies. *T. gondii*-positive serum from mice was used as a reference; negative serum and blank were performed in each plate. Whole formalin-treated *T. gondii* tachyzoite antigen was obtained from the Kerafast Company (Boston, MA, USA. Catalog No. EH2002). Serum dilution of 1:25 is effective for assessing the *T. gondii* antibody, which has been reported in ostriches and other animals [7, 8].

Histopathological examination of ostrich heart and brain tissues for *T. gondii* and *N. caninum*

A total of 370 ostrich tissue samples (293 hearts and 77 brains) were respectively cut into three pieces (1.0 × 1.0 × 0.3 cm), embedded in paraffin, and sectioned at a thickness of 5 μm. These tissue sections were then stained with hematoxylin and eosin (H&E). Immunohistochemical (IHC) staining was used to verify suspected samples by rabbit polyclonal *T. gondii* antibody and mouse polyclonal *N. caninum* antibody. *T. gondii*-positive tissues or *N. caninum*-positive tissues

from mice were used as reference; negative serum and blank were performed in each batch. The sections were examined with an Olympus CX21 optical microscope to search for cysts and determine the infection of *T. gondii* or *N. caninum*.

Isolation of viable *T. gondii* from ostrich hearts by bioassay in mice

Ostrich hearts that tested positive for *T. gondii* antibodies were bioassayed in mice individually (n = 8); sheep hearts containing *T. gondii* cysts were used as controls. Myocardia (50 g) from each heart were homogenized, digested in pepsin, and inoculated subcutaneously into 5 outbred *Kunming* mice, which were given water supplemented with dexamethasone phosphate (10 μg/ml) 3 days before inoculation [3]. The remaining pepsin-digested myocardial samples were stored in 1.5 mL cryotubes at −20 °C until further analysis. Clinical signs in these mice were observed daily. The mice were bled and sacrificed at 64 days post inoculation. Then the sera were diluted 1:25 and 1:200 to test for *T. gondii* antibodies; in addition, squash preparations of the brain were microscopically examined for *T. gondii* cysts. The mouse brains were then inoculated into new groups of mice.

PCR identification of *T. gondii* and *N. caninum* in ostrich heart and brain tissues

DNA was extracted from all tissue samples (293 hearts, 77 brains, and 8 pepsin -digested sediments of the myocardium) using a commercial DNA extraction kit (Tiangen Biotec Company, Beijing, China, DP304). PCR was used to detect the DNA of *T. gondii* (TOX5/TOX8) in amplified fragments of 450 bp [15] and *N. caninum* (NP6/NP21) in fragments of 337 bp [16]. The DNA isolated from *T. gondii* (CT1 strain) or *N. caninum* (NC1 strain) was used as a reference for PCR.

Statistical analysis

Statistical analysis was performed using GraphPad Prism 4.0 (GraphPad Software Inc., San Diego, CA,

Table 1 Samples from Ostriches raised on farms in Henan Province and Hebei Province (n = 402)

Location	Collection time	Samples No.	Positive No. in different titers				Total positive No. and rate (%)	Isolation obtained by mice from samples[a]
			25	50	100	200		
Hebei Province	2015 Summer/fall	118 hearts	0	0	0	0	–	0
Henan Province	2015 Spring[b]	31 hearts	1	0	0	0	1/31 (3.2%)	0/1
	2015 Fall[b]	134 hearts	13	10	8	0	19/166 (11.5%)	0/7
		66 brains	–	–	–			
		32 sera	6	6	6			
	2012–2014	10 hearts[c] 11 brains[c]	–				–	0
Total	2012–2015	293 hearts 77 brains 32 sera	20	16	14	0	20/315 (6.4%)	0/8

[a]Number of antibody-positive groups /Number of inoculated-groups
[b]P-value >0.05 by two-tailed chi-square tests for season factor in Henan Province
[c]formalin fixed samples

USA). Data were analyzed by using the chi-square test or Fisher's exact test. $P < 0.05$ was considered statistically significant.

Results and discussion

T. gondii antibody testing

T. gondii antibodies have been previously detected in the meat juice of pig, sheep, and cattle [17, 18]. In the present study, by using MAT, *T. gondii* antibodies were found in 6.4% (20/315) of the ostriches, with titers of 25 in 20, titers of 50 in 16, titers of 100 in 14 (8 hearts and 6 sera), and none showed a titer >200. The seroepidemiology of *T. gondii* was 10.2% (20/197: 165 hearts, 32 sera) in Henan Province. None of the samples from Hebei Province (118 hearts) were positive (Table 1). Hebei is located north of Henan, drier and colder. The climate of Hebei Province may contribute to the negative toxoplasmosis results involving ostriches from the region. In Henan Province, 11.5% (19/166) of the ostrich samples that were collected in the fall were seropositive for *T. gondii*, whereas 3.2% (1/31) of those collected in the spring were seropositive. The risk of *T. gondii* infection in the fall was thus higher compared to that in the spring, with an odds ratio of 3.878 (95% CI, 0.4995–30.10). However, this difference was not statistically significant ($P > 0.05$). This finding suggests that ostriches from Henan Province had been in contact with *T. gondii* oocysts from cats or from soil, water, or food. Ostriches feed from the ground, are raised much like free-range chickens and have a relatively free activity field. In Henan Province, the seroprevalence of *T. gondii* in free-range chickens was 18.9% (132/700) [19]; in cats, it was 52.3% (102/195) and 51.6% (16/31) [20, 21]; 12.7% (99/779) and 29.3% (83/283) in sheep [22, 23], 23.7% (627/2642) in pig [24]. Compared with these reports, seroprevalence of *T. gondii* was lower among farm-reared ostriches (10.2%, 20/197) in the same location. This result is consistent with other reports. A low prevalence of *T. gondii* antibodies in ostriches has been reported in other countries. The seroprevalence of *T. gondii* was about 74% to 80% among backyard chickens in Brazil [25, 26], but lower among ostriches (about 11% to 17%) [2, 9, 10] (Table 2). A summary of the prevalence of *T. gondii* in ostriches in various countries is shown in Table 2. Prevalence varies from 1% to 48%, depending on the country. In conclusion, this is the first report to show the prevalence of *T. gondii* in ostriches from China.

T. gondii isolation, T. gondii and N. caninum morphological and molecular assays

Viable *T. gondii* had been isolated from ostrich brains, thereby serving as direct evidence that ostriches are intermediate hosts [2]. Isolation of *T. gondii* from the chicken heart or brain by bioassay in mice has been

Table 2 Prevalence of *Toxoplasma gondii* infection in ostriches

Country	No. of samples received	No. of seropositive (%)	Serologic test (cut-off titer)	References
Zimbabwe	50	24 (48%)	MAT (25)	[8]
Canada	973	28 (3%)	MAT (25)	[7]
Brazil	46	8 (17%)	MAT (16)	[9]
	195	28 (14%)	MAT (16)	[10]
	344	38 (11%)	MAT (8)	[2]
Spain	117	1 (1%)	MAT (25)	[11]
Egypt	120	15 (13%)	MAT (25)	[12]
Iran	28	6 (21%)	ELISA	[13]
China	315	20 (6%)	MAT (25)	This study

shown to be effective [3, 27]. A previous study has shown that the density of *T. gondii* cysts in the heart is higher than that in muscle or brain of chickens [27]. Eight ostrich hearts were bioassayed in immunosuppressed *Kunming* mice in an effort to isolate *T. gondii*, but this was unsuccessful. Furthermore, H&E or IHC staining did not detect any tissue cysts of *T. gondii* or *N. caninum*, and no positive DNA of *T. gondii* or *N. caninum* was detected by PCR in a total of 370 ostrich tissue samples and 8 pepsin-digested liquids from myocardia. These results may be explained by (1) the relative low density of *T. gondii* cysts in ostriches from China or (2) false positive on the MAT. Antigen from whole formalin-treated tachyzoites was used in the MAT. The MAT is highly sensitive and has been extensively used to test *T. gondii* antibodies in many animals and birds, including ostriches. The accuracy of the MAT has been validated in ostriches because 14/38 (36.8%) isolation has been achieved [2]. However, we can not rule out the possibility that *T. gondii* antigen cross-reacts with other parasites (*Hammondia hammondi*) [28].

Some birds (chickens, pigeons, sparrows) have been shown to be intermediate hosts for *N. caninum* [29]. However, a recent literature search has found no study on *N. caninum* in ostriches. Ostriches have not been proven to be intermediate hosts for *N. caninum*. An examination of tissue sections was the most straightforward way of observing the parasites and lesions by light microscopy. Mineo found that no serological positivity of *N. caninum* was observed in 294 samples of serum. However, *N. caninum* cysts were found in Psittaciformes muscle by tissue section [30]. PCR is a sensitive method for detecting parasites. The DNA of *N. caninum* in the heart and brain of many animals has detected by PCR, particularly in the brains [31]. The absence of *N. caninum* from these ostrich samples suggests that this parasite occurs at low to negligible frequencies in ostriches from China. Further investigations using samples from different areas may facilitate in better understanding the process of neosporosis in ostriches.

Conclusions

The results of the present study indicate that *T. gondii* has a lower prevalence in ostriches compared to other animals, the cause of this difference is unknown. However, consumers are precautions of eating raw or undercooked ostrich meat to avoid being infected with *T. gondii*. *N. caninum* occurs at low to negligible frequencies in ostriches from China. The establishment of differences in prevalence rates between ostrich and other birds may assist in the design of preventive and control measures against toxoplasmosis.

Abbreviations

H&E: Hematoxylin and eosin staining; IHC: Immunohistochemistry; MAT: Modified agglutination test; PCR: Polymerase chain reaction

Acknowledgments

We thank J. P. Dubey (US Department of Agriculture, Beltsville, MD, USA) and J. Liu (China Agricultural University, Beijing, China) for providing positive serum, primary antibody, positive tissues, and DNA of *T. gondii* or *N. caninum*.

Funding

The China Henan Science and Technology Open and Cooperation Project (Grant No. 152106000056) and China Postdoctoral Science Foundation (Grant No. 2016M600577) supported this study.

Authors' contributions

YJF performed the laboratory tests, data analysis, and wrote the manuscript. YYL, YHW participated in sample collection and laboratory testing. LXZ helped in the writing of the manuscript. YRY designed the study protocol, analyzed the results and helped in the writing of the manuscript. All authors have read and approved the final version of the manuscript.

Consent for publication

All authors consent for publication of this report.

Competing interests

The authors declare that they have no competing interests. None of the authors of this report have financial or personal relationships with other people or organizations that could inappropriately influence its content.

Author details

[1]Laboratory of Veterinary Pathology, College of Animal Science and Veterinary Medicine, Henan Agricultural University, Zhengzhou 450002, People's Republic of China. [2]Center for Animal Disease Control and Prevention of Henan Province, Zhengzhou 450002, People's Republic of China.

References

1. Dubey JP. A review of toxoplasmosis in wild birds. Vet Parasitol. 2002; 106(2):121–53.
2. da Silva RC, Langoni H. Risk factors and molecular typing of *Toxoplasma gondii* isolated from ostriches (*Struthio camelus*) from a Brazilian slaughterhouse. Vet Parasitol. 2016;225:73–80.
3. Dubey JP. Toxoplasmosis of animals and humans. Boca Raton: CRC Press; 2010.
4. Dubey JP. Neosporosis in dogs. Commonw Agric Bur Rev. 2013;8:1–26.
5. Lorenzi H, Khan A, Behnke MS, Namasivayam S, Swapna LS, Hadjithomas M, Karamycheva S, Pinney D, Brunk BP, Ajioka JW, Ajzenberg D, Boothroyd JC, Boyle JP, Dardé ML, Diaz-Miranda MA, Dubey JP, Fritz HM, Gennari SM, Gregory BD, Kim K, Saeij JP, Su C, White MW, Zhu XQ, Howe DK, Rosenthal BM, Grigg ME, Parkinson J, Liu L, Kissinger JC, Roos DS, Sibley LD. Local admixture of amplified and diversified secreted pathogenesis determinants shapes mosaic *Toxoplasma gondii* genomes. Nat Commun. 2016;7:10147.
6. Dubey JP. *Toxoplasma gondii* infections in chickens (*Gallus domesticus*): prevalence, clinical disease, diagnosis and public health significance. Zoonoses Public Health. 2010;57(1):60–73.
7. Dubey JP, Scandrett WB, OCH K, Gajadhar AA. Prevalence of antibodies to *Toxoplasma gondii* in ostriches (*Struthio camelus*). J Parasitol. 2000;86(3):623–4.
8. Hove T, Mukaratirwa S. Seroprevalence of *Toxoplasma gondii* in farm-reared ostriches and wild game species from Zimbabwe. Acta Trop. 2005;94(1):49–53.
9. Almeida AB, Krindges MM, de Barros LD, Garcia JL, Camillo G, Vogel FSF, Araujo DN, Stefani LM, da Silva AS. Occurrence of antibodies to *Toxoplasma gondii* in rheas (*Rhea americana*) and ostriches (*Struthio camelus*) from farms of different Brazilian regions. Rev Bras Parasitol Vet. 2013;22(3):437–9.
10. Contente APA, Domingues PF, da Silva RC. Prevalence of *Toxoplasma gondii* antibodies in ostriches (*Struthio camelus*) from commercial breeding facilities in the state of São Paulo, Brazil. Braz J Vet Res Anim Sci. 2009;46(3):175–80.
11. Martínez-Díaz RA, Simmons B, Ponee-Gordo F. Serologic screening to detect *Toxoplasma gondii* antibodies in farmed ostriches (*Struthio camelus*) in Spain. Braz J Vet Parasitol. 2002;62(3–4):69–71.
12. El-Madawy SR, Metawea FY. Serological assays and PCR for detection of *Toxoplasma gondii* infection in an ostrich farm at Ismailia Provine. Egypt IOSR J Agr Vet Sci. 2013;2(2):56–60.
13. Rahimi E, Yazdanpour S, Dehkordi FS. Detection of *Toxoplasma gondii* antibodies in various poultry meat samples using enzyme linked immuno sorbent assay and its confirmation by polymerase chain reaction. J Pure Appl Microbio. 2014;8(1):421–7.
14. Dubey JP, Desmonts G. Serological responses of equids fed *Toxoplasma gondii* oocysts. Equine Vet J. 1987;19(4):337–9.
15. Su C, Dubey JP. Toxoplasma gondii in molecuar detection of foodborne pathogens. Boca Raton: CRC Press; 2009.
16. Liddell S, Jenkins MC, Dubey JP. A competitive PCR assay for quantitative detection of *Neospora caninum*. Int J Parasitol. 1999;29(10):1583–7.
17. Račka K, Bártová E, Budíková M, Vodrážka P. Survey of *Toxoplasma gondii* antibodies in meat juice of wild boar (*Sus scrofa*) in several districts of the Czech Republic. Ann Agric Environ Med. 2015;22(2):231–5.
18. Berger-Schoch AE, Bernet D, Doherr MG, Gottstein B, Frey CF. Toxoplasma gondii in Switzerland: a serosurvey based on meat juice analysis of slaughtered pigs, wild boar, sheep and cattle. Zoonoses Public Health. 2011;58(7):472–8.
19. Feng YJ, Lu YY, Wang YH, Liu J, Zhang LX, Yang YR. *Toxoplasma gondii* and *Neospora caninum* in free-range chickens in Henan Province of China. Biomed Res Int. 2016;2016:8290536.
20. Wang HY, Pei SL, Hao ZF, Zhou M. Investigation on epidemiology of toxoplasmosis in dogs and cats in Zhengzhou City. J Henan Agr Sci. 2012; 41(11):153–4. In Chinese
21. Yang YR, Ying YQ, Verma SK, Cassinelli ABM, Kwok OCH, Liang HD, Pradhan AK, Zhu XQ, Su CL, Dubey JP. Isolation and genetic characterization of viable *Toxoplasma gondii* from tissues and feces of cats from the central region of China. Vet Parasitol. 2015;211(3–4):283–8.
22. Zhang N, Wang S, Wang D, Li CY, Zhang ZC, Yao ZJ, Li TT, Xie Q, Liu SG, Zhang HZ. Seroprevalence of *Toxoplasma gondii* infection and risk factors in domestic sheep in Henan Province, central China. Parasite. 2016;23:53.
23. Yang YR, Feng YJ, Yao QX, Wang YH, Lu YY, Liang HD, Zhu XQ, Zhang LX. Seroprevalence, isolation, genotyping, and pathogenicity of *Toxoplasma gondii* strains from sheep in China. Front Microbiol. 2017;8:136.
24. Wen QN, Guo YH, Yang JF, Shen H, Du YC. Investigation on epidemiology of toxoplasmosis in pig from Henan Province. Chin J Vet Med. 2015;51(4): 44–5. In Chinese
25. Costa DGC, Marvulo MFV, Silva JSA, Santana SC, Magalhães FJR, Lima Filho CDF, Ribeiro VO, Alves LC, Mota RA, Dubey JP, Silva JCR. Seroprevalence of *Toxoplasma gondii* in domestic and wild animals from the Fernando de Noronha. Brazil J Parasitol. 2012;98(3):679–80.

26. Camillo G, Cadore GC, Ferreira MST, Braünig P, Maciel JF, Pivoto FL, Sangioni LA, Vogel FSF. *Toxoplasma gondii* and *Neospora caninum* antibodies in backyard chickens in Rio Grande do Sul. Brazil Braz J Poultry Sci. 2015;17(2):263–5.
27. Dubey JP, Lehmann T, Lautner F, Kwok OCH, Gamble HR. Toxoplasmosis in sentinel chickens (*Gallus domesticus*) in New England farms: seroconversion, distribution of tissue cysts in brain, heart, and skeletal muscle by bioassay in mice and cats. Vet Parasitol. 2015;214(1–2):55–8.
28. Munday BL, Dubey JP. Serological cross-reactivity between *Hammondia hammondi* and *Toxoplasma gondii* in experimentally inoculated sheep. Aust Vet J. 1986;63:344–5.
29. Donahoe SL, Lindsay SA, Krockenberger M, Phalen D, Šlapeta J. A review of neosporosis and pathologic findings of *Neospora caninum* infection in wildlife. Int J Parasitol Parasites Wildl. 2015;4(2):216–38.
30. Mineo TWP, Carrasco AOT, Raso TF, Werthera K, Pintoa AA, Machado RZ. Survey for natural *Neospora caninum* infection in wild and captive birds. Vet Parasitol. 2011;182(2–4):352–5.
31. Darwich L, Cabezon O, Echeverria I, Pabón M, Marco I, Molina-López R, Alarcia-Alejos O, López-Gatius F, Lavín S, Almería S. Presence of *Toxoplasma gondii* and *Neospora caninum* DNA in the brain of wild birds. Vet Parasitol. 2012;183(3–4):377–81.

8

Relation of antioxidant status at admission and disease severity and outcome in dogs naturally infected with *Babesia canis canis*

Martina Crnogaj[1], José Joaquin Cerón[2], Iva Šmit[1]* (iD), Ivana Kiš[1], Jelena Gotić[1], Mirna Brkljačić[1], Vesna Matijatko[1], Camila Peres Rubio[2], Nada Kučer[1] and Vladimir Mrljak[1]

Abstract

Background: Canine babesiosis is caused by species of the *Babesia* genus and has become an emerging disease worldwide. To the authors' knowledge there are no reports in which antioxidants have been analyzed in different presentations of canine babesiosis or in which the prognostic value of antioxidants has been studied. The aim of this study was to evaluate whether oxidative stress could be related to the severity and outcome of canine babesiosis. For this purpose a profile consisting of four antioxidant biomarkers (superoxide dismutase - SOD, glutathione peroxidase - GPx, catalase, total antioxidant status - TAS) and malondialdehyde - MDA as an oxidant biomarker (previously evaluated, here studied for comparative purposes) were evaluated in dogs with canine babesiosis of different clinical severity and outcomes.

Results: The study was conducted with a sample of 40 dogs suffering from babesiosis (further divided into uncomplicated, one complication and multiple organ dysfunction syndrome - MODS group) and 30 healthy dogs (control group). Additionally, the babesiosis group was divided according to the anaemia into non-anaemic, mildly anaemic, moderately anaemic and severely anaemic dogs. The results of our study showed significantly decreased SOD, catalase and TAS values in diseased dogs compared to controls, while there were no significant differences in GPx between these groups. Dogs that developed MODS showed lower activities of SOD and GPx and higher MDA values compared to dogs with uncomplicated babesiosis as well as with dogs that developed one complication. Superoxide dismutase, catalase and GPx were negatively correlated whereas MDA was positively correlated with the lethal outcome of the disease. Furthermore, this study detected more pronounced decrease in antioxidant biomarkers (SOD, GPx and catalase) in dogs with moderate anaemia compared to those with mild anaemia.

Conclusions: The results of this study showed changes in biomarkers related to the antioxidant status of dogs naturally infected with *B. canis canis*. These biomarkers could be used as indicators of disease severity and outcome in dogs suffering from babesiosis.

Keywords: Babesiosis, Dog, Antioxidant status, Glutathione peroxidase (GPx), Superoxide dismutase (SOD), Catalase, Total antioxidant status (TAS)

* Correspondence: iva.smit@vef.hr
[1]Clinic for Internal Diseases, Faculty of Veterinary Medicine, University of Zagreb, Zagreb, Croatia
Full list of author information is available at the end of the article

Background

Canine babesiosis is a tick born multisystemic disease with worldwide significance [1]. *Babesia spp.* are well-known intraerythrocytic parasites that cause disease in domestic and wild animals. Babesiosis in dogs is caused by species of the *Babesia* genus, which are divided into large babesia including *Babesia canis* and *Babesia sp. (Coco)* and small babesia including *Babesia gibsoni (B. gibsoni), Babesia conradae (B. conradae)* and *Babesia microti*-like piroplasms, also called *Babesia vulpes sp. nov.* There are three genetically distinct subspecies of *Babesia canis*: *Babesia canis canis (B.canis canis), Babesia canis vogeli (B.canis vogeli)* and *Babesia canis rossi (B. canis rossi)* [2–6].

Host response to infection and other forms of tissue injury in humans, as well as in dogs, have been termed the systemic inflammatory response syndrome (SIRS). This inflammatory response can frequently be accompanied by oxidative injury to one or more organ systems in the body leading to multiple organ dysfunction syndrome (MODS), which occurs in canine babesiosis and is related to poor prognosis [2, 7, 8]. Considering the fact that sepsis is defined as SIRS due to a confirmed infection (bacterial, viral, fungal or protozoal) canine babesiosis can be classified as protozoal sepsis [8–13].

Based on clinical manifestations, babesiosis can be classified as uncomplicated (without any organ dysfunction) and complicated form (involving one or various organ dysfunctions such as kidney, liver, lung, etc.) [14, 15]. Although various mechanisms have been suggested to cause both forms of babesiosis, recent studies have indicated that much of the disease process could be explained by host inflammatory responses to the parasite, rather than the parasite itself [16, 17]. The hypothesis that cytokines may also have an influence on the severity of babesiosis in dogs was investigated in several studies with the implication that a mixed cytokine response is present in dogs with babesiosis, and that an excessive pro-inflammatory response may result in a poor outcome [18]. An imbalance in host regulation of the pro-inflammatory systemic response and a compensatory modulating response can frequently be accompanied by oxidative injury in one or more organ systems in the body leading to progression from SIRS to MODS in septic patients with a fatal outcome in certain cases [18–21].

Regardless of its pathogenesis, any tissue damage, if severe enough, induces the release of proinflammatory mediators, including reactive oxygen species (ROS) and reactive nitrogen species (RNS), which are powerful oxidants and nitrating species that can inactivate enzymes and initiate lipid peroxidation and nitration, which in turn leads to free-radical chain reactions that further damage proteins, membranes and nucleic acids [22, 23].

An antioxidant is defined as "any substance that, when presented at low concentration compared to those of an oxidizable substrate (proteins, lipids, carbohydrates and DNA), significantly delays, or prevents oxidation of that substrate", thus protecting the body by elimination of the superoxide anion and hydroperoxides that may oxidize cellular substrates, and preventing a chain reaction of the destructive effects of free radicals [21, 24–26]. Superoxide dismutase (SOD), catalase and glutathione peroxidase (GPx) are the primary intracellular antioxidants and as such act as protective mechanisms during elevated oxidative stress. Total antioxidant status (TAS) evaluates the antioxidant activity of the organism in a global way [27, 28].

Oxidative stress is caused by an imbalance between oxidants and antioxidants and may occur at the level of cells, tissues, or even the whole organism [29]. In recent years, various studies have evaluated the role of oxidative stress and lipid peroxidation in the pathogenesis of babesiosis in different animal species [30–37]. However, to the authors' knowledge there are no studies in which antioxidant biomarkers have been analyzed in different presentations of canine babesiosis or their prognostic value studied. Furthermore, there are no studies in which the antioxidants have been analyzed in canine babesiosis caused by *B. canis canis*.

One of the main features of babesiosis is destruction of red blood cells resulting in hemolytic anaemia. However, the pathogenesis of anaemia in babesiosis has not yet been fully elucidated [38]. The quantity of the destroyed erythrocytes is usually much higher than the degree of parasitaemia, suggesting that non-parasited erythrocytes may also be damaged [39]. Some of the proposed mechanisms responsible for this phenomena could be: sequestration of infected erythrocytes in microcirculation, decreased erythrocyte deformability, hemodilution and destruction of red blood cells due to the effects of oxidative stress [17, 40–43].

The hypothesis of the current study is that the antioxidant response in dogs infected with *B. canis canis* could change depending on the severity of the clinical presentation, and that these changes could be related to the outcome of the disease. For this purpose a profile consisting of four antioxidant biomarkers, GPx, SOD, catalase and TAS, were measured in dogs with canine babesiosis, and changes in these markers were compared between healthy dogs and dogs with babesiosis, between dogs with and without complications, as well as between survivors and non-survivors.

Methods
Animals

This study was performed with 70 dogs that were divided into two groups: babesiosis and control group. All dogs were admitted to the Clinic for Internal Diseases,

Faculty of Veterinary Medicine, University of Zagreb, Croatia and owner consent was obtained for all dogs included in this study as part of a routine clinical protocol.

All dogs included in the study were clinically examined and blood samples were collected from the cephalic vein on the day of admission for haematology and biochemical analysis: blood urea nitrogen (BUN), creatinine, total protein (TP), albumin, alanine aminotransferase (ALT), alkaline phosphatase (AP), aspartate aminotransferase (AST), γ-glutamyl transferase (GGT), glucose, total bilirubin and creatine phosphokinase (CPK).

The babesiosis group consisted of 40 dogs naturally infected by B. canis canis showing clinical signs of acute babesiosis. Dogs in this group were aged between 1 and 13 years, of various breeds and both genders (27 male dogs: 67.5%, 13 female dogs: 32.5%). The diagnosis was confirmed by demonstration of the parasite within infected erythrocytes in blood smears stained with May-Grünwald Giemsa solution and polymerase chain reaction (PCR) analysis performed as previously described [44].

On the basis of clinical manifestations and laboratory data the affected dogs were divided into two groups: uncomplicated and complicated babesiosis, whereas the complicated group was further subdivided into those with one complication and the MODS group, due to the criteria listed in Table 1 [8, 11]. Additionally, the babesiosis group was divided according to the degree of anaemia (on the basis of haematocrit - HCT percentage) into non-anaemic: HCT >37%, mildly anaemic: 30–37%, moderately anaemic: 18–29% and severely anaemic: <18% dogs [45]. All the dogs from the babesiosis group developed SIRS according to a previous described criteria [46].

The control group consisted of 30 clinically healthy dogs of various breeds having a similar age (between 1 and 13 years) and gender distribution (19 male dogs: 63.3%, 11 female dogs: 36.7%) analogous to the infected dogs. The dogs were deemed healthy on the basis of history, clinical examination and laboratory data.

All dogs with confirmed babesiosis received a single dose (6.6 mg/kg of body weight) of imidocarb dipropionate (Imizol® 12%, Schering-Plough), subcutaneously. Dogs with complications received a standard additional therapy, according to clinical condition and type of complication. The therapy included: intravenous fluids (crystalloids ± colloids), number of dogs (N) = 11, oxygen supplementation via intranasal tubes or oxygen cage, N = 3, analgesia (fentanyl transdermal patch, according to patient body weight), N = 5, and intravenous antibiotics (amoxicillin clavulanic acid: 22 mg/kg intravenously every 8 h as monotherapy, or in combination with enrofloxacin 10 mg/kg intravenously every 12 h), N = 7.

Blood analyses

Samples were placed in tubes with ethylenediaminetetraacetic acid (EDTA) for haematological analysis, tubes with lithium heparin for analyzing SOD, GPx and catalase and tubes with no anticoagulant (centrifuged at 1500 × g at 4 °C for 10 min) for analyzing biochemistry profile, TAS and MDA. After sampling, blood was promptly analyzed for haematological analysis and routine biochemistry panel. Since acute pancreatitis has previously been identified as a potential complication of canine babesiosis [47] we also performed a SNAP cPL (canine pancreas-specific lipase) test (Idexx Laboratories, Westbrook) in order to confirm the presence of pancreatitis as a concurrent complication in 14 dogs that showed elevated lipase activity in our routine biochemistry profile.

After the initial analysis samples were stored at −80 °C until antioxidant measurements. The activities of GPx, SOD and catalase were determined in whole blood. Concentrations of TAS and MDA were determined from serum samples.

Table 1 Criteria used for distribution of affected dogs into subgroups

Uncomplicated babesiosis N = 29	Complicated babesiosis dogs that developed at least one of listed complication N = 11	
Dogs without any listed complication	Complication	Criteria
	Renal dysfunction	Creatinine >180 μmol/L
	Respiratory system dysfunction	Dyspnoea with typical nasal discharge or radiographic evidence of pulmonary oedema
	Hepatic dysfunction	ALT >176 U/L, AP >360 U/L, and Bilirubin* >100 μmol/L
	Muscular involvement	CPK > 600 U/L
	Central nervous system dysfunction	a modified Glasgow coma scale <9**
	Additional complication*** — Secondary infection	WBC > 17 × 10⁹/L (neutropenia with lymphopenia)
	Pancreatitis	Positive SNAP cPL test

cPL canine pancreas-specific lipase

*We included a total bilirubin serum concentration greater than 100 μmol/L as an additional criterion for hepatic dysfunction [62]

**Modified Glasgow coma scale: Welzl et al. [12]

***Pancreatitis [13] as well as signs of secondary infection were not considered as main complication, they were only mentioned (since being detected) as an additional complication

Activity of GPx was measured with a commercially available kit (Ransel test kit, Randox Laboratories Ltd. G.B.) based on the method of Paglia and Valentine [48]. SOD activity was measured with a commercial kit (Ransod test kit, Randox Laboratories Ltd. G.B.). Catalase activity was determined according to Johansson and Borg [49]. The activities of GPx and catalase were expressed as liter of whole blood (U/L). The activity of SOD was expressed as milliliter of whole blood (U/mL). Determination of TAS was through use of commercial test reagents (Randox test kit, Randox Laboratories Ltd. GB) according to the manufacturer's instructions. The concentration of TAS was expressed in mmol/L.

The concentration of MDA was measured with the method of Trotta et al. [50]. Absorbance was measured at 523 nm on a Thermospectronic Helios delta spectrophotometer (Unicam, Cambridge, UK). The concentration of MDA was expressed in μmol/L.

Statistical analysis
Pearson X^2 test was used to assess the significance of gender distribution between control and babesiosis groups. In order to test the difference between ages of control and babesiosis groups we conducted t-test for independent samples. In order to assess the normality of data distribution, Kolgomorov-Smirnov test was used. Given the non-parametric distribution of quantitative values, descriptive statistics were performed and the results are presented as median and interquartile range. Differences in analytes between groups were analyzed by Mann-Whitney U-test, with a P value <0.05 considered significant. The correlation between different biomarkers as well as between biomarkers and other laboratory parameters were assessed by Sperman rank correlation test. The relationship between oxidative status markers and outcomes was assessed using Tau-b correlation. The computer software IBM SPSS Statistics version 19.0.0.1. was used for analysis (www.spss.com).

Results
Pearson X^2 value = 0.132 with a P value of 0.716 indicated there were no significant differences in gender between the babesiosis and the control group. T-value = 0.29 with

P value >0.05 indicated there was no significant difference in age between the tested groups.

Depression (37/40), fever (35/40) and anorexia (32/40) were the most prevalent clinical signs at admission. Forty cases fulfilled the selection criteria for acute canine babesiosis and were included in the study. The presence of *B. canis canis* species was confirmed by PCR analysis for all 40 dogs. Uncomplicated babesiosis was diagnosed in 29 (72.5%) and complicated babesiosis in the remaining 11 dogs (27.5%). In dogs with complicated babesiosis, 6 (54.55%) had single organ dysfunction and 5 (45.45%) dogs had MODS. The observed complications were renal dysfunction (5/11), hepatic dysfunction (5/11), muscular involvement (7/11), respiratory system dysfunction (2/11) and central nervous system (CNS) dysfunction (1/11). In dogs that developed MODS, one had developed 4 organ dysfunction (namely: kidney, liver, CNS and muscles), two had 3 organ dysfunction (kidney, muscle and liver; kidney, muscle, respiratory system) while two had 2 organ dysfunction (kidney and muscle; liver and respiratory system). Five out of 14 dogs tested with the SNAP cPL test had positive results, four of which were classified in the MODS group, whereas one was classified in the group with one complication (namely, muscular involvement). Two out of 40 dogs were presented with haematology findings (elevated white blood cell number with marked lymphopenia and neutrophilia) on the basis of which they were considered to have secondary infection. Treatment was successful in all dogs without development of any complications as well as in 7 cases of complicated babesiosis, while 4 dogs with MODS died despite treatment (mortality rate 10%). Anaemia was detected in 23 dogs. Anaemia was severe only in 1/40 (2.5%), moderate in 6/40 (15%) and mild in 16/40 (40%) dogs.

Thirty dogs fulfilled the selection criteria for healthy animals and were included in the study as a control group.

Descriptive statistics of biochemistry parameters (urea, creatinine, bilirubine, ALT, AP, CPK), and haematology parameters (red blood cells - RBC, HCT, white blood cells - WBC and platelets - PLT) are shown in Additional file 1. Descriptive statistics of oxidative biomarkers (SOD,

Table 2 Values of biomarkers of oxidative stress in control and babesiosis group

	Control (N = 30)	Babesiosis (N = 40)
SOD (U/mL)	**0.26^a** (0.23–0.30)	**0.18^b** (0.15–0.22)
GPx (U/L)	**63,761.6^a** (54,664.82–74,960.58)	**60,366.21^a** (44,386.68–73,140.63)
Catalase (U/L)	**7992.15^a** (5944.98–11,082.35)	**4902.49^b** (2000.96–6790.53)
TAS (mmol/L)	**1.25^a** (1.17–1.32)	**0.97^b** (0.9–1.13)
MDA (μmol/L)	**2.31^b** (1.90–2.80)	**4.5^a** (3.11–5.67)

Median (25–75 percentile). Different superscripted small letters (a-b) in each row indicate significant differences (P < 0.001) and the same superscripted letters indicate no statistical difference. Also, a → b signifies highest to lowest value

Table 3 Values of biomarkers of oxidative stress in control and babesiosis subgroups

	Control (N = 30)	Uncomplicated (N = 29)	Complicated (N = 11)	
			One complication (N = 6)	MODS (N = 5)
SOD (U/mL)	**0.26ᵃ** (0.23–0.30)	**0.18ᵇ** (0.17–0.23)	**0.17ᵇ** (0.15–0.24)	**0.07ᶜ** (0.04–0.10)
GPx (U/L)	**63,761.6ᵃ** (54,664.82–74,960.58)	**63,761.79ᵃ** (57,987.78–76,193.72)	**58,446.62ᵃ** (38,885.96–74,709.27)	**29,958.11ᵇ** (11,456.91–36,238.04)
Catalase (U/L)	**7992.15ᵃ** (5944.98–11,082.35)	**5702.03ᵇ** (3338.82–6697.92)	**5319.77ᵃᵇ** (1398.63–9084.15)	**1265.76*ᶜ** (1081.47–2145.59)
TAS (mmol/L)	**1.25ᵃ** (1.17–1.32)	**0.97ᵇ** (0.89–1.08)	**1.02ᵇ** (0.89–1.13)	**1.15ᵇ** (0.85–1.7)
MDA (μmol/L)	**2.31ᶜ** (1.90–2.80)	**4.50ᵇ** (2.99–5.24)	**4.44ᵇ** (2.99–5.54)	**10.5ᵃ** (7.03–13.66)

Median (25–75 percentile). Different superscripted small letters (a-c) in each row indicate significant differences ($P < 0.05$) and the same superscripted letters indicate no statistical difference. Also, a → c signifies highest to lowest value
*There was no significant difference between MODS and one complication group in catalase activity

catalase, GPx, TAS and MDA) are shown in Tables 2, 3, 4 and 5.

The activities of SOD and catalase as well as TAS concentration were significantly lower ($P < 0.001$) in diseased dogs compared with the control group. There was no significant difference ($P > 0.05$) in GPx activity between diseased dogs and controls. The concentration of MDA was significantly increased ($P < 0.001$) in diseased dogs in comparison to the control group (Table 2).

No significant changes were found in investigated biomarkers between dogs with one complication and dogs with uncomplicated babesiosis. However, dogs with MODS showed significantly lower ($P < 0.01$) activities of catalase, SOD and GPx and significantly higher ($P < 0.01$) MDA concentrations compared to dogs with uncomplicated babesiosis. Moreover, dogs with MODS showed significantly lower activities of SOD ($P < 0.01$) and GPx ($P < 0.05$) and significantly higher ($P < 0.05$) MDA concentrations compared to dogs that developed only one complication, however there was no statistical significance detected in catalase activity between these groups (Table 3). Concentrations of TAS were higher in dogs with MODS compared to dogs with uncomplicated babesiosis as well as with dogs that developed only one complication, but detected differences were not statistically significant. Correlations between biochemistry parameters and investigated biomarkers are shown in Table 6. There was a significant negative correlation between antioxidants (SOD, GPx and catalase) and bilirubin but a significant positive correlation between MDA and bilirubin. Furthermore, there was a strong negative correlation of SOD and GPx with CPK and a positive correlation between MDA and urea. In addition, there was a significant negative correlation between GPx and AP.

The lethal outcome of the disease was significantly negatively correlated with SOD, GPx, and catalase, and significantly positively correlated with MDA and TAS (Table 7).

Correlations between the investigated biomarkers are shown in Table 8. There was a significant negative correlation between MDA and antioxidants (SOD, GPx, catalase). A significant positive correlation was detected between GPx and SOD as well as between GPx and catalase.

Values of SOD were significantly lower ($P < 0.001$) whereas values of MDA were significantly higher ($P < 0.001$) in anaemic dogs with babesiosis compared to non-anaemic dogs (Table 4). Furthermore, considering the severity of anaemia, the activities of SOD, GPx and catalase were significantly lower ($P < 0.01$) in moderately anaemic dogs compared to mildly anaemic. There was no significant difference in TAS concentration between anaemic and non-anaemic dogs (Table 4) as well as between different degrees of anaemia (Table 5). Also, there was a significant positive correlation of HCT with GPx and SOD, whereas significant negative correlation of HCT with MDA (Table 6).

Discussion

The aim of this study was to evaluate the possible changes of four antioxidant biomarkers (SOD, GPx, catalase and TAS) depending on the severity of canine babesiosis at admission and their correlation with the outcome. In addition, the relationship of these markers

Table 4 Values of biomarkers of oxidative stress in non-anaemic and anaemic babesiosis group

	Non-anaemic (N 17)	Anaemic (N 23)
SOD (U/mL)	**0.22ᵃ** (0.19–0.25)	**0.16ᵇ** (0.14–0.17)
GPx (U/L)	**63,761.79ᵃ** (59,413.29–76,193.72)	**55,268.09ᵃ** (36,798.41–71,138.54)
Catalase (U/L)	**4983.58ᵃ** (3072.30–7022.41)	**4821.39ᵃ** (1717.07–6350.30)
TAS (mmol/L)	**0.97ᵃ** (0.91–1.13)	**0.98ᵃ** (0.86–1.13)
MDA (μmol/L)	**3.21ᵇ** (2.41–4.50)	**5.18ᵃ** (4.44–6.97)

Median (25–75 percentile). Different superscripted small letters (a-b) in each row indicate significant differences ($P < 0.05$) and the same superscripted letters indicate no statistical difference. Also, a → b signifies highest to lowest value

Table 5 Values of biomarkers of oxidative stress in dogs with babesiosis according to severity of anaemia

*	Non-anaemic (N 17)	Mildly anaemic (N 16)	Moderately anaemic (N 6)
SOD (U/mL)	**0.22**[a] (0.19–0.25)	**0.17**[b] (0.15–0.18)	**0.10**[c] (0.07–0.14)
GPx (U/L)	**63,761.79**[a] (59,413.29–76,193.72)	**64,598.96**[a] (49,248.25–77,186.53)	**36,238.04**[b] (23,134.80–42,991.35)
Catalase (U/L)	**4983.58**[a] (3072.30–7022.41)	**5842.74**[a] (2423.70–7178.58)	**2145.59**[b] (1199.79–5087.84)
TAS (mmol/L)	**0.97**[a] (0.91–1.13)	**0.97**[a] (0.87–1.08)	**1.05**[a] (0.75–1.35)
MDA (µmol/L)	**3.21**[b] (2.41–4.50)	**5.09**[a] (4.41–6.23)	**7.9**[a] (4.39–12.63)

Median (25–75 percentile). Different superscripted small letters (a-c) in each row indicate significant differences ($P < 0.05$) and the same superscripted letters indicate no statistical difference. Also, a → c signifies highest to lowest value
*Since there was only one severely anaemic dog statistic analysis could not be preformed

with anaemia was evaluated. An oxidant biomarker (MDA) previously evaluated in canine babesiosis was studied for comparative purposes [32].

Considering noted marked differences in oxidative stress between males and females in previous studies [51, 52] the gender representation in the control group was purposeful, nonrandom sample. Accordingly, in the current study there was a proportional gender representation between the babesiosis and the control group.

In the present study, in general, a decrease in the antioxidant biomarkers in dogs with babesiosis was observed. These results agree with those reported earlier in sheep suffering from babesiosis [34, 53], in cattle suffering from theileria [31, 54] and in people suffering from malaria [24, 55, 56]. However, Chaudhuri et al. [38] found significantly increased SOD and catalase activity in dogs infected with *B. gibsoni*. Additionally, *B. gibsoni*-infected erythrocytes in vitro showed increased values of SOD and glutathione reductase [30]. Differences in the pathophysiological effects of the parasite species or in the assay used for biomarker measurements could be the cause for these divergences. Generally, it is considered that antioxidant biomarkers are reduced in conditions associated with oxidative stress [57, 58]. Therefore, the significant reduction in antioxidant biomarkers found in diseased dogs in this study could be attributed to the consumption of antioxidants that act as "scavengers" of free radicals during the oxidative processes in

the natural infection with *B. canis canis* in dogs. On the other hand, the increase in MDA concentration in dogs with babesiosis found in this research is consistent with the results of Crnogaj et al. [59] in dogs affected by babesiosis and implies its association with an increase in oxidative compounds.

Anaemia as a common feature of canine babesiosis has been investigated in numerous studies, yet its pathogenesis still remains questionable. Our study detected more pronounced decrease in antioxidant biomarkers (SOD, GPx and catalase) in dogs with moderate anaemia compared to those with mild anaemia. These findings contribute to the presumption that oxidative changes in dogs infected by *B. canis canis* are likely to be closely related to the pathogenesis of anaemia. Since there was just one severely anaemic dog, it was impossible to fully complete the comparison of anaemia with the investigated biomarkers, but it could be postulated that changes in severely anaemic dogs would be more prominent than those in moderately and mildly anaemic dogs. These results agree with those obtained in sheep with babesiosis and cattle suffering from theileriosis [31, 34, 53].

In the early stage of inflammation, it may be possible that endogenous substances such as SOD and reduced glutathione protect tissues from oxidative damage by ROS [60]. The imbalance of the redox state reflects an oxidative stress that may constitute a common pathway for life-threatening conditions and be responsible, at

Table 6 Correlations between oxidative biomarkers and the other analytes measured in dogs with babesiosis

Sperman rank correlation coefficient	TAS (mmol/L)	MDA (µmol/L)	SOD (U/mL)	GPx (U/L)	Catalase (U/L)
HCT (%)	-0.62	**−0.559****	**0.740****	**0.531****	0.190
Urea (mmol/L)	−0.073	**0.500****	−.0280	−0.292	−0.332*
Creatinine (µmol/L)	−0.211	0.209	−0.160	0.086	−0.195
Bilirubine (µmol/L)	−0.107	**0.342***	**−0.330***	**−0.476****	**−0.458****
ALT (U/L)	-0.237	0.026	0.001	0.065	-0.103
AP (U/L)	0.123	−0.084	−0.270	**−0.386***	−0.153
CPK (U/L)	-0.087	0.266	**−0.410****	**−0.438****	−0.219

*$P < 0.05$
**$P < 0.01$

Table 7 Correlations of biomarkers of oxidative stress with the outcome in dogs with babesiosis

Nominal correlation coefficient		TAS (mmol/L)	MDA (µmol/L)	SOD (U/mL)	GPx (U/L)	Catalase (U/L)
Lethal outcome	Tau-b	0.264	0.222	−0.316	−0.301	-0.227
	P	**0.005**	**0.019**	**0.001**	**0.001**	**0.016**

least in part, for tissue damage during a systemic response to injury [23]. Consumption of these substances of the antioxidant system after the persistence of SIRS may reinforce the oxidative stress after the initial inflammatory insult [60]. The existence of correlations between biochemistry parameters and antioxidants noted in this study may suggest that the severity of babesiosis is related to the degree of oxidative stress.

Although TAS did not show significant changes, individual antioxidants (SOD, catalase, GPx) showed significantly lower activity in dogs with MODS. This would imply that although measured antioxidant capacity does not show changes, in canine babesiosis, there are changes in selected components of the total antioxidants that can indicate the presence of MODS. This would be supported by the lack of correlation between TAS and the individual enzymatic antioxidants (SOD, catalase and GPx) in this study. Overall our results could be explained by the fact that the enzymatic antioxidants measured do not contribute greatly to the serum total antioxidant status [61]. Results of the current study concerning SOD, GPx and catalase activity as well as MDA concentration showed that dogs that developed MODS had more severe oxidative stress than dogs from other groups, which allows us to suppose that antioxidants investigated in this study have an influence on babesiosis severity as well as its outcome.

The authors of this research detected a strong negative correlation of the antioxidants measured (SOD, catalase and GPx) whereas a positive correlation of MDA with the lethal outcome of the disease. These results are in agreement with studies in critically ill people admitted to the hospital to intensive care units [35, 36] and they indicate a potential role of these biomarkers as prognostic indicators of disease severity and outcome in dogs

suffering from babesiosis. However these data should be interpreted with caution since the dogs received different treatments.

Conclusion
The results of this study demonstrated changes in antioxidant biomarkers associated with the presence of oxidative stress in dogs naturally infected with *B. canis canis*. These biomarkers could be used as indicators of disease severity and outcome in dogs suffering from babesiosis.

Acknowledgements
The authors are grateful to Blanka Beer Ljubić, Jadranka Foršek, Dora Ivšić Škoda (Faculty of Veterinary Medicine, University of Zagreb) and Relja Beck (Croatian Veterinary Institute, Zagreb) for the help with laboratory analyses. Part of this work was presented on Fifth Croatian veterinary congress with international participation, Tuheljske toplice, 10-13, October 2012.

Funding
This research was carried out at laboratories of Faculty of Veterinary Medicine, University of Zagreb and Croatian Veterinary Institute and partly financial supported by Clinic for Internal Diseases, Faculty of Veterinary Medicine, University of Zagreb, whereas party by the FP7 ERA Chair project "VetMedZg" (Grant Agreement No 621394).

Authors' contributions
MC participated in the design of the study, in the sample collection, drafted the main parts of the manuscript as well as revised the manuscript. IK and IŠ participated in design of the study and drafted the manuscript. MB participated in the sample collection as well as in critical reading and in revising of the manuscript. JG participated in the sample collection and in the statistical analysis and table creation. NK and VM (Vesna Matijatko) participated in the sample collection and helped to draft the manuscript. JJC and RC participated in the critical reading and revising of the manuscript. VM participated in the design of the study and in writing and revising the manuscript. All authors read, commented on, and approved the final manuscript.

Competing interests
The authors declare that they have no competing interests.

Consent for publication
All data generated or analysed during this study are included in this article and its supplementary information files.

Table 8 Correlations between biomarkers of oxidative stress in dogs with babesiosis

Sperman rank correlation coefficient	TAS (mmol/L)	MDA (µmol/L)	SOD (U/mL)	GPx (U/L)	Catalase (U/L)
TAS (mmol/L)	X	−0.021	−0.135	−0.149	0.118
MDA (µmol/L)		X	**−.435****	**−.328***	**−.321***
SOD (U/mL)			X	**.526****	0.285
GPx (U/L)				X	**.380***
Catalase (U/L)					X

*P < 0.05
**P < 0.01

Author details
[1]Clinic for Internal Diseases, Faculty of Veterinary Medicine, University of Zagreb, Zagreb, Croatia. [2]Department of Animal Medicine and Surgery, Faculty of Veterinary Medicine, University of Murcia, 30100 Espinardo, Murcia, Spain.

References

1. Mrljak V, Kučer N, Kuleš J, Tvarijonaviciute A, Brkljačić M, Crnogaj M, et al. Serum concentrations of eicosanoids and lipids in dogs naturally infected with Babesia canis. Vet Parasitol. 2014;201:24–30.
2. Matijatko V, Torti M, Schetters TP. Canine babesiosis in Europe: how many diseases? Trends Parasitol. 2012;28:99–105.
3. Baneth G, Florin-Christensen M, Cardoso L, Schnittger L. Reclassification of Theileria annae as Babesia vulpes sp. nov. Parasit Vectors. 2015;8:207.
4. Uilenberg G, Franssen FF, Perie NM, Spanjer AA. Three groups of Babesia canis distinguished and a proposal for nomenclature. Vet Q. 1989;11:33–40.
5. Taboada J, Merchant SR. Babesiosis of companion animals and man. Vet Clin North Am Small Anim Pract. 1991;21:103–23.
6. Camacho AT, Pallas E, Gestal JJ, Guitian FJ, Olmeda AS, Goethert HK, et al. Infection of dogs in north-west Spain with a Babesia microti-like agent. Vet Rec. 2001;149:552–5.
7. Taboada J, Lobetti R. Babesiosis. In: Green CE, editor. Infectious diseases of the dog and cat. 3rd ed. St Louis: WB Saunders Co; 2006. p. 722–35.
8. Matijatko V, Kiš I, Torti M, Brkljačić M, Kučer N, Rafaj RB, et al. Septic shock in canine babesiosis. Vet Parasitol. 2009;162:263–70.
9. Bone RC, Balk RA, Cerra FB, Dellinger RP, Fein AM, Knaus WA, et al. Definitions for sepsis and organ failure and guidelines for the use of innovative therapies in sepsis. The ACCP/SCCM Consensus Conference Committee. American College of Chest Physicians/Society of Critical Care Medicine. Chest. 1992;101:1644–55.
10. Jacobson LS, Lobetti RG, Becker P, Reyers F, Vaughan-Scott T. Nitric oxide metabolites in naturally occurring canine babesiosis. Vet Parasitol. 2002;104: 27–41.
11. Jacobson LS, Clark IA. The pathophysiology of canine babesiosis: new approaches to an old puzzle. J S Afr Vet Assoc. 1994;65:134–45.
12. Welzl C, Leisewitz AL, Jacobson LS, Vaughan-Scott T, Myburgh E. Systemic inflammatory response syndrome and multiple-organ damage/dysfunction in complicated canine babesiosis. J S Afr Vet Assoc. 2001;72:158–62.
13. Koster LS, Steiner JM, Suchodolski JS, Schoeman JP. Serum canine pancreatic-specific lipase concentrations in dogs with naturally occurring Babesia rossi infection. J S Afr Vet Assoc. 2015;86:E1–7.
14. Lobetti RG. Canine babesiosis: comp cont Educ; 1998. p. 20.
15. Jacobson LS. The South African form of severe and complicated canine babesiosis: clinical advances 1994-2004. Vet Parasitol. 2006;138:126–39.
16. Matijatko V, Mrljak V, Kiš I, Kučer N, Foršek J, Živicnjak T, et al. Evidence of an acute phase response in dogs naturally infected with Babesia canis. Vet Parasitol. 2007;144:242–50.
17. Schetters TP, Moubri K, Cooke BM. Comparison of Babesia rossi and Babesia canis isolates with emphasis on effects of vaccination with soluble parasite antigens: a review. J S Afr Vet Assoc. 2009;80:75–8.
18. Zygner W, Gojska-Zygner O, Baska P, Dlugosz E. Increased concentration of serum TNF alpha and its correlations with arterial blood pressure and indices of renal damage in dogs infected with Babesia canis. Parasitol Res. 2014;113:1499–503.
19. Goddard A, Leisewitz AL, Kjelgaard-Hansen M, Kristensen AT, Schoeman JP. Excessive pro-inflammatory serum cytokine concentrations in virulent canine Babesiosis. PLoS One. 2016;11:e0150113.
20. Paim FC, Da Silva AS, Paim CB, Franca RT, Costa MM, Duarte MM, et al. Increased cytokine and nitric oxide levels in serum of dogs experimentally infected with Rangelia vitalii. Korean J Parasitol. 2013;51:133–7.
21. Rubio CP, Hernandez-Ruiz J, Martinez-Subiela S, Tvarijonaviciute A, Ceron JJ. Spectrophotometric assays for total antioxidant capacity (TAC) in dog serum: an update. BMC Vet Res. 2016;12:166.
22. Muller S, Liebau E, Walter RD, Krauth-Siegel RL. Thiol-based redox metabolism of protozoan parasites. Trends Parasitol. 2003;19:320–8.
23. Alonso de Vega JM, Diaz J, Serrano E, Carbonell LF. Oxidative stress in critically ill patients with systemic inflammatory response syndrome. Crit Care Med. 2002;30:1782–6.
24. Erel O, Kocyigit A, Avci S, Aktepe N, Bulut V. Oxidative stress and antioxidative status of plasma and erythrocytes in patients with vivax malaria. Clin Biochem. 1997;30:631–9.
25. Halliwell B, Gutteridge JM. Free radicals in biology and medicine. 3rd ed. Midsomer Norton: Oxford University Press; 1999.
26. Halliwell B. Antioxidants in human health and disease. Annu Rev Nutr. 1996; 16:33–50.
27. Aytekin I, Onmaz AC, Alp H, Ulucan A. Effects of 2,4-D (dichlorophenoxyacetic acid) on blood anti-oxidant oxidant balance and on tissues in lambs. Rev Med Vet-Toulouse. 2010;161:283–7.
28. Aytekin I, Onmaz AC, Ulucan A, Alp H. Effects of accidental ammonium Sulphate poisoning on antioxidant/oxidant status in lambs. Rev Med Vet-Toulouse. 2011;162:346–51.
29. Sies H, Cadenas E. Oxidative stress: damage to intact cells and organs. Philos Trans R Soc Lond Ser B Biol Sci. 1985;311:617–31.
30. Otsuka Y, Yamasaki M, Yamato O, Maede Y. Increased generation of superoxide in erythrocytes infected with Babesia gibsoni. J Vet Med Sci. 2001;63:1077–81.
31. Asri Rezaei S, Dalir-Naghadeh B. Evaluation of antioxidant status and oxidative stress in cattle naturally infected with Theileria annulata. Vet Parasitol. 2006;142:179–86.
32. Crnogaj M, Petlevski R, Mrljak V, Kiš I, Torti M, Kučer N, et al. Malondialdehyde levels in serum of dogs infected with Babesia canis. Vet Med (Praha). 2010;55:163–71.
33. Kumar A, Varshney JP, Patra RC. A comparative study on oxidative stress in dogs infected with Ehrlichia canis with or without concurrent infection with Babesia gibsoni. Vet Res Commun. 2006;30:917–20.
34. Esmaeilnejad B, Tavassoli M, Asri-Rezaei S, Dalir-Naghadeh B, Malekinejad H, Jalilzadeh-Amin G, et al. Evaluation of antioxidant status, oxidative stress and serum trace mineral levels associated with Babesia ovis parasitemia in sheep. Vet Parasitol. 2014;205:38–45.
35. Kucukkurt I, Cigerci IH, Ince S, Kozan E, Aytekin I, Eryavuz A, et al. The effects of Babesiosis on oxidative stress and DNA damage in Anatolian black goats naturally infected with Babesia ovis. Iran J Parasitol. 2014;9:90–8.
36. Deger S, Deger Y, Bicek K, Ozdal N, Gul A. Status of lipid peroxidation, antioxidants, and oxidation products of nitric oxide in Equine Babesiosis: status of antioxidant and oxidant in Equine Babesiosis. J Equine Vet Sci. 2009;29:743–7.
37. Saleh MA. Erythrocytic oxidative damage in crossbred cattle naturally infected with Babesia bigemina. Res Vet Sci. 2009;86:43–8.
38. Chaudhuri S, Varshney JP, Patra RC. Erythrocytic antioxidant defense, lipid peroxides level and blood iron, zinc and copper concentrations in dogs naturally infected with Babesia gibsoni. Res Vet Sci. 2008;85:120–4.
39. Murase T, Maede Y. Increased erythrophagocytic activity of macrophages in dogs with Babesia gibsoni infection. Jpn J Vet Sci. 1990;52:321–7.
40. Maegraith B, Gilles HM, Devakul K. Pathological processes in Babesia canis infections. Z Tropenmed Parasitol. 1957;8:485–514.
41. Murase T, Ueda T, Yamato O, Tajima M, Maede Y. Oxidative damage and enhanced erythrophagocytosis in canine erythrocytes infected with Babesia gibsoni. J Vet Med Sci. 1996;58:259–61.
42. Reyers F, Leisewitz AL, Lobetti RG, Milner RJ, Jacobson LS, van Zyl M. Canine babesiosis in South Africa: more than one disease. Does this serve as a model for falciparum malaria? Ann Trop Med Parasitol. 1998; 92:503–11.
43. Schetters TP, Kleuskens J, Scholtes N, Gorenflot A. Parasite localization and dissemination in the Babesia-infected host. Ann Trop Med Parasitol. 1998;92:513–9.
44. Beck R, Vojta L, Mrljak V, Marinculić A, Beck A. Živicnjak, et al. diversity of Babesia and Theileria species in symptomatic and asymptomatic dogs in Croatia. Int J Parasitol. 2009;39:843–8.
45. Kraft W, Dürr UM, Fürll M, Bostedt H, Heinritzi K. Hämatologie. In: Kraft W, Dürr UM, editors. Klinische Labordiagnostik in der Tiermedizin. 6th ed. Stuttgart: Schattauer; 2005. p. 49–92.
46. Okano S, Yoshida M, Fukushima U, Higuchi S, Takase K, Hagio M. Usefulness of systemic inflammatory response syndrome criteria as an index for prognosis judgement. Vet Rec. 2002;150:245–6.
47. Mohr AJ, Lobetti RG, van der Lugt JJ. Acute pancreatitis: a newly recognised potential complication of canine babesiosis. J S Afr Vet Assoc. 2000;71:232–9.
48. Paglia DE, Valentine WN. Studies on the quantitative and qualitative characterization of erythrocyte glutathione peroxidase. J Lab Clin Med. 1967; 70:158–69.
49. Johansson LH, Borg LA. A spectrophotometric method for determination of catalase activity in small tissue samples. Anal Biochem. 1988;174:331–6.
50. Trotta RJ, Sullivan SG, Stern A. Lipid peroxidation and haemoglobin degradation in red blood cells exposed to t-butyl hydroperoxide. Effects of the hexose monophosphate shunt as mediated by glutathione and ascorbate. Biochem J. 1982;204:405–15.
51. Vajdovich P, Gaal T, Szilagyi A, Harnos A. Changes in some red blood cell and clinical laboratory parameters in young and old beagle dogs. Vet Res Commun. 1997;21:463–70.

52. Todorova I, Simeonova G, Kyuchukova D, Dinev D, Gadjeva V. Reference values of oxidative stress parameters (MDA, SOD, CAT) in dogs and cats. Comp Clin Pathol. 2005;13:190–4.
53. Esmaeilnejad B, Tavassoli M, Asri-Rezaei S, Dalir-Naghadeh B. Evaluation of antioxidant status and oxidative stress in sheep naturally infected with Babesia ovis. Vet Parasitol. 2012;185:124–30.
54. Razavi SM, Nazifi S, Bateni M, Rakhshandehroo E. Alterations of erythrocyte antioxidant mechanisms: antioxidant enzymes, lipid peroxidation and serum trace elements associated with anemia in bovine tropical theileriosis. Vet Parasitol. 2011;180:209–14.
55. D'Souza V, Swagata H, Vijayalaxmi K, Namratha AS. Erythrocyte antioxidant enzymes and their correlation with malondialdehyde in malaria. Biomed Res. 2009;20:25–7.
56. Akpotuzor JO, Udoh AE, Etukudo MH. Total antioxidant status, vitamins a, C and beta-carotene levels of children with *P. falciparum* infection in University of Calabar Teaching Hospital (UCTH), Calabar. Pak J Nutr. 2007;6:485–9.
57. Woodford FP, Whitehead TP. Is measuring serum antioxidant capacity clinically useful? Ann Clin Biochem. 1998;35:48–56.
58. Peng J, Jones GL, Watson K. Stress proteins as biomarkers of oxidative stress: effects of antioxidant supplements. Free Radic Biol Med. 2000;28:1598–606.
59. Crnogaj M, Kiš I, Kučer N, Šmit I, Mayer I, Brkljačić M, et al. Lipid peroxidation in dogs naturally infected with Babesia canis canis. Vet Arhiv. 2015;85:37–48.
60. Robinson MK, Rounds JD, Hong RW, Jacobs DO, Wilmore DW. Glutathione deficiency increases organ dysfunction after hemorrhagic shock. Surgery. 1992;112:140–7.
61. Nemec A, Drobnič-Košorok M, Skitek M, Pavlica Z, Galac S, Butinar J. Total antioxidant capacity (TAC) values and their correlation with individual antioxidants in serum of healthy beagles. Acta Vet Brno. 2000;69:297–303.
62. Weiser MG. Diagnosis of immunohemolytic disease. Semin Vet Med Surg. 1992;7:311–4.

9

Avian infectious bronchitis virus disrupts the melanoma differentiation associated gene 5 (MDA5) signaling pathway by cleavage of the adaptor protein MAVS

Liping Yu, Xiaorong Zhang, Tianqi Wu, Jin Su, Yuyang Wang, Yuexin Wang, Baoyang Ruan, Xiaosai Niu and Yantao Wu[*] (ID)

Abstract

Background: Melanoma differentiation associated gene 5 (MDA5) and retinoic acid-inducible gene-I (RIG-I) selectively sense cytoplasmic viral RNA to induce an antiviral immune response. Infectious bronchitis virus (IBV) is one of the most important infectious agents in chickens, and in chicken cells, it can be recognized by MDA5 to activate interferon production. RIG-I is considered to be absent in chickens. However, the absence of RIG-I in chickens raises the question of whether this protein influences the antiviral immune response against IBV infection.

Results: Here, we showed that chicken cells transfected with domestic goose RIG-I (dgRIG-I) exhibited increased IFN-β activity after IBV infection. We also found that IBV can cleave MAVS, an adaptor protein downstream of RIG-I and MDA5 that acts as a platform for antiviral innate immunity at an early stage of infection.

Conclusions: Although chicken MDA5 (chMDA5) is functionally active during IBV infection, the absence of RIG-I may increase the susceptibility of chickens to IBV infection, and IBV may disrupt the activation of the host antiviral response through the cleavage of MAVS.

Keywords: Infectious bronchitis virus, Melanoma differentiation associated gene 5, Retinoic acid-inducible gene-I, Mavs

Background

Infectious bronchitis (IB) is a serious and highly contagious disease in chickens that is caused by the infectious bronchitis virus (IBV) [1]. Although the host uses multiple mechanisms to thwart viral invasion, the overall clearance and outcome of IBV infection in chickens are critically dependent on the early protection provided by the innate immune system [2]. To enable its survival, IBV has evolved to disrupt the activation of the host antiviral signaling pathway using a number of mechanisms, such as delaying the activation of the IFN response during the early stages of IBV infection [3, 4].

The innate immune system plays a critical role in the detection and elimination of invading pathogens, especially the IFN antiviral immune response [5]. To activate the antiviral immune response, pattern recognition receptors (PRRs) recognize specific pathogen-associated molecular patterns (PAMPs) [6, 7]. The PRRs include Toll-like receptors (TLRs), retinoic acid-inducible gene I (RIG-I)-like receptors (RLRs), and nucleotide-binding oligomerization domain (NOD)-like receptors (NLRs). RLRs include RIG-I [8], melanoma differentiation associated gene 5 (MDA5) [9] and laboratory of genetics and physiology 2 (LGP2) [10]. RIG-I and MDA5 interact with the mitochondrial antiviral signaling gene (MAVS, also called IPS-1/VISA/CARDIF) [11], a critical downstream adaptor protein located at the mitochondrial membrane, via caspase activation and recruitment domains (CARD)-CARD domains at their N-terminal [12]. Activated MAVS can recruit downstream interferon regulatory factor-3/7 (IRF3/IRF7) and the transcriptional factor nuclear factor κB (NF-

* Correspondence: ytwu@yzu.edu.cn
Jiangsu Co-Innovation Center for Prevention of Animal Infectious Diseases and Zoonoses, College of Veterinary Medicine, Yangzhou University, Yangzhou, Jiangsu 225009, China

κB) [13], leading to the rapid production of type I IFNs and proinflammatory cytokines [11, 14, 15].

Although both RIG-I and MDA5 are closely related, exhibiting 25% and 40% identities in their N-terminal CARD and C-terminal helicase domains [16, 17], they can recognize different types of ligands and distinct subsets of RNA viruses. RIG-I has been reported to recognize short dsRNA produced during the replication of RNA viruses and uncapped 5′-triphosphate (5′-ppp) ssRNA [18]. MDA5 can be activated by long dsRNA, including the synthetic dsRNA analogue poly I:C [16, 19]. Overexpression of MDA5 and RIG-I inhibits the growth of encephalomyocarditis virus (EMCV) and vesicular stomatitis virus (VSV) [19], and overproduction of MDA5 but not RIG-I leads to enhanced IFN-β promoter activity in measles virus (MV)-infected A549 cells [9]. It has also been demonstrated that expression of MDA5 and RIG-I resulted in the activation of the IFN-β promoter in influenza A virus-infected epithelial cells [20]. Barber et al. suggested that the lack of RIG-I observed in chickens results in a deficiency of the antiviral innate immune response, possibly explaining the high susceptibility of chickens compared to ducks during Avian influenza virus (AIV) infection [21]. Similarly, the absence of RIG-I in chickens may contribute to the susceptibility of only chickens to IBV.

To explore the mechanisms that control the chicken immune response to IBV infection with regard to the RIG-like helicase, we have cloned chicken MDA5 (chMDA5) and domestic goose RIG-I (dgRIG-I) and demonstrated that they act as positive regulators in the activation of IFN-β induced by IBV. Furthermore, the knockdown or overexpression of chMDA5 has no effect on IBV replication. In this study, we also investigated the potential role of MAVS in the MDA5-mediated antiviral signaling pathway after IBV infection and demonstrated a positive regulatory role of MAVS.

Methods
Virus and cells
The JS/2010/12 strain of IBV was previously characterized as nephropathogenic by our laboratory, and its genomic sequence was determined (GenBank accession No. JQ900122.1). In this study, the stock of JS/2010/12 strain propagated in 10-day-old SPF Line 22 of White Leghorn chicken embryos for 5 passages (P5) was used. The 50% tissue culture infective dose (TCID50) of the IBV strain was determined by identifying the cytopathic effect (CPE) induced by the virus in CEK cells. The DF1 chicken fibroblast cell line was used for all transfection-based assays. The cells were maintained in Dulbecco's modified Eagle's medium (DMEM, HyClone) containing 10% FBS. CEK cells were aseptically generated from 20-day-old SPF chicken embryos. The cell suspension was obtained by

trypsinization of kidneys for 30 min at 37 °C and subsequent filtration with a 100-μm mesh. Then, the cells were cultured in M199 media (HyClone) containing 3% FBS (HyClone).

Plasmid and small interfering RNA (siRNA)
The chMDA5 ORF was amplified from CEK cells by overlap PCR with primers chMDA5-F1/R1 and chMDA5-F2/R2, producing a 3006 bp MDA5 PCR product (GenBank accession No. GU570144.1). The PCR product was digested with EcoR V and Xba I, then was inserted into the pcDNA-5′-Flag plasmid that had been digested with the same enzymes. The chTLR3 ORF was PCR amplified from CEK cells with the primer pair chTLR3 F/R, and the product was cloned into the p3 × flag-CMV-7.1 vector (Invitrogen) at the Not I and EcoR V sites. The dgRIG-I ORF (GenBank accession No. JF804977) was amplified from goose splenic cDNA using primers dgRIG-I F/R, and the fragment was inserted into the p3 × flag-CMV-7.1 vector at the EcoR I and BamH I sites. The small interfering RNAs (siRNA) targeting the chicken chMDA5, chTLR3, and chMAVS mRNAs as well as control siRNA were synthesized by Santa Cruz Biotechnology and have been previously described [22].

Transfection
Plasmids and siRNA were transfected into cells with Lipofectamine 2000 (Invitrogen) according to the manufacturer's instructions. Briefly, plasmid DNA (2 μg for a 6-well plate) and siRNA (20 nM, Santa Cruz Biotechnology) were diluted with opti-MEM. Lipofectamine 2000 (5 μl for a 6-well plate) was also diluted with opti-MEM. Diluted DNA was added to the diluted Lipofectamine 2000 reagent (1:1) and was incubated for 5 min, then inoculated into cells and incubated for 24 h before further treatments.

RNA isolation and real-time PCR
To quantitate gene expression and IBV replication from IBV-infected CEK cells and chicken embryos, primers and probes specific for chMDA5 [23], chIFN-β [24], chIFN-λ, chMx [25] and IBV 5′-UTR (Table 1) were used for real-time PCR as previously described [26]. Briefly, RNA was extracted using an RNA extraction kit (MiniBEST Universal RNA Extraction Kit, Takara, China) according to the manufacturer's instructions. A total of 1 μg of RNA was then reverse transcribed to cDNA using a reverse transcription kit (HiScript Q RT SuperMix for qPCR, Vazyme, China) according to the manufacturer's instructions, after which the transcribed products were diluted and stored at −20 °C. Gene expression was quantitated using a LightCycler 2.0 System (Roche Diagnostics Ltd., Switzerland). The relative expression ratios of the target genes chMDA5,

Table 1 SiRNA for silencing as well as primers for plasmid construction and real-time PCR used in this study

Purpose	Name	Sequence(5′ to3′)	Accession no.	References
Cloning of chMDA5	chMDA5-F1	AAAGATATCTATGTCGGAGGAGTGCCGA (EcoRV)	GU570144.1	
	chMDA5-R1	AATGGATCCCTTCTTTTGTCATC		
Cloning of chMDA5	chMDA5-F2	ACAAAAGAAGGGATCCATTTAGAG (overlap sequence)		
	chMDA5-R2	CTAGTCTAGATTAATCTTCATCACTTGAAGGACAA (XbaI)		
Cloning of chTLR3	chTLR3-F	ATAAGAATGCGGCCGCTAAACTAATGGGATGCTCTATTCCTTGCT (NotI)	NM_001011691	
	chTLR3-R	AAAGATATCAATCAGCGCACTTTACTATTAGATTTAAG (EcoRV)		
Cloning of dgRIG- I	dgRIG-I-F	GGAATTCC ATGACGGCGGAGGAAAAG (EcoRI)	JF804977.1	
	dgRIG-I-R	GAGGATCCTCAAATGGTGGGTACAAGTTGGAC (BamHI)		
Silencing	SiMDA5	GAACGUGAAGAUGUAAAUATT		[22]
Silencing	SiTLR3	GCAGAUUGUAGUCACCUAATT		[22]
Silencing	SiMAVS	UACAGGAGGCUUCAAGGAGGUGUCA		[22]
Silencing	siRNA control	AUUACGGGCCAGUAAUCUAT		
Real-time PCR	chIFN-β F	CAGCTCTCACCACCACCTTCTC		[24]
	chIFN-β R	GGAGGTGGAGCCGTATTCTG		
Real-time PCR	chβ-actin F	CAACACAGTGCTGTCTGGTGGTA		[27]
	chβ-actin R	ATCGTACTCCTGCTTGCTGATCC		
Real-time PCR	chIFN-λ F	TGAGCTGGACCTCACCATCA	NM_001128496.1	
Real-time PCR	chIFN-λ R	GGGCTGTTGGCACGTCTCT		
Real-time PCR	chMda5 F	TGGAGCTGGGCATCTTTCAG		[23]
	chMda5 R	GTTCCCACGACTCTCAATAACAGT		
Real-time PCR	chMx F	TTGTCTGGTGTTGCTCTTCCT		[25]
	chMx R	GCTGTATTTCTGTGTTGCGGTA		
Real-time PCR	IBV-GL533	GCCATGTTGTCACTGTCTATTG		[26]
	IBV-GU391	GCTTTTGAGCCTAGCGTT		
	IBV-Probe	FAM-CACCACCAGAACCTGTCACCTC-BHQ		

The underlined nucleotides are restriction enzyme sequences. Restriction enzymes are indicated in parentheses

chIFN-β, chIFN-λ and chMx were calculated using the $\triangle\triangle$Ct method. To assess IBV replication *in ovo* and in vitro, real-time PCR was performed by absolute quantitation PCR [26].

Selection of appropriate reference genes

Eight housekeeping were screened to identify the most stably expressed reference genes in different chicken embryo tissues: β-actin (ACTB) [27], testis-specific alpha-tubulin mRNA (TUBAT) [28], Mitochondrial ribosomal protein S30 (MRPS30) [29], Eukaryotic translation elongation factor 1 alpha 2 (EFF1) [29], Guanine nucleotide binding protein (G protein), ribosomal protein L32 [30], β-glucuronidase (GUSB) [31], glyceraldehyde-3-phosphate dehydrogenase (GAPDH) [31] and Ribosomal protein L5 (RPL5) [29]. To calculate the stability of reference genes, three different analysis methods (geNorm, NormFinder and Best-Keeper) were used [30–32]. (Additional file 1: Methods and Table S1).

Western blot

CEK cells were infected with IBV, and at different time points post-infection, the cells were lysed with RIPA lysis buffer (Beyotime Institute of Biotechnology, China). The cell lysates were analyzed for N proteins by Western blot with anti-N antibody (1:1000) (Prepared by our laboratory). Actin was detected using a β-actin antibody (1:5000, Sigma) as a protein loading control. An anti-MAVS antibody (1:1000, Cell Signaling Technology) was used to detect the MAVS protein.

Animal experiment

Eleven-day-old SPF chicken embryos were inoculated with IBV at 10^3 EID$_{50}$ via allantoic cavity. Three embryos inoculated with PBS served as a negative control. Three embryos from each group were killed at 72 h post-inoculation to determine chMDA5, chIFN-β, chIFN-λ and antiviral protein chMx transcription levels in the trachea, lung, liver, kidney, muscle and intestine of embryos, with all tissues being immediately processed for RNA extraction.

Cell experiment

CEK cells were infected with JS/2010/12 and harvested at 72 h post-inoculation. Viral stocks were prepared by freezing/thawing cells three times; the initial JS/2010/12 stock inoculated CEK cells for 5 passages. Then, DF1 cells were infected with this viral stock, and RNA was extracted at different time points. The viral genome copy number was quantified by qPCR. Although no CPE was observed, an increase in the viral genome copy number can be seen over time. CEK cells in 24-well plates were infected with IBV at an MOI of 1 and were incubated at 37 °C for 1 h. Cells that were inoculated with PBS served as a negative control. At different time points post-infection (Figs. 1 and 2), supernatants from three different wells for each group were harvested for RNA extraction to determine the level of virus replication (Fig. 1) and chMDA5, chIFN-β, chIFN-λ and chMx expression. After reaching 90% confluence, CEK cells in 6-well plates were infected with IBV at an MOI of 1. Then, cells were harvested at different time points and

subsequently lysed with lysis buffer. The level of IBV replication was assessed via a Western blot assay.

Statistical analysis

All statistical analysis were performed in GraphPad Prism 5.0. To identify significant differences between different groups, mean comparisons were performed using one-way ANOVA or student t-tests. Results were considered significant at $p < 0.05$.

Results

IBV induces IFN response in different tissues of chicken embryos

IBV could replicate sufficiently in 9–11 day old chicken embryos, to evaluate the relationship between antiviral response and viral replication in different embryo tissues, chicken embryos were inoculated with IBV, then the trachea, intestine, kidney, lung, liver, and muscle of the embryos were collected 72 h post-infection. The replication

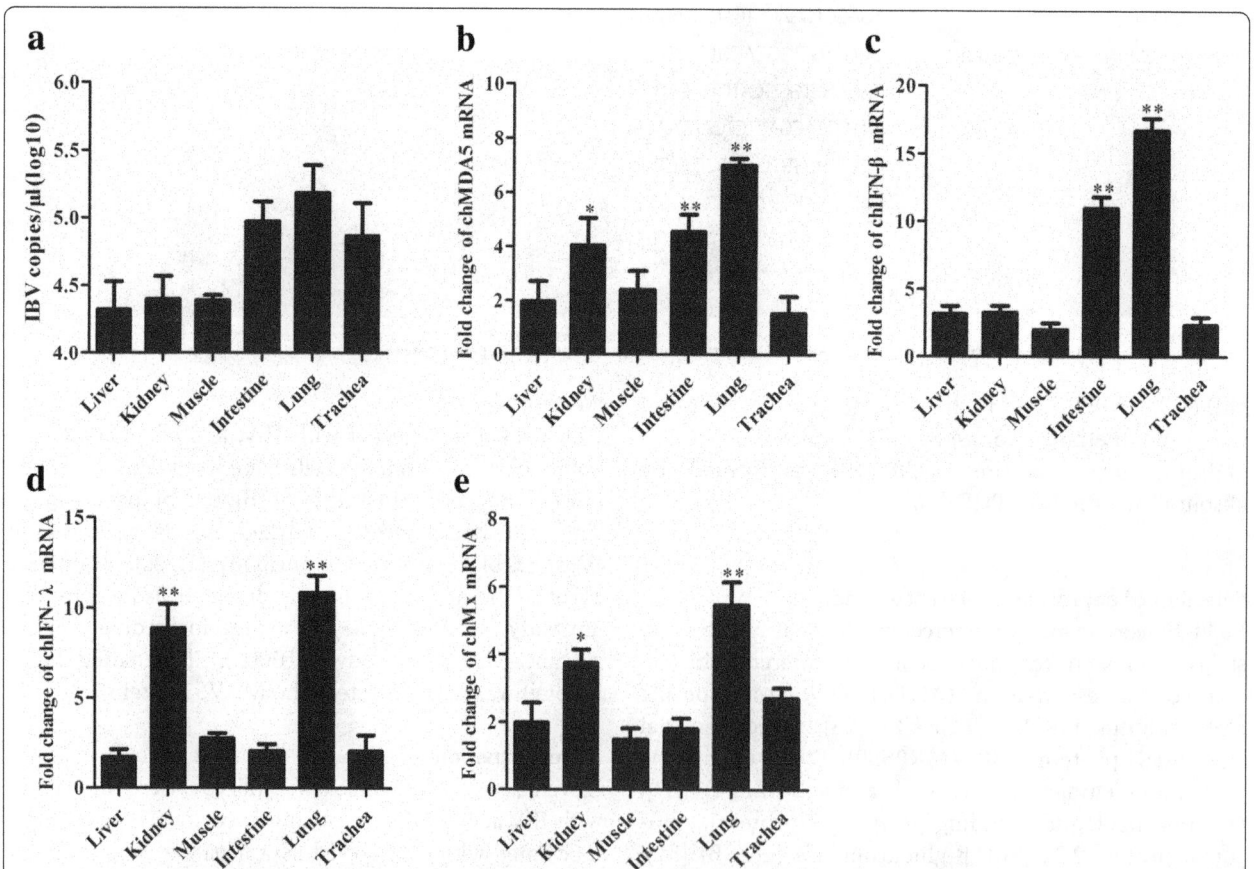

Fig. 1 IBV induces chMDA5, chIFN-β, chIFN-λ and chMx expression in chicken embryos. In this experiment three embryos were inoculated with IBV, and three embryos were inoculated with PBS served as negative control; then, the trachea, intestine, kidney, lung, liver, and muscle tissues were collected from the embryos 72 h post-infection. a The IBV genome loads were quantified by RT-qPCR. b chMDA5, (c) chIFN-β, (d) chIFN-λ and (e) chMx were calculated as fold change of the infected group relative to the uninfected group and normalized against β actin. Data are shown as the mean ± SD (n = 3, 3 embryos) (* P ≤ 0.05; ** P ≤ 0.01). The representatives of three independent experiments showed similar results. Values represent the average of the results from three independent experiments with standard error bars

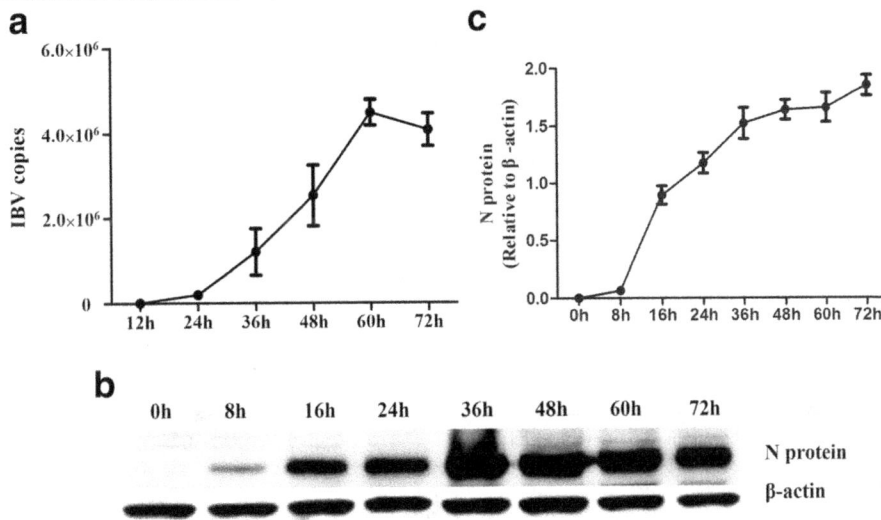

Fig. 2 IBV replication has a time-dependent activity in CEK cells. CEK cells were infected with IBV at an MOI of 1. At the indicated times post-infection, (**a**) viral RNA was quantified by RT-qPCR. Data are presented as the mean ± SD (* $P \leq 0.05$; ** $P \leq 0.01$); (**b**) The cellular IBV N proteins were quantified by Western blot. **c** The graph indicating the fold change of the N proteins. The fold change of N proteins is expressed as densitometric units (Image-Pro-plus 6.0) of bands normalized to the β-actin, results from three independent experiments

ability of IBV was determined by absolute quantification real-time PCR. IBV can be detected in all tissues, and the viral genome load was higher in the lung and trachea compared with other tissues (Fig. 3a). Eight housekeeping genes were selected for screening stably expressed reference genes in different chicken embryo tissues to be used in comparison to the determined cytokine expression studies (Additional file 2: Figure S1). The transcription of the antiviral cytokines chMDA5, chIFN-β, chIFN-λ and chMx in different tissues was normalized using three different reference genes (Additional file 2: Figure S1). We found that variability in expression for each gene was similar when normalized to different stable reference genes (Additional file 3: Figure S2). Therefore, β-actin was selected as an internal reference gene in this study. The data showed that chMDA5 (Fig. 3b) was expressed in all tissues, and stronger expression was observed in the intestine and lung ($P \leq 0.01$) and kidney ($P \leq 0.05$). IBV induced higher chIFN-β (Fig. 3c), chIFN-λ (Fig. 3d) and chMx (Fig. 3e) transcription in the lung; chMx and chIFN-λ transcription in kidneys than the negative control group ($P \leq 0.01$).

Accumulation of a large amount of dsRNA in IBV-infected CEK cells results in a strong IFN response

To investigate the replication ability of IBV in vitro, CEK cells were infected with IBV at an MOI of 1. The replication of IBV was quantified by RT-qPCR to detect the IBV genome load in cell culture supernatants, and N protein was detected by a Western blot assay. We observed a significant increase in the IBV genome load in cell culture supernatants, with the highest level occurring at 60 h

post-infection for the IBV-infected cells compared to the other time points (Fig. 1a). The IBV N protein expression data are illustrated in Fig. 1b and c. The highest expression level of N protein occurred at 72 h post-infection.

To monitor the kinetics of the chMDA5 and IFN response in relation to IBV replication in vitro, the transcription of chMDA5, chIFN-β, chIFN-λ and chMx was quantified in IBV-infected CEK cells (Fig. 2a–d). The expression of chMDA5, chIFN-β, chIFN-λ and chMx peaked at 60 h post-infection. The chIFN-β transcription level was significantly down regulated at 12 h post-infection and upregulated from 24 h to 60 h post-infection. IBV-infected CEK cells exhibited a significant induction of innate immunity gene transcription (chMDA5, chIFN-β, chIFN-λ and chMx) compared with the negative control group at 48 h, 60 h and 72 h ($P \leq 0.05$) post-infection, consistent with IBV replication.

Dose-dependent antiviral cytokine potency of IBV

To determine the relationship between the antiviral immune response and virus titer, CEK cells were infected with IBV at 10^{-2}, 10^{-1}, 10^{0}, 10^{1} and 10^{2} MOI for 36 h. As shown in Fig. 4, IBV induced chMDA5 (Fig. 4b), chIFN-β (Fig. 4c), chIFN-λ (Fig. 4d) and chMx (Fig. 4e) transcription in CEK cells at different infectious doses. We also found that IBV induced chMDA5, chIFN-β, chIFN-λ and chMx transcription in CEK cells to a greater extent than in mock-infected cells at infectious doses of 10^{1} and 10^{2} MOI ($P \leq 0.01$). Overall, IBV significantly induced the activation of chMDA5, chIFN-β, chIFN-λ and chMx in a dose-dependent manner.

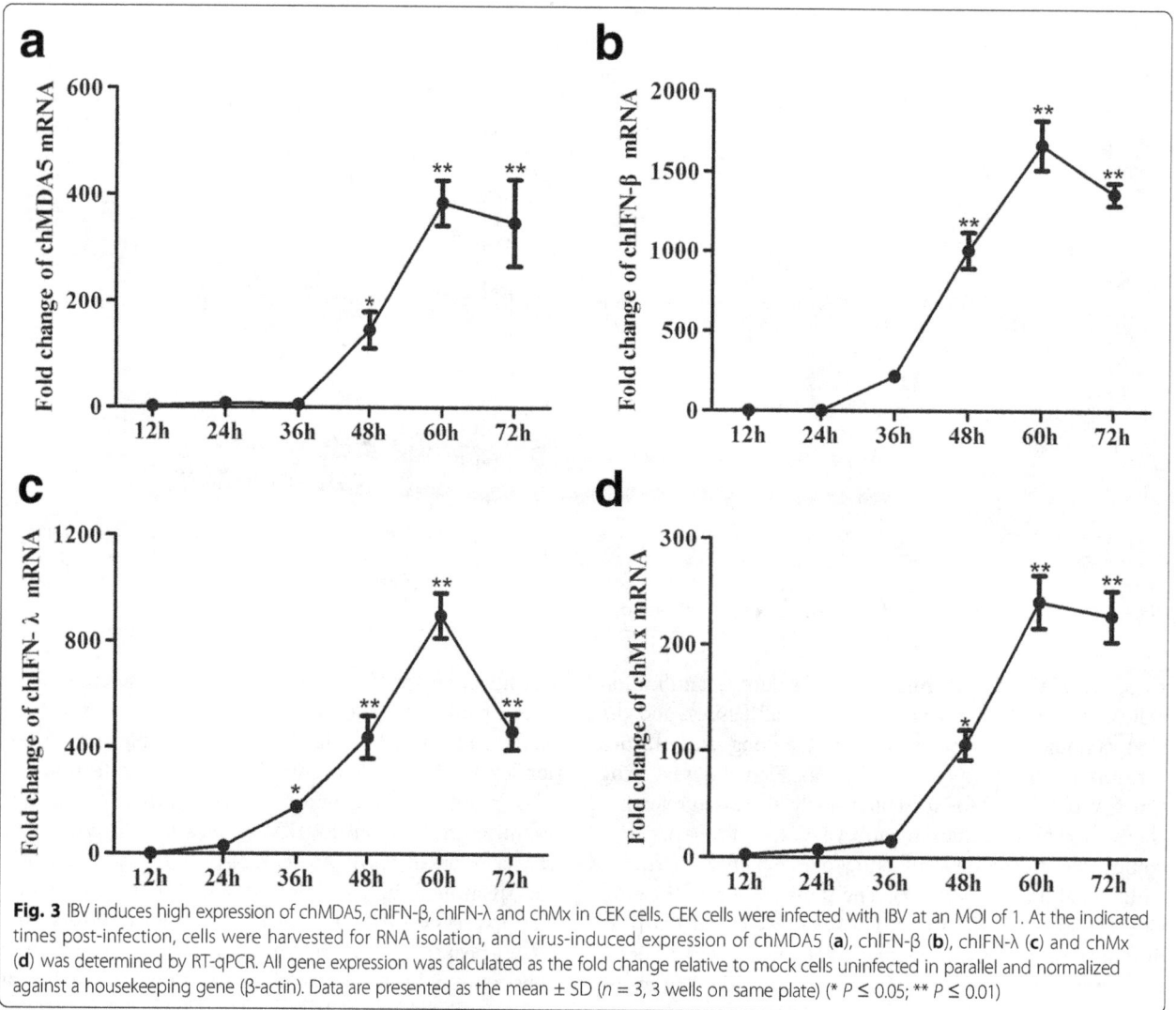

Fig. 3 IBV induces high expression of chMDA5, chIFN-β, chIFN-λ and chMx in CEK cells. CEK cells were infected with IBV at an MOI of 1. At the indicated times post-infection, cells were harvested for RNA isolation, and virus-induced expression of chMDA5 (**a**), chIFN-β (**b**), chIFN-λ (**c**) and chMx (**d**) was determined by RT-qPCR. All gene expression was calculated as the fold change relative to mock cells uninfected in parallel and normalized against a housekeeping gene (β-actin). Data are presented as the mean ± SD ($n = 3$, 3 wells on same plate) (* $P \leq 0.05$; ** $P \leq 0.01$)

ChMDA5 and dgRIG-I enhance the transcription of chIFN-β induced by IBV in CEK cells

The PRRs RIG-I and MDA5 are critical regulators of the host antiviral response and share a similar homology in their overall primary structure. This similarity prompted us to investigate whether dgRIG-I has the same role as chMDA5 in the IBV-induced IFN response in chicken cells. The expression of chMDA5 in DF1 cells enhanced chIFN-β transcription after the cells were infected with IBV compared with the control group transfected with vector and primed by IBV infection ($P \leq 0.05$) (Fig. 5a). We also found that infection with IBV induced higher chIFN-β transcription in dgRIG-I-expressing cells to a greater extent than the control group ($P \leq 0.01$), and dgRIG-I induced chIFN-β expression after IBV infection to a greater extent than chMDA5. Expression of chTLR3 did not enhance chIFN-β transcription after being infected with IBV. These results appear to indicate

that IBV stimulates chIFN-β transcription via MDA5. Similarly, the IBV-induced chIFN-β transcription was further increased by the overexpression of dgRIG-I. These data show that chMDA5 and dgRIG-I act as positive regulators of the IBV-induced chIFN-β signaling pathway (Fig. 5a).

To investigate whether chMDA5 and dgRIG-I can influence the replication of IBV, DF1 cells were transfected with chMDA5 or dgRIG-I, then were infected with IBV at an MOI of 1. The supernatants were harvested and titrated onto CEK cells. The test results indicated that neither the expression of chMDA5 nor dgRIG-I in CEK cells affected viral replication (Fig. 5b and c).

IBV cleaves MAVS at an early stage of infection

RIG-I and MDA5 interact with MAVS via CARD-CARD domains at their N-terminal, which is essential for the activation of the NF-κB and IRF3/7

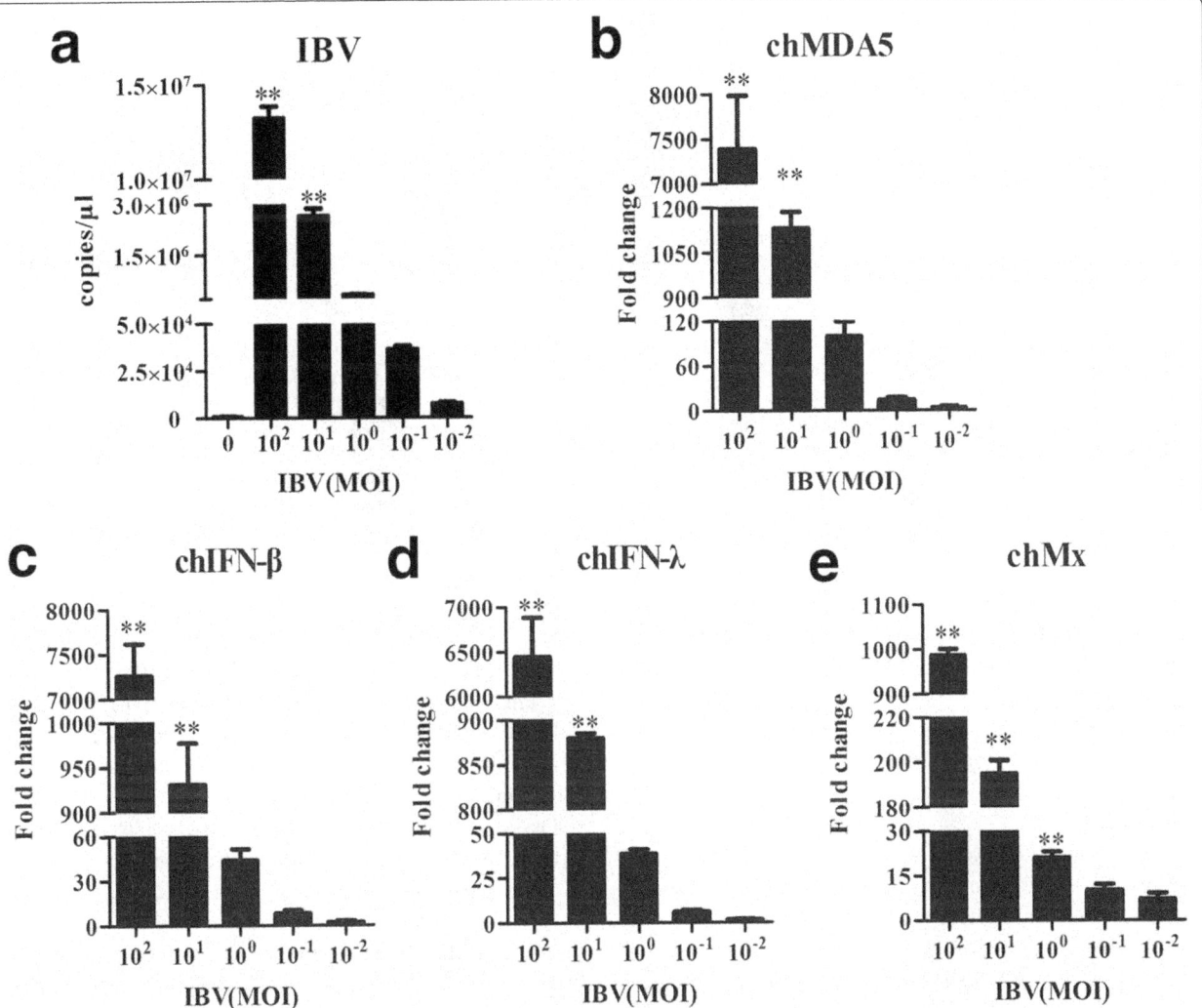

Fig. 4 Dose-dependent antiviral cytokine potency of IBV. CEK cells were inoculated with 10^{-2}, 10^{-1}, 10^{0}, 10^{1} and 10^{2} MOI of IBV, then the cells were harvested at 36 h post-treatment for RNA extraction. The IBV genome load (**a**) was quantified by RT-qPCR. The mRNA levels of chMDA5 (**b**), chIFN-β (**c**), chIFN-λ (**d**) and chMx (**e**) were evaluated by RT-qPCR. All gene expression was calculated as the fold change relative to uninfected control cells and normalized against a housekeeping gene (β-actin). Data are presented as the mean ± SD (n = 3, 3 wells on same plate) (* $P \leq 0.05$; ** $P \leq 0.01$)

downstream signaling pathway. MAVS plays a critical role in antiviral activity. To determine whether chMAVS is involved in the antiviral immune response to IBV infection, the expression level of chMAVS in IBV-infected CEK cells was investigated. We found that the cleavage of MAVS was induced by IBV at 8 h and 12 h post-infection but was not cleaved after 24 h (Fig. 6). We inferred that at the early stage of IBV infection, IBV-induced cleavage of MAVS allows IBV to evade the MDA5-mediated innate immunity signaling pathway.

Knockdown of chMDA5 and chMAVS influences IBV-induced IFN-β transcription

A gene silencing technique was also used to identify whether chMDA5, chTLR3 and chMAVS influence the

antiviral immune response mediated by IBV. First, to assess the effect of chMDA5, chTLR3 and chMAVS on IBV-induced IFN-β transcription, the expression of chMDA5, chTLR3 and chMAVS was knocked down. Compared with the control group, silencing of chMAVS or chMDA5 mRNA in DF1 cells significantly reduced IBV-induced IFN-β transcription. The simultaneous silencing of chMDA5, chTLR3 and chMAVS reduced the transcription of IFN-β significantly (Fig. 7a). These results suggest that both chMDA5 and chMAVS are involved in the activation of IFN-β in DF1 cells following IBV infection.

To further understand the role of chMDA5 and chMAVS during IBV infection, chMDA5 and chMAVS were knocked down in CEK cells, then the cells were infected with IBV at an MOI of 1. IBV in supernatants

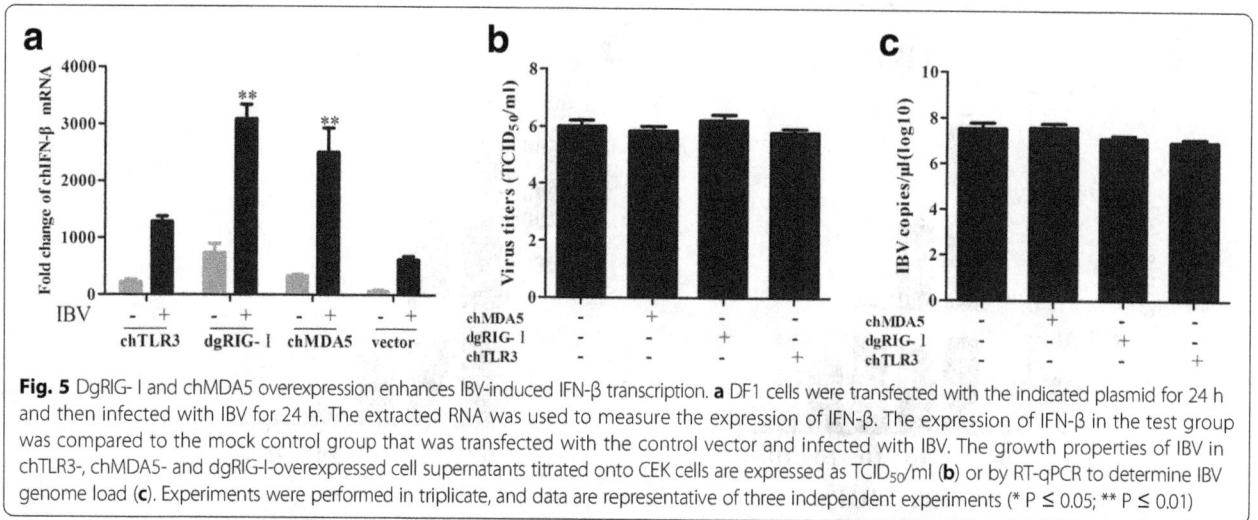

Fig. 5 DgRIG-I and chMDA5 overexpression enhances IBV-induced IFN-β transcription. **a** DF1 cells were transfected with the indicated plasmid for 24 h and then infected with IBV for 24 h. The extracted RNA was used to measure the expression of IFN-β. The expression of IFN-β in the test group was compared to the mock control group that was transfected with the control vector and infected with IBV. The growth properties of IBV in chTLR3-, chMDA5- and dgRIG-I-overexpressed cell supernatants titrated onto CEK cells are expressed as TCID$_{50}$/ml (**b**) or by RT-qPCR to determine IBV genome load (**c**). Experiments were performed in triplicate, and data are representative of three independent experiments (* P ≤ 0.05; ** P ≤ 0.01)

was titrated onto CEK cells at 48 h post-infection while the IBV genome loads were quantitated by real-time PCR. The results indicated that the observed viral replication in chMDA5 and chMAVS knockdown cells was the same as in the control group (Fig. 7b and c). Overall, inhibition of chMDA5 and chMAVS expression has no effect on the replication of IBV.

Discussion

In ovo and in vitro study, we show that infection with IBV leads to a considerable activation of the type I IFN and antiviral immune response [33]. Among birds, the RIG-I and MDA5 genes are present in ducks, geese and pigeons, but only MDA5 gene can be identified in chickens [34]. RIG-I and MDA5 share a similar homology in their overall primary structure and induce the downstream signaling pathway involving MAVS [7, 11, 12]. In this study, to investigate the effect of dgRIG-I in the chicken immune system response to IBV infection, we identified and cloned dgRIG-I. We found that dgRIG-I plays a similar role to chMDA5 in upregulating the transcription of chIFN-β in response to IBV infection. It has been

previously demonstrated that IBV can delay the transcription of chIFN-β in the early stages of infection [35]. In this study, we found that through the cleavage of the chMAVS protein, IBV can downregulate chIFN-β transcription, and the knockdown of chMAVS had a dramatic effect on chIFN-β activation, indicating a more predominant role of MAVS in the innate immune response against IBV infection.

Tissue distribution is an important characteristic of MDA5 function, as it influences the capacity of MDA5 to capture different viruses as they enter and proliferate in different tissues [22, 23]. Understanding the distribution patterns of MDA5 will enable us to explain the relationship between the immune system and viral infection, and help to identify the relationship between IBV and the host. Previous reports found that expression of the chMDA5 gene could be detected in all tissues examined [22, 23, 34]. Wenxin Zhang demonstrated that IBV failed to increase the MDA5 promoter activity and the expression of endogenous MDA5, which may be explained by the differences in virulence and adaptability of the IBV strain [36]. The expression of MDA5 was significantly upregulated in chicken intestine and lung after being infected with IBV, which in turn upregulated the expression of IFN-β and IFN-λ. Based on this distribution, chMDA5 can respond to invading pathogens as early as possible.

MDA5 and RIG-I are the two major PRRs for detecting RNA viruses. They can both detect RNA viruses and activate a signaling pathway that leads to the production of type I interferon and the initiation of antiviral activities [17, 37]. Considerable attention has recently been given to the role of chMDA5 in IBV infections in chickens, which appear to lack RIG-I [34]. Our results confirm the findings that chMDA5 is the receptor that mediates the antiviral response to IBV infection. Upregulation of chIFN-β following IBV infection in chMDA5-overexpression cells

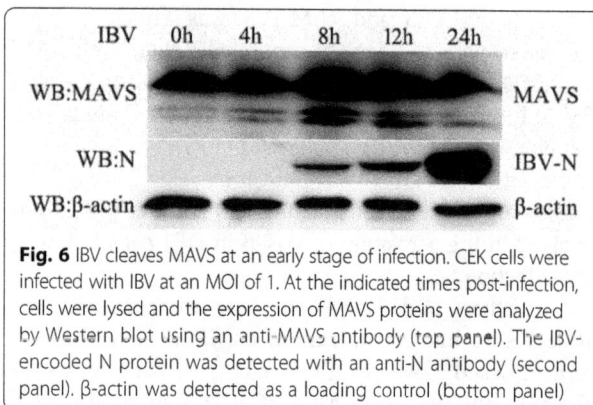

Fig. 6 IBV cleaves MAVS at an early stage of infection. CEK cells were infected with IBV at an MOI of 1. At the indicated times post-infection, cells were lysed and the expression of MAVS proteins were analyzed by Western blot using an anti-MAVS antibody (top panel). The IBV-encoded N protein was detected with an anti-N antibody (second panel). β-actin was detected as a loading control (bottom panel)

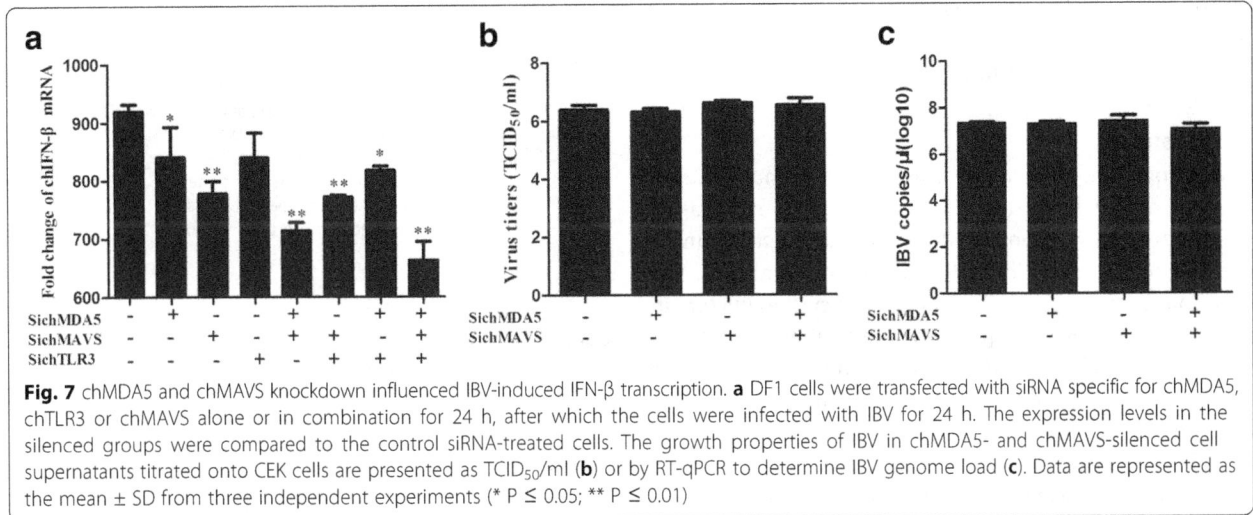

Fig. 7 chMDA5 and chMAVS knockdown influenced IBV-induced IFN-β transcription. **a** DF1 cells were transfected with siRNA specific for chMDA5, chTLR3 or chMAVS alone or in combination for 24 h, after which the cells were infected with IBV for 24 h. The expression levels in the silenced groups were compared to the control siRNA-treated cells. The growth properties of IBV in chMDA5- and chMAVS-silenced cell supernatants titrated onto CEK cells are presented as TCID$_{50}$/ml (**b**) or by RT-qPCR to determine IBV genome load (**c**). Data are represented as the mean ± SD from three independent experiments (* P ≤ 0.05; ** P ≤ 0.01)

suggests that chMDA5 interacts with the proteins induced by IBV infection [25]. The silencing of chMDA5 expression resulted in a reduction of IBV-induced chIFN-β transcription and highlights the role that chMDA5 may play in antiviral defense. The absence of RIG-I in chickens may lead to insufficient antiviral responses to IBV infections, resulting in only chickens being susceptible to IBV infections, whereas ducks and geese, which possess RIG-I, are not infected with IBV [38]. chIFN-β was upregulated in response to IBV infection in dgRIG-I-overexpressed chicken cells, which is similar to observations made in mammalian models [23, 38]. Our study implies that dgRIG-I plays a similar role as chMDA5 in IBV-infected chicken cells, inducing the interferon response.

Although chMDA5 was found to be capable of sensing IBV, leading to the induction of chIFN-β expression in chicken cells, the overexpression of chIFN-β induced by chMDA5 and dgRIG-I did not affect the viral replication in our experiment. Silencing of chMDA5 also had little impact on IBV replication, and a subtle role for chMDA5 may be masked by incomplete silencing of chMDA5, resulting in trace levels of IFN activity. Nevertheless, our data gave a similar result as mammalian models showing that MDA5 is not critical to combat the influenza virus [23]. It is known that type I IFNs are induced by the infection of host cells with viruses and that secreted type I IFNs cause cells to express various antiviral proteins, such as myxovirus-resistance protein (Mx) GTPase, ribonuclease L (RNase L), RNA-dependent protein kinase (PKR), oligoadenylate synthetase (OAS), and interferon stimulated gene (ISG) by autocrine and paracrine mechanisms [27]. Previous studies have suggested that IBV replication was reduced by 50%, as measured by syncytia formation, after a treatment with 100 U/ml of IFN [39, 40]. This implies that even in cells responding to type I IFN, the autocrine

and paracrine effects of IFNs from virus-infected cells may not be sufficient to suppress viral replication. IBV delays the IFN response at an early stage of infection in chicken cells, since it needs time to infect neighboring cells before the establishment of an antiviral state induced by IFN [25], which is secreted paracrinely by chMDA5 and dgRIG-I mediated induction in IBV-infected cells. The data in Fig. 4 also support this conclusion, which suggests that the expression level of IFN in the group infected with a higher dose of IBV was higher than in the group that received a lower dose.

Infectious diseases are a manifestation of constant battles between the host and pathogenic microbes. This host-pathogen antagonism is demonstrated by the interaction between viruses and MAVS, a critical molecule that is downstream of MDA5 and RIG-I [11, 41]. For example, MAVS can orchestrate a strong immune response against hepatitis C virus (HCV), but HCV counterattacks by cleaving MAVS, thus crippling the immune response [42, 43]. MAVS activity was proposed to be linked to both peroxisomes and mitochondrial location in the assembly of a macromolecular signaling complex [13]. When MAVS was cleaved and released to the outside of mitochondria, such as the endoplasmic reticulum or cytoplasm, it failed to signal [13, 44]. IBV can efficiently cleave MAVS in the early stages of infection, leading to the blockage of IFN expression. Furthermore, chIFN-β expression, induced by IBV infection, was effectively inhibited by blocking the expression of MAVS using siRNA. More significant results were observed when MAVS was silenced together with siMDA5. In conclusion, we showed that chMAVS acts as a key modulator of antiviral signaling by regulating chMDA5-mediated signaling in IBV-infected cells.

Future studies should focus on more detailed aspects of host-pathogen interactions that involve chMAVS to gain control of the host immune system.

Conclusions

Taken together, our study represents a comprehensive analysis of the host antiviral immune response against IBV infection. We show that IBV induces activation of the IFN response in CEK cells and chicken embryos. We also found that chMAVS acts as a key modulator in antiviral signaling by positively regulating chMDA5-mediated signaling. dgRIG-I and chMDA5 have similar roles in the IBV-induced IFN-β signaling pathway, the absence of RIG-I may increase the susceptibility of chickens to IBV infection. The exact contributions of these PRRs and MAVS are worth exploring in future studies.

Additional files

> **Additional file 1:** Supplementary information, selection of appropriate reference genes. (DOCX 36 kb)
>
> **Additional file 2: Figure S1.** Transcriptional stability of eight candidate reference genes in different chicken embryo tissues. Three eleven-day-old SPF chicken embryos were inoculated with PBS. Then, the kidney (A and B), liver (C and D), muscle (E and F), intestine (G and H), lung (I and J) and trachea (K and L) tissues were collected from the embryos 72 h post-inoculation, and RNA was extracted. Candidate reference gene mRNA was amplified by real-time PCR. The transcriptional stability of the candidate reference genes was measured using geNorm and NormFinder software. (A), (C), (E), (G), (I) and (K) are the geNorm analysis results. Average expression stability M of all eight reference genes. The most stably expressed genes have lower M values. (B), (D), (F), (H), (J) and (L) are the NormFinder analysis results. The lower stability value indicates a gene that is more stable. (TIFF 730 kb)
>
> **Additional file 3: Figure S2.** IBV induces chMDA5, chIFN-β, chIFN-λ and chMx expression in chicken embryos. In this experiment three embryos were inoculated with IBV, and three embryos were inoculated with PBS, which served as negative controls. Then, the trachea, intestine, kidney, lung, liver, and muscle tissues were collected from the embryos 72 h post-infection. (A) chMDA5, (B) chIFN-β, (C) chIFN-λ and (D) chMx were calculated as fold change of the infected group relative to the uninfected group and normalized against three different reference genes. In the kidney, liver and muscle tissues chMDA5, chIFN-β, chIFN-λ and chMx transcription was normalized to ACTB (1), EFF1 (2) and RPL5 (3) respectively. In the intestine chMDA5, chIFN-β, chIFN-λ and chMx transcription was normalized to ACTB (1), GAPDH (2) and RPL32 (3) respectively. In the lung chMDA5, chIFN-β, chIFN-λ and chMx transcription was normalized to ACTB (1), TUBAT (2) and RPL5 (3) respectively. In the trachea chMDA5, chIFN-β, chIFN-λ and chMx transcription was normalized to ACTB (1), EFF1 (2) and RPL32 (3) respectively. Data are shown as the mean ± SD. (n=3) (* $P \leq 0.05$; ** $P \leq 0.01$). (TIFF 1330 kb)
>
> **Additional file 4:** The datasets analysed during the current study. (XLSX 20 kb)

Abbreviations

ACTB: β-actin; AIV: Avian influenza virus; CARD: Caspase activation and recruitment domains; CEK: Chicken embryonic kidney; CPE: Cytopathic effect; EFF1: Eukaryotic translation elongation factor 1 alpha; EMCV: Encephalomyocarditis virus; GAPDH: Glyceraldehyde-3-phosphate dehydrogenase; GUSB: β-glucuronidase; HCV: Hepatitis C virus; IBV: Infectious bronchitis virus; IFN: Interferon; IFN-λ: Interferon-lambda; IRF3/IRF7: Interferon regulatory factor-3/7; ISG: Interferon stimulated gene; LGP2: Laboratory of genetics and physiology 2; MAVS: Mitochondrial antiviral signaling gene, also called IPS-1/VISA/CARDIF; MDA5: Melanoma differentiation associated gene 5; MOI: Multiplicity of infection; MRPS30: Mitochondrial ribosomal protein S30; MV: Measles virus; Mx: Myxovirus-resistance protein; NLRs: Nucleotide-binding oligomerization domain (NOD)-like receptors; OAS: Oligoadenylate synthetase; PAMPs: Pathogen-Associated molecular patterns; PKR: RNA-dependent protein kinase; PRRs: Pattern recognition receptors; RIG-I: Retinoic acid-inducible gene-I; RLRs: Retinoic acid-inducible gene I -like receptors; RNase L: Ribonuclease L; RPL32: Guanine nucleotide binding protein (G protein), ribosomal protein L32; RPL5: Ribosomal protein L5; siRNA: Small interfering RNA; SPF: Specific pathogen free; TCID50: 50% tissue culture infective dose; TUBAT: Testis-specific alpha-tubulin mRNA; VSV: Vesicular stomatitis virus

Acknowledgements

We are grateful to Yage Hu for the necropsy and collection of tissue samples.

Funding

This work was supported by China Agriculture Research System (CARS-40-K16), the Yangzhou University Funding for Scientific Research (KYLX16_1405), the National Natural Science Foundation of China (31101815) and the Priority Academic Program Development of Jiangsu Higher Education Institutions.

Authors' contributions

LPY and XRZ contributed to the study design, data evaluation and the manuscript writing; TQW collected samples, measured viral load with qRT-PCR, and analyzed the data; JS developed the experiment of chMDA5 and chMAVS influences on IBV-induced IFN-β transcription; YYW helped to draft and modify the manuscript; YXW, BYR and XSN helped with experimental design of IBV infected chicken embryos, carried out RNA isolation, qRT-PCR and data analysis; YTW conceived of the study, participated in the design of the study and helped prepare the final manuscript. All authors read and approved the final manuscript.

Consent for publication

Not applicable

Competing interests

All authors declare that they have no competing interests.

References

1. Cavanagh D. Coronavirus avian infectious bronchitis virus. Vet Res. 2007; 38(2):281–97.
2. Oudshoorn D, van der Hoeven B, Limpens RW, Beugeling C, Snijder EJ, Barcena M, Kikkert M. Antiviral Innate Immune Response Interferes with the Formation of Replication-Associated Membrane Structures Induced by a Positive-Strand RNA Virus. MBio. 2016;7(6):e01991–16.
3. Kint J, Dickhout A, Kutter J, Maier HJ, Britton P, Koumans J, Pijlman GP, Fros JJ, Wiegertjes GF, Forlenza M. Infectious bronchitis Coronavirus inhibits STAT1 signaling and requires accessory proteins for resistance to type I interferon activity. J Virol. 2015;89(23):12047–57.
4. Kint J, Langereis MA, Maier HJ, Britton P, van Kuppeveld FJ, Koumans J, Wiegertjes GF, Forlenza M. Infectious bronchitis Coronavirus limits interferon production by inducing a host shutoff that requires accessory protein 5b. J Virol. 2016;90(16):7519–28.
5. Takeuchi O, Akira S. Recognition of viruses by innate immunity. Immunol Rev. 2007;220:214–24.
6. Akira S, Uematsu S, Takeuchi O. Pathogen recognition and innate immunity. Cell. 2006;124(4):783–801.
7. Meylan E, Curran J, Hofmann K, Moradpour D, Binder M, Bartenschlager R, Tschopp R. Cardif is an adaptor protein in the RIG-I antiviral pathway and is targeted by hepatitis C virus. Nature. 2005;437(7062):1167–72.

8. Hornung V, Ellegast J, Kim S, Brzozka K, Jung A, Kato H, Poeck H, Akira S, Conzelmann KK, Schlee M, et al. 5 '-triphosphate RNA is the ligand for RIG-I. Science. 2006;314(5801):994–7.

9. Berghall H, Siren J, Sarkar D, Julkunen I, Fisher PB, Vainionpaa R, Matikainen S. The interferon-inducible RNA helicase, mda-5, is involved in measles virus-induced expression of antiviral cytokines. Microbes Infect. 2006;8(8):2138–44.

10. Komuro A, Horvath CM. RNA- and virus-independent inhibition of antiviral signaling by RNA helicase LGP2. J Virol. 2006;80(24):12332–42.

11. Lin RT, Lacoste J, Nakhaei P, Sun Q, Yang L, Paz S, Wilkinson P, Julkunen I, Vitour D, Meurs E, et al. Dissociation of a MAVS/IPS-1/VISA/Cardif-1KK epsilon molecular complex from the mitochondrial outer membrane by hepatitis C virus NS3-4A proteolytic cleavage. J Virol. 2006;80(12):6072–83.

12. Kawai T, Takahashi K, Sato S, Coban C, Kumar H, Kato H, Ishii KJ, Takeuchi O, Akira S. IPS-1, an adaptor triggering RIG-I- and Mda5-mediated type I interferon induction. Nat Immunol. 2005;6(10):981–8.

13. Seth RB, Sun LJ, Ea CK, Chen ZJJ. Identification and characterization of MAVS, a mitochondrial antiviral signaling protein that activates NF-kappa B and IRF3. Cell. 2005;122(5):669–82.

14. Soulat D, Burckstummer T, Westermayer S, Goncalves A, Bauch A, Stefanovic A, Hantschel O, Bennett KL, Decker T, Superti-Furga G. The DEAD-box helicase DDX3X is a critical component of the TANK-binding kinase 1-dependent innate immune response. EMBO J. 2008;27(15):2135–46.

15. Xu LG, Wang YY, Han KJ, Li LY, Zhai ZH, Shu HB. VISA is an adapter protein required for virus-triggered IFN-beta signaling. Mol Cell. 2005;19(6):727–40.

16. Kang DC, Gopalkrishnan RV, Wu Q, Jankowsky E, Pyle AM. Fisher PB: mda-5: an interferon-inducible putative RNA helicase with double-stranded RNA-dependent ATPase activity and melanoma growth-suppressive properties. Proc Natl Acad Sci U S A. 2002;99(2):637–42.

17. Barral PM, Sarkar D, Su ZZ, Barber GN, DeSalle R, Racaniello VR, Fisher PB. Functions of the cytoplasmic RNA sensors RIG-I and MDA-5: key regulators of innate immunity. Pharmacol Ther. 2009;124(2):219–34.

18. Yoneyama M, Kikuchi M, Natsukawa T, Shinobu N, Imaizumi T, Miyagishi M, Taira K, Akira S, Fujita T. The RNA helicase RIG-I has an essential function in double-stranded RNA-induced innate antiviral responses. Nat Immunol. 2004;5(7):730–7.

19. Yoneyama M, Kikuchi M, Matsumoto K, Imaizumi T, Miyagishi M, Taira K, Foy E, Loo YM, Gale M Jr, Akira S, et al. Shared and unique functions of the DExD/H-box helicases RIG-I, MDA5, and LGP2 in antiviral innate immunity. J Immunol. 2005;175(5):2851–8.

20. Siren J, Imaizumi T, Sarkar D, Pietila T, Noah DL, Lin R, Hiscott J, Krug RM, Fisher PB, Julkunen I, et al. Retinoic acid inducible gene-I and mda-5 are involved in influenza a virus-induced expression of antiviral cytokines. Microbes Infect. 2006;8(8):2013–20.

21. Barber MR, Aldridge JR Jr, Webster RG, Magor KE. Association of RIG-I with innate immunity of ducks to influenza. Proc Natl Acad Sci U S A. 2010; 107(13):5913–8.

22. Hayashi T, Watanabe C, Suzuki Y, Tanikawa T, Uchida Y, Saito T. Chicken MDA5 senses short double-stranded RNA with implications for antiviral response against avian influenza viruses in chicken. J Innate Immun. 2014;6(1):58–71.

23. Karpala AJ, Stewart C, McKay J, Lowenthal JW, Bean AG. Characterization of chicken Mda5 activity: regulation of IFN-beta in the absence of RIG-I functionality. J Immunol. 2011;186(9):5397–405.

24. Rebel JM, Peeters B, Fijten H, Post J, Cornelissen J, Vervelde L. Highly pathogenic or low pathogenic avian influenza virus subtype H7N1 infection in chicken lungs: small differences in general acute responses. Vet Res. 2011;42:10.

25. Kint J, Fernandez-Gutierrez M, Maier HJ, Britton P, Langereis MA, Koumans J, Wiegertjes GF, Forlenza M. Activation of the chicken type I interferon response by infectious bronchitis coronavirus. J Virol. 2015;89(2):1156–67.

26. Callison SA, Hilt DA, Boynton TO, Sample BF, Robison R, Swayne DE, Jackwood MW. Development and evaluation of a real-time Taqman RT-PCR assay for the detection of infectious bronchitis virus from infected chickens. J Virol Methods. 2006;138(1–2):60–5.

27. Boo KH, Yang JS. Intrinsic cellular defenses against virus infection by antiviral type I interferon. Yonsei Med J. 2010;51(1):9–17.

28. Nascimento CS, Barbosa LT, Brito C, Fernandes RP, Mann RS, Pinto AP, Oliveira HC, Dodson MV, Guimaraes SE, Duarte MS. Identification of suitable reference genes for real time quantitative polymerase chain reaction assays on Pectoralis major muscle in chicken (Gallus Gallus). PLoS One. 2015;10(5):e0127935.

29. Cedraz de Oliveira H, AAJ PG, Gonzaga Gromboni JG, Vasconcelos Farias Filho R, Souza do Nascimento C, Arias Wenceslau A. Influence of heat stress, sex and genetic groups on reference genes stability in muscle tissue of chicken. PLoS One. 2017;12(5):e0176402.

30. Bages S, Estany J, Tor M, Pena RN. Investigating reference genes for quantitative real-time PCR analysis across four chicken tissues. Gene. 2015;561(1):82–7.

31. Borowska D, Rothwell L, Bailey RA, Watson K, Kaiser P. Identification of stable reference genes for quantitative PCR in cells derived from chicken lymphoid organs. Vet Immunol Immunopathol. 2016;170:20–4.

32. Batra A, Maier HJ, Fife MS. Selection of reference genes for gene expression analysis by real-time qPCR in avian cells infected with infectious bronchitis virus. Avian Pathol. 2017;46(2):173–80.

33. He Y, Xie Z, Dai J, Cao Y, Hou J, Zheng Y, Wei T, Mo M, Wei P. Responses of the toll-like receptor and melanoma differentiation-associated protein 5 signaling pathways to avian infectious bronchitis virus infection in chicks. Virol Sin. 2016;31(1):57–68.

34. Lee CC, Wu CC, Lin TL. Characterization of chicken melanoma differentiation-associated gene 5 (MDA5) from alternative translation initiation. Comp Immunol Microbiol Infect Dis. 2012;35(4):335–43.

35. Vervelde L, Matthijs MG, van Haarlem DA, de Wit JJ, Jansen CA. Rapid NK-cell activation in chicken after infection with infectious bronchitis virus M41. Vet Immunol Immunopathol. 2013;151(3–4):337–41.

36. Zhang WX, Zuo EW, He Y, Chen DY, Long X, Chen MJ, Li TT, Yang XG, Xu HY, Lu SS, et al. Promoter structures and differential responses to viral and non-viral inducers of chicken melanoma differentiation-associated gene 5. Mol Immunol. 2016;76:1–6.

37. Deddouche S, Matt N, Budd A, Mueller S, Kemp C, Galiana-Arnoux D, Dostert C, Antoniewski C, Hoffmann JA, Imler JL. The DExD/H-box helicase Dicer-2 mediates the induction of antiviral activity in drosophila. Nat Immunol. 2008;9(12):1425–32.

38. Guo Z, Chen LM, Zeng H, Gomez JA, Plowden J, Fujita T, Katz JM, Donis RO, Sambhara S. NS1 protein of influenza a virus inhibits the function of intracytoplasmic pathogen sensor, RIG-I. Am J Respir Cell Mol Biol. 2007;36(3):263–9.

39. Pei J, Sekellick MJ, Marcus PI, Choi IS, Collisson EW. Chicken interferon type I inhibits infectious bronchitis virus replication and associated respiratory illness. J Interf Cytokine Res. 2001;21(12):1071–7.

40. Otsuki K, Maeda J, Yamamoto H, Tsubokura M. Studies on avian infectious bronchitis virus (IBV). III. Interferon induction by and sensitivity to interferon of IBV. Arch Virol. 1979;60(3–4):249–55.

41. Yoneyama M, Fujita T. RNA recognition and signal transduction by RIG-I-like receptors. Immunol Rev. 2009;227(1):54–65.

42. Ferreira AR, Magalhaes AC, Camoes F, Gouveia A, Vieira M, Kagan JC, Ribeiro D. Hepatitis C virus NS3-4A inhibits the peroxisomal MAVS-dependent antiviral signaling response. J Cell Mol Med. 2016;20(4):750–7.

43. Cao X, Ding Q, Lu J, Tao W, Huang B, Zhao Y, Niu J, Liu YJ, Zhong J. MDA5 plays a critical role in interferon response during hepatitis C virus infection. J Hepatol. 2015;62(4):771–8.

44. Chen Z, Benureau Y, Rijnbrand R, Yi J, Wang T, Warter L, Lanford RE, Weinman SA, Lemon SM, Martin A, et al. GB virus B disrupts RIG-I signaling by NS3/4A-mediated cleavage of the adaptor protein MAVS. J Virol. 2007;81(2):964–76.

10

Seroprevalence of *Toxoplasma gondii* infection in feral cats in Qatar

Sonia Boughattas[1], Jerzy Behnke[2], Aarti Sharma[1] and Marawan Abu-Madi[1*]

Abstract

Background: Cats are essential in the life cycle of *Toxoplasma gondii* as they can shed the environmentally resistant oocysts after acquiring infection. Human populations living in cities with high densities of feral cats are therefore likely to be at risk of infection. The current study is the first to estimate the seroprevalence of *T. gondii* in the feral cat population in Qatar. We investigated the seroprevalence of *T. gondii* among 495 adult cats from urban and suburban districts in Qatar. Using results from the Modified Agglutination Test, we fitted statistical models with host sex, area and season as explanatory factors and seropositivity as the outcome.

Results: The analysis revealed an overall seroprevalence of 82%. Seroprevalence was significantly higher in the summer season ($P = 0.006$). No significant difference was detected ($P > 0.05$) between seroprevalence in female and male cats and in cats from urban and suburban districts of Qatar.

Conclusions: Despite the seasonal difference, the observed seroprevalence of *T. gondii* suggests high environmental contamination throughout the year, with some female cats generating more intense responses compared to males. Both findings merit further investigations.

Keywords: Serosurvey, Antibodies, Toxoplasmosis, Felids, Middle East, Season, Sex

Background

Toxoplasmosis is a widespread zoonotic parasitic infection. It is estimated that about one third of the world population is chronically infected with *Toxoplasma gondii*.

Felids are the only definitive hosts of the parasite and can shed millions of environmentally resistant oocysts in their feces if they become infected [1]. The oocysts can remain infectious for more than 1 year in unfrozen and moist soil [2] and can cause outbreaks of toxoplasmosis. This is evidenced by the large waterborne outbreak of toxoplasmosis in Canada in 1995 that was epidemiologically linked to oocyst contamination of a water reservoir in British Columbia [3].

Cats were introduced to Qatar in the 1960s to control the high rodent population in the country, but subsequently they in turn reproduced rapidly [4]. The current density of cats in Qatar may pose a risk for humans, as cats are natural hosts for a wide range of zoonotic pathogens, including *T. gondii*. The overall seroprevalence of *T. gondii* among the Qatari human population has been estimated at 29.8% with a progressive rise from <4% in the 1 year old group to 41.2% at >45 years of age [5]. Such observations provide further evidence for the increased risk of infection with increasing age through longer exposure time.

As cats shed *Toxoplasma* oocysts for only a short period of time after initial infection, detection of patent infections in cat populations (based on faecal oocyst counts) is likely to underestimate the number of animals that have been exposed to infection [1]. However, *T. gondii* elicits strong antibody responses in its hosts and therefore assessment of seroprevalence is an alternative approach for studying the epidemiology of this pathogen. Estimates of antibody prevalence in the cat population also provide another useful indicator of environmental contamination [6]. The current study is the first to estimate the seroprevalence of *T. gondii* in the feral cat population in Qatar.

Methods
Sample collection
Feral cats were caught live as part of the routine activities of the Qatar Cat Control Unit as described previously [4].

* Correspondence: abumadi@qu.edu.qa
[1]Department of Biomedical Science, College of Health Sciences, Biomedical Research Center, Qatar University, P.O. Box 2713, Doha, Qatar
Full list of author information is available at the end of the article

Briefly, trapped adult cats that were eligible for the trap-neuter-return program were transported to a shelter for sterilization. For each animal the sex, the area, and the season of sampling were recorded. In the current study, sampling began in September 2014, and ended in September 2015 (394 samples in summer and 101 samples in winter).

Cats from both urban ($n = 216$) and sub-urban ($n = 279$) areas were investigated in this study. Within each sector, traps were set out in places most likely to be frequented by cats at night, i.e. in alleyways, in back yards close to houses, and near to rubbish bins and municipal garbage containers.

Blood was drawn by experienced veterinarians complying strictly with animal welfare guidelines as stipulated by the National Institutional Animal Care and Use Committee of Qatar. Blood samples were then centrifuged at $5000 \times g$ for 20 min at room temperature and the resulting supernatants were collected and used for serology.

Serology

A total number of 495 sera (234 males and 261 females) were tested for *T. gondii* IgG antibodies using commercially available *Toxoplasma gondii* antigen (#EH2001, Kerafast® Boston, USA). Two-fold serial dilutions, in phosphate buffered saline (pH 7.2), were made from 1:25 to 1:200 and tested with a Modified Agglutination Test (MAT), as previously described [7]. Samples that were positive at a dilution of 1:200 were further diluted in a second run to a dilution of 1:3,200 for antibody titration, and those positive at 1:3,200 were diluted in a third run until no further agglutination was evident.

Positive controls (provided by the Department of Laboratory Medicine and Pathology at Hamad General Hospital) and negative controls (serum dilution buffer without serum) were included in each test. Agglutination in at least half of the "U" well bottoms of a microplate was accepted as a positive reaction. In the case of complete sedimentation on the well bottom with no sign of agglutination, the sample was recorded as negative, i.e. no evidence of *T. gondii* antibodies in the serum. A titer (inverse of a dilution) of 25 or higher was considered positive.

Statistical analysis

Prevalence values (percentage of animals infected) are given with 95% confidence limits (CL_{95}), calculated by bespoke software based on the tables of Rohlf and Sokal [8]. For analysis of seroprevalence, we used maximum likelihood techniques based on log linear analysis of contingency tables in the software package IBM SPSS Statistics Version 21 (IBM Corporation). Initially, full factorial models were fitted, incorporating as factors SEX (at 2 levels, males and females), AREA (at 2 levels, 1 for urban areas [Al Hilal, Bin Omran, Al Sadd, Umm-Ghwailina,

Al Salata, Madinat Khalifa, Al Nasr, Al Maamoura, Al Dafna, Al Muntzah, Al Markhiya, Al Najma, Old Airport, Al Asiri] and 2 for suburban areas [Al Azizia, Al Rayyan, Al Luqta, Al Waab, Abu Hamour, Al Wakrah, Muaither, Um Al Amad, Shahaniya, Al Gharrafa, Al Kharaitiyat, Umm Salal, Al Zaghwa, Al Wajba, Al Khor, Al Khissa]) and SEASON (at 2 levels, summer [May-October] and winter [November-April]). INFECTION, reflecting the presence or absence of antibodies to *T. gondii* (overall or at specific dilutions) was coded as a binary factor, and the cut-off for statistical significance was considered to be a *P* value of 0.05 (two tailed) [4].

For analysis of quantitative data we first ranked the titers on a scale from 0 to 8, where 0 = no agglutination, 1 = maximum agglutination at 1:25 and so on to 8 = agglutination at dilutions higher than 1:3,200. We used a zero-inflated model in R version 2.2.1 (R Core Development Team and the *pscl* package) that analyzed a binomial process (0, 1 for the high responders versus the rest with a binomial model with logit link) and a Poisson (Poisson model with log link) for the rest.

Results

Of the 495 feral cats (234 males and 261 females) tested, 406 (82.0%, CL_{95} = 76.11–86.79) were positive for *T. gondii* antibodies. Four samples presented prozone effects with negative results at the low dilution of 1:25 and positive agglutination at higher dilutions $\geq 1:1,600$. The frequency distribution of antibody titers among the sampled cats is shown in Fig. 1, and the bimodal distribution of antibody titres, with peaks in the lower and top ends of the positive range can be clearly seen.

Seroprevalence of *T. gondii* was similar in males and females: 82.5% (CL_{95} = 78.58–85.84) and 81.6% (CL_{95} = 77.45–85.17) respectively. With SEASON and AREA taken into account, the difference between the sexes was not significant (for SEX x INFECTION χ_1^2 = 0.216, $P > 0.05$). However, when the prevalence of antibodies in male and female cats was plotted separately against serum dilution (Fig. 2a), there was a significant effect of host SEX at high antibody titers (models taking SEASON and AREA taken into consideration, at a serum dilution of 1:400, for SEX x INFECTION χ_1^2 = 11.69, $P = 0.001$; and in serum dilutions higher than 1:3,200; $\chi_1^2 = 7.30$, $P = 0.007$).

Seroprevalence was similar in cats from urban and sub-urban areas (82.4%, CL_{95} = 78.64–85.67, and 81.7%, CL_{95} = 77.42–85.37, respectively) and no significant difference between areas was detected whether testing overall positivity (for AREA x INFECTION χ_1^2 = 0.42, $P > 0.05$), or positivity at specific dilutions of serum.

The number of cats sampled in the summer was 394, and 101 in the winter months. There was a significant effect of SEASON on seropositivity (with host SEX and

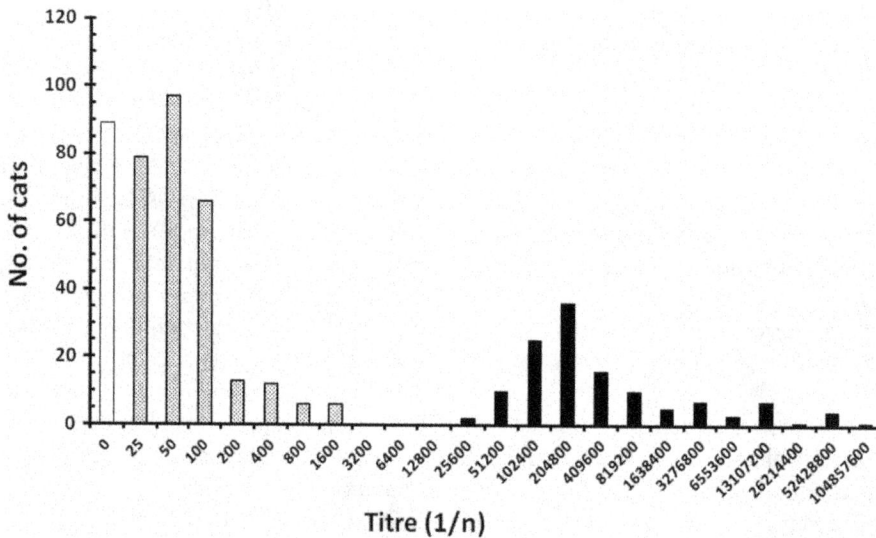

Fig. 1 Frequency distribution of antibody titres among the sampled cats. The figure shows the number of cats for which no antibody was detected (first column filled in white) and those that had detectable antibody. Titres for the latter are given as the reciprocal of the maximum dilution (n) at which agglutination was detected and these fall into two peaks. Columns filled with stippled shading indicate the numbers of cats with titres in the lower intensity antibody range and those filled in black represent cats with the higher titres

AREA taken into account, for SEASON x INFECTION $\chi^2_1 = 7.52$, $P = 0.006$). Seroprevalence was higher in the summer months (84.5%, $CL_{95} = 79.62–88.46$) in contrast to the winter (72.3%, $CL_{95} = 65.53–78.14$ and see Fig. 2b).

Quantitative analysis was in general in agreement with these conclusions. Based on the zero-inflated model and a binomial process in which the high responders (cats showing titers in excess of 1:3,200) were coded as 1, and the rest as zero, the occurrence of the highest titers (>1:3,200) was affected significantly only by host sex ($z = 2.534$, $P = 0.0113$). Males (mean rank = 0.201 ± 0.025, $n = 234$) had a lower frequency of high titers than females (mean rank = 0.307 ± 0.029, $n = 251$), as found in the earlier log linear model given above.

Discussion

This study demonstrated a high overall seroprevalence of T. gondii antibodies in the feral cat population in Qatar. Seroprevalence was higher than values reported from neighboring countries, as for example 19.6% in Kuwait [9] and 30.4% in Iraq [10]. Similar seroprevalences to those recorded in this study have been observed mainly among cats from tropical areas: Ethiopia with 85.4% [11] and the Amazon with 87.3% [12].

While the present work did not find an overall significant difference in seroprevalence between male and female cats as observed elsewhere [13, 14], higher antibody titers were detected in female cats when analysis was restricted to the high dilutions (>1/400) which is in accordance with other reports [6, 15]. However our observation of some female cats expressing more intense antibody

responses than male cats contrasts with the conclusions reached by Miro et al. [16], who reported in their study that stray male cats had significantly higher seroprevalence. The authors linked their findings to differences in the territorial habits of male and female cats, as male cats are more likely to wander and thus experience more access to contaminated sources [17]. Although ecological, social and epidemiological factors may account for some of the female biased antibody responses in our study, hormone-influenced immunological mechanisms have been proposed as the more likely mechanism underlying sex-biased parasitism with T. gondii [18].

Cat bioassays have not provided any clear evidence of sex-bias in the occurrence of toxoplasmosis [19]. However, experimental studies in mice have shown that females are more susceptible than males to T. gondii infection and develop more severe cerebral inflammation. They are more likely to die following infection than males [20]. Female mice that survived the acute phase and developed chronic infections harbored more cysts in their brains than did surviving males. Gonadectomy of female mice was shown to reduce the development of tissue cysts caused by T. gondii infection, whereas estrogen administration was found to exacerbate the infection [21].

It remains unknown when the cats that tested positive had acquired the infection. The low intensity responses (≤1/400) which were recorded in more than half of the cats in our study suggest antibodies from a past infection but may also include cats that have very recently been exposed to the parasite, and have not yet developed

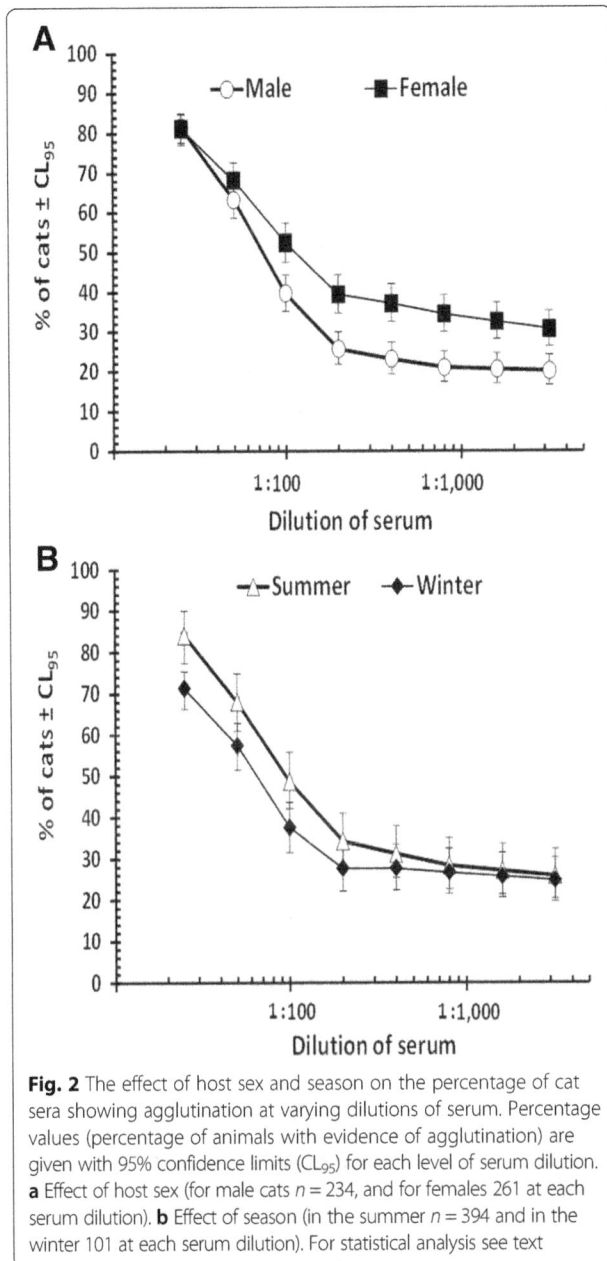

Fig. 2 The effect of host sex and season on the percentage of cat sera showing agglutination at varying dilutions of serum. Percentage values (percentage of animals with evidence of agglutination) are given with 95% confidence limits (CL$_{95}$) for each level of serum dilution. **a** Effect of host sex (for male cats $n = 234$, and for females 261 at each serum dilution). **b** Effect of season (in the summer $n = 394$ and in the winter 101 at each serum dilution). For statistical analysis see text

environment, especially given that some reports have documented cats travelling up to 45 km in just 2 days [23]. Domestic and stray/feral cats are the same species (*Felis catus*) and the main difference between them is their lifestyle. In contrast to domestic animals, feral cats are unowned and live in the streets, alleys, farm buildings, factories, wharves or abandoned vehicles. They may be semi dependent on humans from whom they may receive some food. It has been reported elsewhere that 76.5% of cats fed table leftovers are *Toxoplasma* seropositive with a majority showing high IgG antibodies titers [24]. These free-roaming cats are exposed to a wide variety of pathogens, and have been shown to be excellent sentinels of infectious and parasitic diseases. Consequently they provide useful information on circulation of pathogens in domestic and wild ecosystems [13]. Most cats are thought to become infected with *T. gondii* after weaning when they begin to hunt for food. Outdoor access facilitates hunting behavior, as in the Netherlands where 93% of the cats with free outdoor access exhibited hunting behavior [22]. Stray cats and cats with outdoor access usually acquire the infection from hunting rather than from the ingestion of oocysts [25]. Hence the recommendation to pet owners that to protect their cats from *T. gondii* infection the hunting of small prey should be discouraged/prevented, and that all meat served to their pet cats should be thoroughly cooked and/or frozen before cooking [26].

In a study conducted in Italy, it was suggested that infected intermediate hosts that are prey for cats are more available in the summer season [27]. A recent analysis reported a correlation between the geolatitude (which strongly correlates with temperature and quantity and quality of sunlight) and humidity (which favors the survival of *Toxoplasma* oocysts in soil) and occurrence of toxoplasmosis [28]. The efficiency of transmission may therefore differ between seasons in Qatar, with a higher risk of exposure in the summer months (where the climate is more suitable for survival of the oocysts). Qatar typically experiences two seasons. In the summer season, daytime temperatures frequently exceed 45 °C and seldom fall below 18 °C at night. Humidity peaks in August at 90%, before subsiding to 70% towards the end of October [4]. The latter months of the summer season certainly fall within this definition of the optimal climatic conditions for transmission. During the winter season temperatures peak at about 28 °C and may fall as low as 7 °C at night and the mean humidity is usually in the range 75–86%. These conditions are less suitable for survival of oocysts of *T. gondii* in the external environment. Thus, the tenacity and infectivity of oocysts in winter may be less than in summer, and hence transmission to cats and potential intermediate hosts such as rodents may be less efficient in winter months. However, this

the maximum response. The cats that showed intense antibody responses (≥1/800 dilution) are more likely to be cats that had acquired the infection recently but after a sufficient time to mount the response [22]. Since the prevalence of high intensity antibody responses was almost identical in both winter and summer months, this indicates that there is a persistent source of *T. gondii* infection in the environment in which the cats live. Moreover, the consistently high seroprevalence in both urban and sub-urban areas of Qatar suggests a high level of *T. gondii* contamination throughout the country.

The large home ranges of feral cats, which can stretch to 10 km^2, implies widespread contamination of the requires further studies, for instance by environmental sampling for *T. gondii* oocysts and thorough assessment of the resilience of oocysts of local isolates of *T. gondii* to typical summer and winter conditions in Qatar. Unfortunately, most people are unaware that they can acquire toxoplasmosis from the environment by direct contact with soil or water [29].

Conclusions

The seroprevalence of *T.gondii* in cats in Qatar is high. Our data showed that female cats were more likely to have high antibody responses compared with males, and that seroprevalence is higher in the summer months. Overall, our data imply high contamination of the local environment in Qatar and we recommend further investigation of food/water sources through which transmission may occur.

Acknowledgments
We would like to thank the Biomedical Research Center at Qatar University and the Cat Control Unit at the Ministry of Municipality and Environment for providing facilities for this work.

Funding
This publication was made possible by NPRP grant number NPRP 4-164-4-001 from Qatar National Research Fund. The contents of this report are solely the responsibility of the authors and do not necessarily represent the official views of Qatar University and QRNF.

Authors' contributions
SB carried out the serology and drafted the manuscript. AS collected the cat samples and contributed to the serology. JMB carried out the statistical analysis and participated in the preparation and refinement of the manuscript. MAM conceived the study, collected the background information on the samples and revised the manuscript critically for important intellectual content. All authors read and approved the final manuscript.

Competing interests
The authors declare that they have no competing interests.

Consent for publication
Not applicable.

Author details
[1]Department of Biomedical Science, College of Health Sciences, Biomedical Research Center, Qatar University, P.O. Box 2713, Doha, Qatar. [2]School of Biology, University of Nottingham, University Park, Nottingham NG7 2RD, UK.

References
1. Dubey JP. Oocyst shedding by cats fed isolated bradyzoites and comparison of infectivity of bradyzoites of the VEG strain *Toxoplasma gondii* to cats and mice. J Parasitol. 2001;87:215–9.
2. Mancianti F, Nardoni S, Mugnaini L, Zambernardi L, Guerrini A, Gazzola V, Papini RA. A retrospective molecular study of select intestinal protozoa in healthy pet cats from Italy. J Feline Med Surg. 2015;17:163–7.
3. Bowie WR, King AS, Werker DH, Isaac-Renton JL, Bell A, Eng SB, Marion SA. Outbreak of toxoplasmosis associated with municipal drinking water. The BC *Toxoplasma* Investigation Team. Lancet. 1997;350:173–7.
4. Abu-Madi MA, Behnke JM. Feline patent *Toxoplasma*-like coccidiosis among feral cats (*Felis catus*) in Doha city, Qatar and its immediate surroundings. Acta Parasitol. 2014;59:390–7.
5. Abu-Madi MA, Al-Molawi N, Behnke JM. Seroprevalence and epidemiological correlates of *Toxoplasma gondii* infections among patients referred for hospital-based serological testing in Doha, Qatar. Parasit Vectors. 2008;1:39.
6. Silaghi C, Knaus M, Rapti D, Kusi I, Shukullari E, Hamel D, Pfister K, Rehbein S. Survey of *Toxoplasma gondii* and *Neospora caninum*, haemotropic mycoplasmas and other arthropod-borne pathogens in cats from Albania. Parasit Vectors. 2014;7:62.
7. Dubey JP, Desmonts G. Serological responses of equids fed *Toxoplasma gondii* oocysts. Equine Vet J. 1987;19:337–9.
8. Rohlf FJ, Sokal RR. Statistical Tables (3rd Edition) W.H. Freeman and Company, San Francisco 1995.
9. Abdou NE, Al-Batel MK, El-Azazy OM, Sami AM, Majeed QA. Enteric protozoan parasites in stray cats in Kuwait with special references to toxoplasmosis and risk factors affecting its occurrence. J Egypt Soc Parasitol. 2013;43:303–14.
10. Switzer AD, McMillan-Cole AC, Kasten RW, Stuckey MJ, Kass PH, Chomel BB. *Bartonella* and *Toxoplasma* infections in stray cats from Iraq. Am J Trop Med Hyg. 2013;89:1219–24.
11. Tiao N, Darrington C, Molla B, Saville WJ, Tilahun G, Kwok OC, Gebreyes WA, Lappin MR, Jones JL, Dubey JP. An investigation into the seroprevalence of *Toxoplasma gondii*, *Bartonella spp.*, feline immunodeficiency virus (FIV), and feline leukaemia virus (FeLV) in cats in Addis Ababa, Ethiopia. Epidemiol Infect. 2013; 141: 1029–33.
12. Cavalcante GT, Aguiar DM, Chiebao D, Dubey JP, Ruiz VL, Dias RA, Camargo LM, Labruna MB, Gennari SM. Seroprevalence of *Toxoplasma gondii* antibodies in cats and pigs from rural Western Amazon, Brazil. J Parasitol. 2006;92:863–4.
13. Adams PJ, Elliot AD, Algar D, Brazell RI. Gastrointestinal parasites of feral cats from Christmas Island. Aust Vet J. 2008;86:60–3.
14. Cong W, Meng QF, Blaga R, Villena I, Zhu XQ, Qian AD. *Toxoplasma gondii*, *Dirofilaria immitis*, feline immunodeficiency virus (FIV), and feline leukemia virus (FeLV) infections in stray and pet cats (*Felis catus*) in northwest China: co-infections and risk factors. Parasitol Res. 2016;115:217–23.
15. Jittapalapong S, Nimsupan B, Pinyopanuwat N, Chimnoi W, Kabeya H, Maruyama S. Seroprevalence of *Toxoplasma gondii* antibodies in stray cats and dogs in the Bangkok metropolitan area, Thailand. Vet Parasitol. 2007; 145:138–41.
16. Miro G, Montoya A, Jimenez S, Frisuelos C, Mateo M, Fuentes I. Prevalence of antibodies to *Toxoplasma gondii* and intestinal parasites in stray, farm and household cats in Spain. Vet Parasitol. 2004;126:249–55.
17. Rahimi MT, Daryani A, Sarvi S, Shokri A, Ahmadpour E, Teshnizi SH, Mizani A, Sharif M. Cats and *Toxoplasma gondii*: A systematic review and meta-analysis in Iran. Onderstepoort J Vet Res. 2015;82:823.
18. Flegr J, Lindova JL, Kodym P. Sex-dependent toxoplasmosis associated differences in testosterone concentration in humans. Parasitology. 2008;135: 427–31.
19. Dubey JP, Hoover EA, Walls KW. Effect of age and sex on the acquisition of immunity to toxoplasmosis in cats. J Protozool. 1977;24:184–6.
20. Klein SL. Hormonal and immunological mechanisms mediating sex differences in parasite infection. Parasite Immunol. 2004;26:246–64.
21. Roberts CW, Cruickshank SM, Alexander J. Sex-determined resistance to *Toxoplasma gondii* is associated with temporal differences in cytokine production. Infect Immun. 1995;63:2549–55.
22. Opsteegh M, Haveman R, Swart AN, Mensink-Beerepoot ME, Hofhuis A, Langelaar MF, van der Giessen JW. Seroprevalence and risk factors for *Toxoplasma gondii* infection in domestic cats in The Netherlands. Prev Vet Med. 2012;104:317–26.
23. Fancourt BA, Jackson RB. Regional seroprevalence of *Toxoplasma gondii* antibodies in feral and stray cats (*Felis catus*) from Tasmania. Aust J Zool. 2014;62:272–83.
24. Galván Ramírez ML, Sánchez Vargas G, Vielma Sandoval M, Soto Mancilla JL. Presence of anti-*Toxoplasma* antibodies in humans and their cats in the urban zone of Guadalajara. Rev Soc Bras Med Trop. 1999;32:483–8.

25. Deksne G, Petruséviča A, Kirjušina M. Seroprevalence and factors associated with *Toxoplasma gondii* infection in domestic cats from urban areas in Latvia. J Parasitol. 2013;99:48–50.

26. Jokelainen P, Simola O, Rantanen E, Näreaho A, Lohi H, Sukura A. Feline toxoplasmosis in Finland: cross-sectional epidemiological study and case series study. J Vet Diagn Invest. 2012;24:1115–24.

27. Papini R, Sbrana C, Rosa B, Saturni AM, Sorrentino AM, Cerretani M, Raffaelli G, Guidi G. Serological survey of *Toxoplasma gondii* infections in stray cats from Italy. Rev Med Vet. 2006;157:193–6.

28. Flegr J, Prandota J, Sovičková M, Israili ZH. Toxoplasmosis – A Global Threat. Correlation of latent toxoplasmosis with specific disease burden in a set of 88 countries. PLoS One. 2014;9:e90203.

29. Torrey EF, Yolken RH. *Toxoplasma* oocysts as a public health problem. Trends Parasitol. 2013;29:380–4.

11

Implementation of an extended ZINB model in the study of low levels of natural gastrointestinal nematode infections in adult sheep

M. Atlija[1†], J. M. Prada[2,3*†], B. Gutiérrez-Gil[1,4], F. A. Rojo-Vázquez[4,5], M. J. Stear[2], J. J. Arranz[1] and M. Martínez-Valladares[4]

Abstract

Background: In this study, two traits related with resistance to gastrointestinal nematodes (GIN) were measured in 529 adult sheep: faecal egg count (FEC) and activity of immunoglobulin A in plasma (IgA). In dry years, FEC can be very low in semi-extensive systems, such as the one studied here, which makes identifying animals that are resistant or susceptible to infection a difficult task. A zero inflated negative binomial model (ZINB) model was used to calculate the extent of zero inflation for FEC; the model was extended to include information from the IgA responses.

Results: In this dataset, 64 % of animals had zero FEC while the ZINB model suggested that 38 % of sheep had not been recently infected with GIN. Therefore 26 % of sheep were predicted to be infected animals with egg counts that were zero or below the detection limit and likely to be relatively resistant to nematode infection. IgA activities of all animals were then used to decide which of the sheep with zero egg counts had been exposed and which sheep had not been recently exposed. Animals with zero FEC and high IgA activity were considered resistant while animals with zero FEC and low IgA activity were considered as not recently infected. For the animals considered as exposed to the infection, the correlations among the studied traits were estimated, and the influence of these traits on the discrimination between unexposed and infected animals was assessed.

Conclusions: The model presented here improved the detection of infected animals with zero FEC. The correlations calculated here will be useful in the development of a reliable index of GIN resistance that could be of assistance for the study of host resistance in studies based on natural infection, especially in adult sheep, and also the design of breeding programs aimed at increasing resistance to parasites.

Keywords: Gastrointestinal nematodes, Sheep, Prevalence, Egg count, IgA, ZINB

Background

Infection by gastrointestinal nematodes (GIN) is common in ruminants worldwide, causing major economic losses due to decreased growth and milk production [1, 2]. Grazing ruminants are infected by a variety of species of GIN with different pathogenicities and geographical distributions [3].

The control of GIN in ruminants is largely based on the use of anthelmintics, combined with grazing management strategies. However, anthelmintic resistance has appeared worldwide [4–6]. In northwest (NW) Spain, a recent survey showed that GIN in 63.6 % of the sampled flocks were resistant to at least one of the most commonly used drugs [7]. The increasing prevalence of anthelmintic resistance has led to the search for alternative control methods, such as selective breeding for resistance to GIN. However, for this purpose, the identification of an appropriate method to measure resistance to infection is necessary, especially

* Correspondence: joaquin.prada@princeton.edu
[†]Equal contributors
[2]Institute of Biodiversity, Animal Health and Comparative Medicine, University of Glasgow, Bearsden Road, Glasgow G61 1QH, UK
[3]Department of Ecology and Evolutionary Biology, Princeton University, Princeton, NJ 08540, USA
Full list of author information is available at the end of the article

in conditions where the worm burden is low. Hence, a sensitive method for detecting infections is needed.

Faecal egg counts (FEC) have been the traditional indicator trait used to assess the level of infection, based on the number of eggs per gram (epg) of faeces, and it is related to both the worm burden and the fecundity of female adults in the host [8–10]. Faecal egg counts have been used to measure genetic resistance to GIN, although in natural infections they can be quite variable both within and between populations [11]. However, FEC are not particularly sensitive and should be interpreted in conjunction with information about the nutritional status, age and management of sheep flocks [12]. As adult sheep are in general more resistant than naïve young animals, their FECs tend to be lower, adding an additional limitation to the sensitivity problem of the technique.

Other phenotypes related to GIN infections, such as the levels of IgA in serum may be taken into account with the goal of defining resistant animals under natural conditions. IgA is a secreted antibody that plays a major role in gut infections. Animals that display high IgA activity have been shown to present lower FEC and shorter adult female *Teladorsagia circumcincta* among experimentally and naturally infected sheep [9, 13, 14].

The distribution of FEC in naturally infected populations is characteristically over-dispersed within domestic and wild animals [15, 16], as well as in human populations [17]. The negative binomial (NB) distribution has been widely used to describe parasite eggs distribution. However, when there are more zero FEC values than expected, zero-inflated negative binomial (ZINB) models are more appropriate [15, 18]. A zero-inflated distribution is a mixture of two distributions and can arise if some animals with zero egg counts have been exposed and are resistant to the infection while other animals with zero egg counts have not been exposed or recently infected e.g. no established worms since the last anthelmintic treatment. Resistant animals tend to have few parasite eggs in their faeces. Due to the McMaster measurement technique, small egg numbers are difficult to detect and will be counted as zero, whether the animal has really zero eggs or just a small number of them. We hypothesize that by exploiting additional information, such as that provided by parasite-specific IgA activity, we could improve the ability to discriminate animals with low level of infection with zero egg counts from unexposed/recently uninfected animals. Therefore, the objective of the study was to determine the prevalence of GIN infections in naturally infected adult sheep showing low levels of infection by combining information from the two widely used indicator traits previously mentioned (FEC and IgA). For this purpose, we applied a ZINB model and extended it to include data from IgA responses. For the subset of animals that were considered as exposed to the infection based on the ZINB model, we calculated the correlations among the two

indicator traits related to the infection by GIN (FEC, IgA) and the hidden variable of animal status (i.e. the parameter that determines if the animal has been recently infected or not). The aim was to test whether we could improve the value of mixture and enhance the utility of the ZINB model in animals naturally infected with low doses of parasites.

Methods
Study area and animal sampling
The study was carried out in the region of Castilla y León, in the NW of Spain, and included 17 commercial dairy flocks distributed in seven out of the nine provinces of the region (Burgos, León, Palencia, Segovia, Valladolid, Salamanca and Zamora) (Fig. 1). In the study area, the flocks are reared under a semi-extensive system in which sheep graze on natural pasture for six hours per day and are kept indoors for the rest of the day. The average size of the sampled flocks was 912, ranging from 302 to 2121 animals per flock.

The survey was conducted from December 2011 to June 2012. This period was extremely dry (Additional file 1). Two conditions had to be met to include a flock in the study: first, the last anthelmintic treatment must have been administered at least 2 months before collecting the samples, and second, the sheep had to be grazing at the time of sampling. The animals included in this study were ewes obtained by artificial insemination from farms belonging to the Selection Nucleus of the National Association of Churra Breeders (ANCHE). Moreover, these animals were a subset of those previously genotyped with the *Illumina* OvineSNP50 BeadChip by [19] which were still alive during the sampling period and for which both phenotypes related to parasite resistance were available. Faecal samples were collected for each ewe directly from the rectum and blood samples were obtained by venipuncture of the jugular vein. Serum samples were stored at -20 °C until processing. This study is based on 529 adult Churra sheep with faecal and blood serum samples. The mean number of sheep sampled per flock was 31 (range: 11–60 individuals). The age of the sheep included in the study varied between 4 and 11 years. All of the sheep were undergoing milking at the time of sampling and were experiencing at least their third lactation.

Parasitological measures
A modified McMaster technique [20] using zinc sulphate as a flotation solution was used to determine the number of eggs in faeces. The minimum detection limit of this technique was 15 eggs per gram (epg). Faecal egg counts were determined by multiplying the number of eggs observed microscopically (Neggs) by 15.

In each flock, pooled faeces were cultured to recover and identify third-stage larvae (L3) following standard parasitological techniques [20]. A total of 100 L3 were

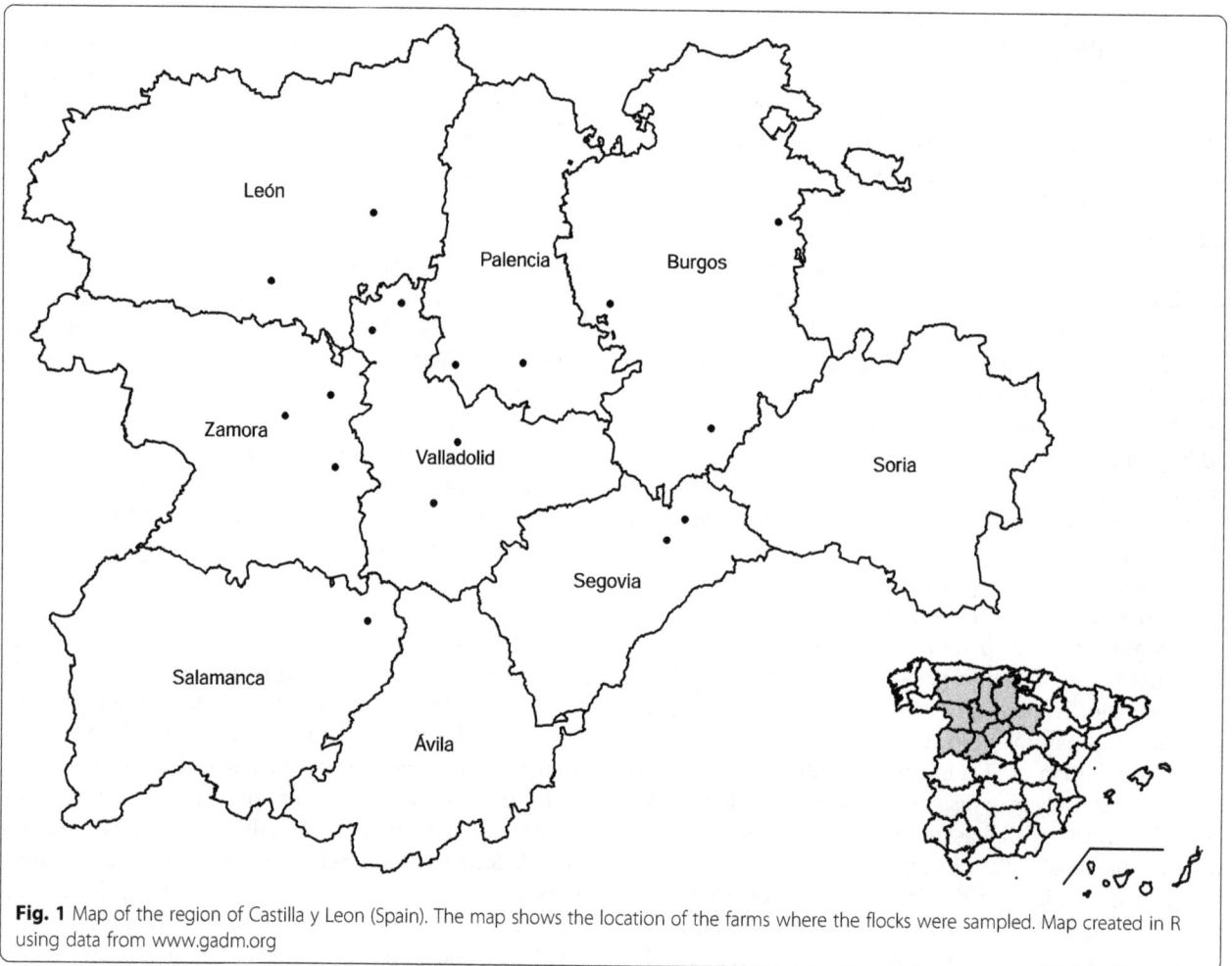

Fig. 1 Map of the region of Castilla y Leon (Spain). The map shows the location of the farms where the flocks were sampled. Map created in R using data from www.gadm.org

identified per flock to estimate the percentage of each species.

Titre of IgA

An indirect ELISA was carried out to determine the activity of IgA in the serum, results were scored as optical density (OD). The preparation of somatic antigen from fourth-stage larvae (L4) of *T. circumcincta* was conducted as previously described by [21]. Microtitre plates (Sigma) were coated with 100 µl of PBS containing 2.5 µg/ml of *T. circumcincta* L4 somatic antigen, after which the plates were stored overnight at 4 °C. After discarding their contents, the plates were blocked with 250 µl of PT-Milk (4 g powdered milk + 100 ml PBS-Tween; PBS-Tween: 1 L PBS pH 7.4 + 1 ml Tween) for 30 min at 37 °C. Then, the blocking buffer was discarded, and 100 µl of serum was added, followed by incubation for 30 min at 37 °C. After washing the plates four times with PBS-Tween, 100 µl of a rabbit anti-sheep IgA antibody, conjugated to horseradish peroxidase (Serotec), at a dilution of 1/500 in PT-Milk, was added, followed by incubation for 30 min at 37 °C. The plates were then washed again four times with PBS-

Tween and subsequently incubated in a peroxidase substrate and tetramethylbenzidine solution to produce a colour reaction, which was stopped by the addition of 50 µl of 2 M H_2SO_4. Finally, the absorbance was measured at 450 nm in a microplate reader (Titertek Multiskan). Positive and negative controls were included in every plate. Positive controls were obtained from a pool of serum from experimentally infected sheep with *T. circumcincta* and negative controls from non-infected sheep that were kept indoors. The results were expressed as the optical density ratio (ODR):

$$ODR = (sample\ OD\text{-}negative\ OD)/(positive\ OD\text{-}negative\ OD)$$

(1)

Descriptive statistics

Descriptive statistical analysis for the two traits was conducted for the 529 sampled animals with the 'pastecs' package [22] in R [23]. The Shapiro-Wilk test was carried out to determine if the data for each trait was normally distributed. Due to the large number of zero counts in the FEC data and the fact that the animals graze during short periods of time (semi-extensive rearing system), we decided to use a ZINB model to estimate the zero-inflation parameter and then extended it to discriminate between exposed and unexposed animals. The zero inflated model with IgA data was compared to a simpler negative binomial model using a likelihood ratio test. Moreover, in this particular study, a zero inflated model is a biologically meaningful description of the system; the adverse climatic conditions for larval development of the year studied will reduce pasture contamination, and the short grazing periods due to the semi-extensive rearing system will reduce exposure, which means that some animals would not have been infected at the time of sampling, and may not have been infected since the last anthelmintic treatment. The zero inflated model also allows for a more natural extension into discriminating between infected and uninfected animals.

Estimation of zero-inflation

In the zero inflated model, positive FEC are derived from a NB distribution, while a zero count can arise from either the NB distribution or the zero distribution (a binary distribution that generates structural zeros). The probability of belonging to the zero distribution is called the zero-inflation parameter. The animals that have zero counts arising from the zero distribution are assumed to have not been infected since the last anthelmintic treatment, so these animals can be excluded

from further analysis. A Markov Chain Monte Carlo model similar to the one described in Denwood et al. [15] using the '*runjags*' package [24] was employed to estimate the zero-inflation parameter.

In this model, the negative binomial distribution arises from a gamma-Poisson mixture distribution. Uninformative priors were used for the parameters of the gamma distribution. The posterior distribution of the zero-inflation parameter is shown in Fig. 2.

Extending the ZINB model

A zero-inflation model does not determine which animals are exposed and resistant (as opposed to unexposed). The classical ZINB model was therefore extended to accommodate IgA data as additional information for the animal status, i.e. infected or not recently infected. The animal status is calculated as,

$$\text{Status} = \begin{cases} 0; & \text{not recently infected} \quad \text{with probability } 1-P^{\text{exp}}, \\ 1; & \text{infected} \quad \text{with probability } P^{\text{exp}} \end{cases}$$

$$(2)$$

where status = 0 means that the animal has not been recently infected and status = 1 means that the animal is infected. P is the probability of being recently exposed and is equivalent to one minus the zero-inflation parameter. The raw egg counts (FEC/15) were used and it is assumed that for each animal i, the number of eggs counted arises from the following,

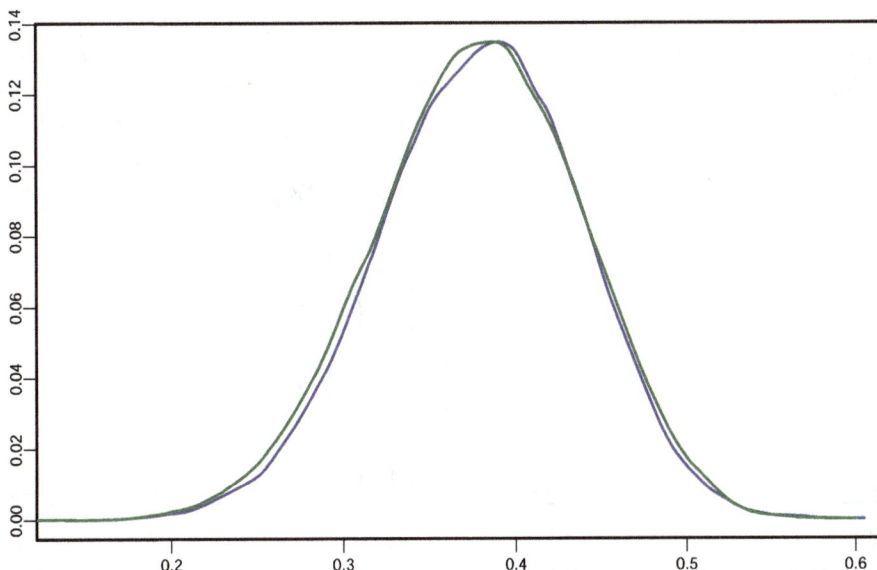

Fig. 2 Posterior distribution obtained from the extended ZINB model. Each colour represents a different chain. Both chains have a mean around 0.38 and no sample was recovered from either of the chains with a zero-inflation parameter equal to zero (minimum value recovered = 0.12)

$$\text{Neggs}_i \sim \begin{cases} 0 & \text{if Status} = 0, \\ \text{Poisson}(\lambda_i) & \text{if Status} = 1 \end{cases} \quad (3)$$

where λ_i is the number of eggs arising from the gamma distribution (equation 4).

$$\lambda_i \sim \text{gamma(shape, rate)} \quad (4)$$

with the shape and the rate parameters of the gamma being calculated by the model. Similarly the IgA data can be partitioned in 2 gamma distributions (equation 5) based on the animal status.

$$\text{IgA}_i \sim \begin{cases} \text{gamma}(\text{sh}_1, , \text{rt}_1) & \text{if Status} = 0, \\ \text{gamma}(\text{sh}_2, , \text{rt}_2) & \text{if Status} = 1 \end{cases} \quad (5)$$

with sh_1, sh_2, rt_1 and rt_2 being the two shapes and two rates respectively that parametrize the two gamma distributions. In the model, samples are drawn for sh_1 and sh_2 as well as for mn_1 and mn_2, which are the two means of the two gamma distributions. The rates are calculated by rate = shape/mean and the mean for the animals not recently infected (mn_1) is always smaller than the mean of the infected (mn_2). The fully annotated R code of the model is given in the Additional file 2.

The number of iterations sampled was 50,000, with the first 5,000 being discarded (burn in), and assessed convergence with the Gelman-Rubin statistic from the 'coda' package [25] being under 1.05.

Using the realisations of the animal status across the iterations (unexposed animals have status = 0, exposed and infected have status = 1), it is possible to calculate the probability for each animal to be in one status or the other, P_i^{exp}; animals without zero FEC will always be in the infected status. The animals that were estimated to be unexposed, i.e. the animals with status = 0, in each sample of the Markov Chain were excluded from further analyses, allowing the use of simple statistical tools to analyse the remaining dataset for each sample.

Correlations between phenotypes

Considering FEC, IgA and the realisations of animal status, P_i^{exp}, the Kendall's rank correlation coefficient was used to estimate the relationships among these three parameters. We used Kendall's rank because it is an appropriate non-parametric hypothesis test. Correlations were calculated in R, using the 'ltm' package [26], for each sample of the Markov Chain and the average across the samples is reported below.

Results

Descriptive statistics of the phenotypic data

Faecal egg counts and larval identification: Faecal egg counts of GIN ranged from 0 to 1,290 epg. In 64 % of the faecal samples no eggs were detected. The FEC mean and total variance were 38.2 (±105.9) and 11,218.9 respectively. The FEC distribution was heavily skewed to the right and showed a high level of over-dispersion (Fig. 3a). The Shapiro-Wilk test for the FEC data indicated a clear deviation from normality (p-value < 2.2 x10^{-16}). Most of the eggs detected in positive samples were strongyle-type.

Apart from the GIN eggs, other parasite eggs were detected in faeces: 13.3 % of the sheep sampled had *D. dendriticum* eggs, with a range of 0–1,035 epg; 2.9 % had *Trichuris* spp. eggs (0–30 epg), two animals (0.9 %), had *Moniezia* spp. eggs (0–1,035 epg) and one ewe had *Capillaria* spp eggs at a concentration of 15 eggs per gram.

After collecting L3 from coprocultures, we identified the following genera of GIN: *Trichostrongylus* spp. (49.3 %), *T. circumcincta* (48.6 %), *Nematodirus* spp. (1.4 %) and *Cooperia* spp. (0.7 %). In all flocks, we confirmed the presence of *T. circumcincta*. We also observed a number of lungworm larvae, though they were not identified to the species level.

IgA activity in the serum samples: For individual animals, the mean ODR was 4.1 (±4.3), showing a range between 0.09 and 32.9; the ODR variance was 18.4. The distribution of IgA activities was positively skewed (Fig. 3b)

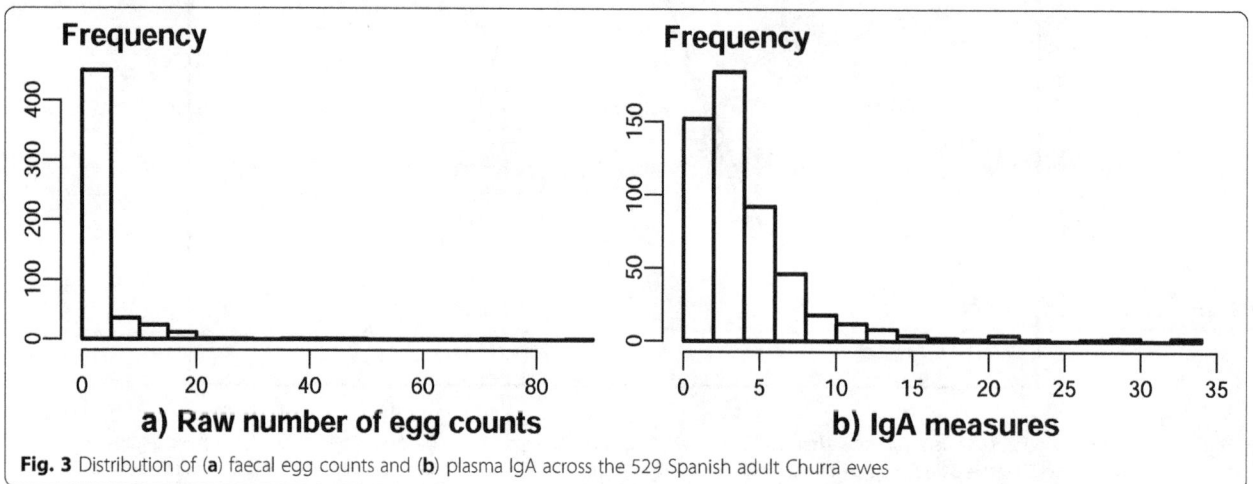

Fig. 3 Distribution of (**a**) faecal egg counts and (**b**) plasma IgA across the 529 Spanish adult Churra ewes

with most of the sheep displaying relatively low IgA values, and only a few sheep presenting particularly high levels of IgA.

The Shapiro-Wilk test indicated a clear deviation from the normality (p-value < 2.2 x10^{-16}). The Kolmogorov-Smirnov test indicated that the IgA was not gamma distributed (p-value = 0.0088), however this is due to the long tail of high IgA values. If the analysis is done with 10 animals less (effectively cutting the max IgA values to 20), the test indicates that the data is indeed gamma distributed (p-value = 0.21).

Zero-inflation parameter and extension of the ZINB model for FEC data

To verify that the data is zero inflated, a likelihood ratio test was performed comparing the ZINB model to a simpler NB model, with a p-value of the likelihood ratio test = 6.62 x10^{-5}, which indicates that the zero-inflated model provides a better fit to the data. The mean of the zero-inflation parameter was 0.38, this indicates that on average, 38 % of all the animals were not exposed and infected since the last anthelmintic treatment (2 months before the samples were taken), therefore it was estimated that 328 ewes were infected at sampling, even though only 190 had non-zero FEC. The zero-inflation parameter credible interval was much narrower when using the extended ZINB model as opposed to the ZINB model using FEC data only (from 0.013–0.46 to 0.25–0.49). The distribution of the probability of being exposed across all the animals in the data is shown in Fig. 4.

Associations between phenotypes

The associations between phenotypes was calculated for the subset of animals that were considered exposed to the infection based on the implementation of the extended ZINB model (status = 1) in each sample of the Markov Chain. The correlations between Neggs, IgA and the estimated probability of being exposed to infection (P_i^{exp}) are shown in Table 1. The phenotypic correlation between plasma IgA and number of eggs was close to zero and not statistically significant, while animal status was positively correlated to the number of eggs and IgA.

Discussion

Adult female sheep play a key role in the epidemiology of GIN infection because eggs deposited during the periparturient period influence the severity of the infection during the grazing season. However, outside the periparturient period, egg counts in adult sheep are typically low [27]. In general, GIN populations in naturally infected sheep are usually over-dispersed, with the majority of sheep showing low epg values and only a few sheep presenting a high level of infection [28]. In addition, some infected sheep will have low egg counts [8]. Therefore, supplementary information is needed as well as egg counts to determine which sheep are infected in adult sheep flocks.

In this study, the mean FEC per flock was quite low (38.2 epg) compared with other studies carried out in

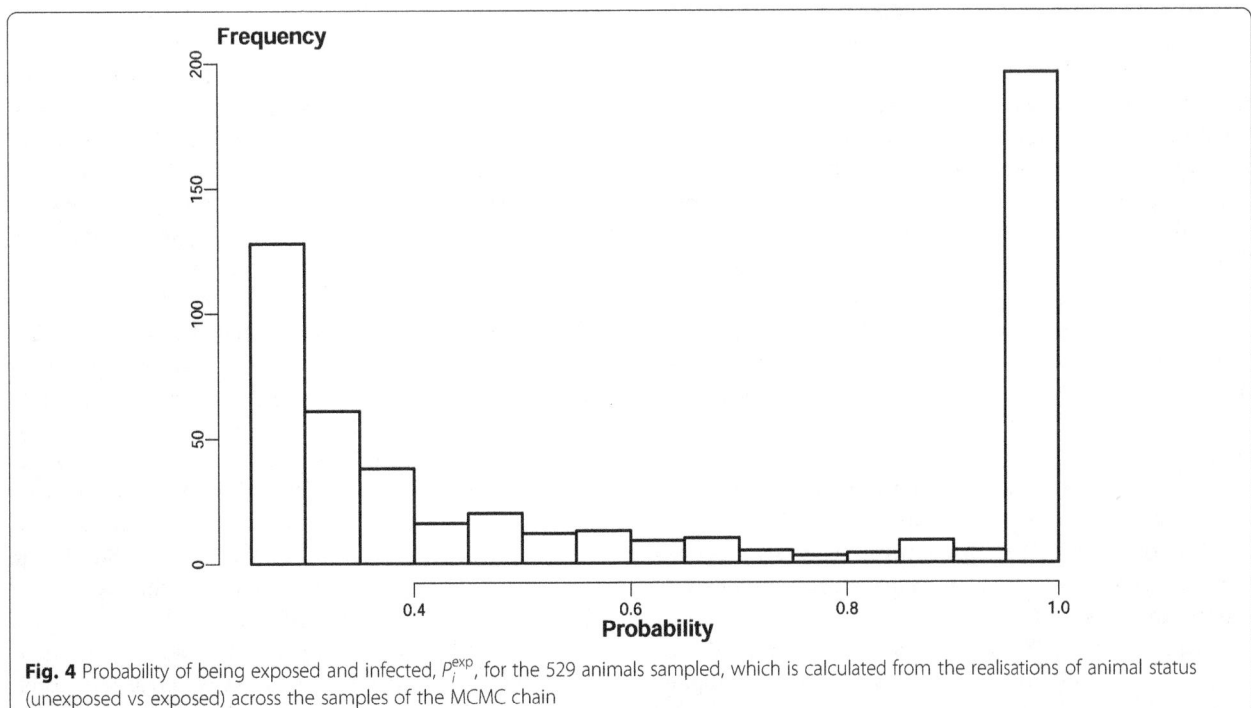

Fig. 4 Probability of being exposed and infected, P_i^{exp}, for the 529 animals sampled, which is calculated from the realisations of animal status (unexposed vs exposed) across the samples of the MCMC chain

Table 1 Estimated correlations in the Churra sheep population

	Neggs	IgA	P_i^{exp}
Neggs	1	0.012	0.67**
IgA		1	0.18**
P_i^{exp}			1

Neggs is the number of eggs counted, IgA is the activity of IgA in serum (Optical density ratio) and P_i^{exp} is the probability of being exposed
**$P < 0.001$

the same area (NW of Spain). Gutiérrez-Gil et al. [29] reported that the mean FEC was 260 epg between the years 1999 and 2003. Similar records were described by Martínez-Valladares et al. [30], who showed that the prevalence of GIN, based solely on the presence or absence of FEC, in sheep flocks was 100 %, and the mean epg was 237.2 (±375.9) between the years 2006 and 2011. In the current study, the low levels of infection are likely a consequence of the exceptional climatic conditions during this study since the longevity of infective trichostrongylid L3 nematodes is related to temperature and humidity [30, 31]. The table in Additional file 1 displays the mean temperature and precipitation for the period between December-June of the last 5 years (2007/2008–2011/2012) in the region of Castilla y León, highlighting the fact that the year 2011/2012 was extremely dry. According to Martínez-Valladares et al. [30], there is a direct relationship between GIN infection levels and the humidity of ambient air.

Faecal egg count, which has been for many years the traditional diagnostic tool for assessing GIN infection, has a low sensitivity [32], especially for very low counts as is the case in this study. Therefore, when the excretion of eggs in faeces is low, it is necessary to use other, more sensitive, diagnostic methods that might provide a more reliable indicator of infection.

IgA activity in the current study is moderately high, and this is presumed to be due to the fact that the antibodies persist for some time after GIN infection. The experimental studies of different breeds of sheep infected with GIN showed IgA activity for prolonged periods of time post infection. In an experiment carried out by Henderson and Stear [33], the peak of IgA was at 6–10 days after a deliberate infection with *T. circumcincta* in sheep although detectable IgA was evident 6 weeks later. Furthermore in an experiment with Churra sheep, Martínez-Valladares et al. [34] also showed that the elevated level of IgA in blood and nasal secretions was maintained 4 weeks post infection with this same parasite species. In the study by MacKinnon et al. [35] IgA activity was also evident 4 weeks post infection with *Haemonchus contortus* in Caribbean hair sheep.

In this study, a ZINB model was used to calculate the extent of zero inflation. This approach has been applied to several parasitic infections [15, 17, 18]. This model

was then extended to identify the animals that are likely to be uninfected. This was done by adding the IgA information to the model. In a ZINB model using only FEC data, the model would not be able to assign animals with zero FEC as infected or uninfected. (Additional file 3).

There is heterogeneity among animals in the intensity of infection. Some infected animals will be exposed to more parasites than others. Both genetic variation in resistance and variation in exposure will contribute to the observed variation in IgA activity and FEC in exposed animals. Among animals that have not been exposed to parasites, FEC will be zero and parasite-specific IgA will be very low or zero. Animals with zero FEC and zero or low IgA activity are therefore more likely to be unexposed but it is possible that some of these animals have been exposed to low intensities of infection. Therefore the extension of the ZINB model to include additional data does not guarantee that every animal will be correctly assigned. It does however significantly improve the discrimination between exposed and unexposed animals and make subsequent analyses based on exposed animals more reliable (Fig. 4, Additional file 3).

To our knowledge, this is the first description of a ZINB model for the analysis of multiple traits with the aim of discerning which animals are infected and which have not been recently exposed or exposed to a very low infection level. This procedure is relatively straightforward and allows the study of nematode infections in adult animals and in flocks with low prevalence of infection, such as in Mediterranean dairy farms where animals are under a semi-extensive management system. The approach improves our ability to identify animals that have been infected with GIN, even at low FEC, which is needed for the study of host resistance in naturally infected individuals and the breeding of resistant sheep.

Because the over-dispersion pattern of GIN (number of eggs and adult worms found in the host) is also observed in other hosts such as cattle, free-range pigs, chickens, humans and wild animals [36–38], the approach described here could also be useful in other systems.

The correlations between the number of eggs and IgA and animal status were calculated using the non-parametric Kendall's test. Although the number of eggs has been found negatively correlated with IgA in young lambs [39, 40], in the case of adult sheep, this correlation is not as clear and both Coltman et al. [39] and Gutiérrez-Gil et al. [29] reported non-significant correlations in naturally infected adult sheep after comparing logFEC and IgA against somatic antigen from *T. circumcinta* L4. Our results are similar, and suggest that this correlation is indeed close to zero in adult sheep. In experimentally infected adult sheep, Martinez-Valladares et al. [9] showed negative correlations between IgA in gastric mucus and FEC whereas the correlation between FEC and the serum IgA levels (which are lower than in the gastric mucus) were not significant. The absence of a clear correlation between plasma IgA and FEC may be a consequence of the fact that plasma IgA shows a complex relationship with mucosal IgA [41]. Alternatively, adult sheep may show greater IgE activity; reduced numbers of established parasites would decrease IgA responses and the relative importance of IgA on egg output would be lowered [42].

The extension of the ZINB model has allowed us to combine the information from two different traits that can indicate resistance or susceptibility to GIN. The IgA response was added to the model to help discriminate between unexposed and infected animals with zero FEC. Recent research has produced an index of the intensity of nematode infection in young lambs [43] and the observed correlations among the parasitological variable are necessary for this process. As mentioned previously, the use of a reliable indicator trait may be of interest not only for the management of parasite infections but also for the design of breeding programs aimed at achieving resistance to parasites.

Conclusions

In summary, in the current study, two different phenotypes related to GIN infection (FEC and IgA against somatic antigen from L4 of *T. circumcincta*) were analysed. There was a high percentage of sheep without eggs in faeces (64 %) and a zero inflated model was used to detect the amount of zero inflation in the data. The ZINB model suggested that 38 % of sampled sheep had not been exposed to nematode infection in the previous 2 months, since the last anthelmintic treatment. Therefore, in addition to FEC data, the evaluation of IgA in serum may help to distinguish adult animals with low level of infection from resistant animals assist selective breeding for resistance to GIN.

Additional files

Additional file 1: Mean temperatures (ºC) and precipitation (mm) from December to June during the sampling period (highlighted in gray), and during the four previous years. (PDF 24 kb)

Additional file 2: Annotated R code for the ZINB model. (PDF 20 kb)

Additional file 3: Exposed probability in a classic ZINB model. Histogram of probabilities of being exposed for the data (a) and zoom of only the zero FEC (b) using only FEC data in the ZINB model. Animals with non-zero FEC will always have an "infected" status in the model (= 1) while animals with zero FEC can be exposed or unexposed. If only the FEC data is used, each animal with zero FEC will have a probability of being infected similar to one minus the zero-inflation parameter (b). (PDF 34 kb)

Additional file 4: Raw data used. (TXT 5 kb)

Abbreviations
ANCHE, National Association of Churra Breeders (Spain); FEC, faecal egg counts; GIN, gastrointestinal nematodes; IgA, immunoglobulin A; OD/ODR, optical density (ratio); ZINB/NB, (zero-inflated) negative binomial

Acknowledgements
We would like to thank our funding sources and the National Association of Churra Breeders in Spain.

Funding
This work was supported by a competitive grant from the Castilla and León regional government (Junta de Castilla y León) (Ref. LE245A12-2); the EC-funded Innovative Training Network (ITN) NematodeSystemHealth (M. A. and J. M. P., P7-KBBE-2009-3-245140); the BBSRC grant BB/L004004070/1; the Spanish "Ramón y Cajal" Programme from the Spanish Ministry of Economy and Competitiveness (B. G. G., RYC-2012-10230) and a postdoctoral Jae-Doc contract from the Consejo Superior de Investigaciones Científicas (CSIC) and co-funded by the European Social Fund (M. M. V.).

Authors' contributions
MA analyzed the samples in the wetlab and helped in the statistical analysis. JMP created the mathematical model and performed the statistical analysis. MS and JMP conceived the mathematical study. BG G, JJA and MMV designed the data sourcing and sample collection. MA, JMP, BGG and MMV drafted the manuscript. MJS, JJA and FARV coordinated the study and critically corrected the manuscript. All authors read and approved the final manuscript.

Competing interests
The authors declare that they have no competing interests.

Consent for publication
Not applicable.

Author details
[1]Departamento de Producción Animal, Universidad de León, Campus de Vegazana s/n, 24071 León, Spain. [2]Institute of Biodiversity, Animal Health and Comparative Medicine, University of Glasgow, Bearsden Road, Glasgow G61 1QH, UK. [3]Department of Ecology and Evolutionary Biology, Princeton University, Princeton, NJ 08540, USA. [4]Instituto de Ganadería de Montaña, CSIC-ULE, 24346 Grulleros, León, Spain. [5]Departamento de Sanidad Animal, Universidad de León, Campus de Vegazana s/n, 24071 León, Spain.

References
1. Stear MJ, Bishop SC, Mallard BA, Raadsma H. The sustainability, feasibility and desirability of breeding livestock for disease resistance. Res Vet Sci. 2001;71:1–7.
2. Suarez VH, Cristel SL, Busetti MR. Epidemiology and effects of gastrointestinal nematode infection on milk productions of dairy ewes. Parasite. 2009;16:7.
3. Dobson RJ, LeJambre L, Gill JH: Management of anthelmintic resistance: inheritance of resistance and selection with persistent drugs. Int J Parasitol. 1996; 26(8):993-1000. ISSN 0020-7519. http://dx.doi.org/10.1016/S0020-7519(96)80078-6.
4. Papadopoulos E, Gallidis E, Ptochos S. Anthelmintic resistance in sheep in Europe: A selected review. Vet Parasitol. 2012;189:85–8 [Special Issue: Update on Parasitic Diseases of Sheep].
5. Torres-Acosta JFJ, Mendoza-de-Gives P, Aguilar-Caballero AJ, Cuéllar-Ordaz JA. Anthelmintic resistance in sheep farms: Update of the situation in the American continent. Vet Parasitol. 2012;189:89–96 [Special Issue: Update on Parasitic Diseases of Sheep].
6. Roeber F, Jex AR, Gasser RB. Impact of gastrointestinal parasitic nematodes of sheep, and the role of advanced molecular tools for exploring epidemiology and drug resistance - an Australian perspective. Parasit Vectors. 2013;6:153.
7. Martinez-Valladares M, Martinez-Perez JM, Robles-Perez D, Cordero-Perez C, Famularo MR, Fernandez-Pato N, Castanon-Ordonez L, Rojo-Vazquez FA: The present status of anthelmintic resistance in gastrointestinal nematode infections of sheep in the northwest of Spain by in vivo and in vitro techniques. Vet Parasitol. 2013;191(1-2):177-81. doi:10.1016/j.vetpar.2012.08.009.

8.   Bishop SC, Stear MJ. The use of a gamma-type function to assess the relationship between the number of adult Teladorsagia circumcincta and total egg output. Parasitology. 2000;121(Pt 4):435–40.

9.   Martínez-Valladares M, Vara-Del Río MP, Cruz-Rojo MA, Rojo-Vázquez FA. Genetic resistance to Teladorsagia circumcincta: IgA and parameters at slaughter in Churra sheep. Parasite Immunol. 2005;27:213–8.

10.   Villanua D, Perez-Rodrigues L, Gortazar C, Hofle U, Vimuela J. Avoiding bias in parasite excretion estimates: the effect of sampling time and type of faeces. Parasitology. 2006;133:251–9.

11.   Stear MJ, Bairden K, Duncan JL, Gettinby G, McKellar QA, Murray M, Wallace DS. The distribution of faecal nematode egg counts in Scottish Blackface lambs following natural, predominantly Ostertagia circumcincta infection. Parasitology. 1995;110:573–81.

12.   McKenna PB. Faecal egg counts as a guide for drench use. N Z Vet J. 2002;50:123–4.

13.   Stear MJ, Bishop SC, Doligalska M, Duncan JL, Holmes PH, Irvine J, McCririe L, McKellar QA, Sinski E, Murray M: Regulation of egg production, worm burden, worm length and worm fecundity by host responses in sheep infected with Ostertagia circumcincta. Regulation. 1995;17(12):643–52.

14.   Strain S, Bishop SC, Henderson NG, Kerr A, McKellar QA, Mitchell S, Stear MJ. The genetic control of IgA activity against Teladorsagia circumcincta and its association with parasite resistance in naturally infected sheep. Parasitology. 2002;124(Pt 5):545–52.

15.   Denwood MJ, Stear MJ, Matthews L, Reid SWJ, Toft N, Innocent GT. The distribution of the pathogenic nematode Nematodirus battus in lambs is zero-inflated. Parasitology. 2008;135:1225–35.

16.   Ziadinow I, Deplazes P, Mathis A, Mutunova B, Abdykerimov K, Nurgaziev R, Torgerson P. Frequency distribution of Echinococcus multilocularis and other helminths of foxes in Kyrgyzstan. Vet Parasitol. 2010;171:286–92.

17.   Walker M, Hall A, Anderson RM, Basanez M: Density-dependent effects on the weight of female Ascaris lumbricoides infections of humans and its impact on patterns of egg production. Parasite Vectors. 2009;2:11. doi:10.1186/1756-3305-2-11.

18.   Nodtvedt A, Dohoo I, Sanchez J, Conboy G, DesCjteaux L, Keefe G, Leslie K, Campbell J. The use of negative binomial modelling in a longitudinal study of gastrointestinal parasite burdens in Canadian dairy cows. Can J Vet Res. 2002;66:249–57.

19.   García-Gámez E, Gutiérrez-Gil B, Sahana G, Sánchez J-P, Bayón Y, Arranz J-J. GWA analysis for milk production traits in dairy sheep and genetic support for a QTN influencing milk protein percentage in the LALBA gene. PLoS One. 2012;7:e47782.

20.   Ministry of Agriculture F, (MAFF) F: Manual of Veterinary Parasitological Laboratory Techniques. HMSO; 1986.

21.   Strain SAJ, Stear MJ. The recognition of molecules from fourth-stage larvae of Ostertagia circumcincta by IgA from infected sheep. Parasite Immunol. 1999;21:163–8.

22.   Grosjean P, Ibanez F: pastecs: Package for Analysis of Space-Time Ecological Series. R Package Version 13-18 2014.

23.   Team RDC: R: A Language and Environment for Statistical Computing. R Found Stat Comput Vienna Austria 2011.

24.   Denwood MJ: runjags: Interface utilities, parallel computing methods and additional distributions for MCMC models in JAGS. Httpcranr-Proj 2014.

25.   Plummer M, Best N, Cowles K, Vines K. CODA: Convergence Diagnosis and Output Analysis for MCMC. R News. 2006;6:7–11.

26.   Rizopoulos D. ltm: An R package for latent variable modeling and item response theory analyses. J Stat Softw. 2006;17:1–25.

27.   Stear MJ, Fitton L, Innocent GT, Murphy L, Rennie K, Matthews L. The dynamic influence of genetic variation on the susceptibility of sheep to gastrointestinal nematode infection. J R Soc Interface R Soc. 2007;4:767–76.

28.   Barger IA: The statistical distribution of trichostrongylid nematodes in grazing lambs. Int J Parasitol. 1985;15(6):645-649.

29.   Gutiérrez-Gil B, Pérez J, de la Fuente LF, Meana A, Martínez-Valladares M, San Primitivo F, Rojo-Vázquez FA, Arranz JJ. Genetic parameters for resistance to trichostrongylid infection in dairy sheep. Anim Int J Anim Biosci. 2010;4:505–12.

30.   Martinez-Valladares M, Robles-Perez D, Martinez-Perez JM, Cordero-Perez C, Famularo MR, Fernandez-Pato N, Gonzalez-Lanza C, Castanon-Ordonez L, Rojo-Vazquez FA: Prevalence of gastrointestinal nematodes and Fasciola hepatica in sheep in the northwest of Spain: relation to climatic conditions and/or man-made environmental modifications. Parasite Vector. 2013;6(1): 282. doi:10.1186/1756-3305-6-282.

31.   O'Connor LJ, Walkden-Brown SW, Kahn LP. Ecology of the free-living stages of major trichostrongylid parasites of sheep. Vet Parasitol. 2006;142:1–15.

32.   Raadsma H, Gray GD, Woolaston RR. Breeding for disease resistance in Merino sheep in Australia. Rev Sci Tech Int Off Epizoot. 1998;17:315–28.

33.   Henderson NG, Stear MJ. Eosinophil and IgA responses in sheep infected with Teladorsagia circumcincta. Vet Immunol Immunopathol. 2006;112:62–6.

34.   Martínez-Valladares M, Vara-Del Río MP, Cruz-Rojo MA, Rojo-Vázquez FA. Effect of a low protein diet on the resistance of Churra sheep to Teladorsagia circumcincta. Parasite Immunol. 2005;27:219–25.

35.   MacKinnon KM, Zajac AM, Kooyman FNJ, Notter DR. Differences in immune parameters are associated with resistance to Haemonchus contortus in Caribbean hair sheep. Parasite Immunol. 2010;32:484–93.

36.   Boes J, Coates S, Medley GF, Varady M, Eriksen L, Roepstorff A, Nansen P. Exposure of sows to Ascaris suum influences worm burden distributions in experimentally infected suckling piglets. Parasitology. 1999;119(Pt 5):509–20.

37.   Vercruysse J, Dorny P. Integrated control of nematode infections in cattle: a reality? A need? A future? Int J Parasitol. 1999;29:165–75. discussion 183–4.

38.   Weyher AH, Ross C, Semple S. Gastrointestinal Parasites in Crop Raiding and Wild Foraging Papio anubis in Nigeria. Int J Primatol. 2006;27:1519–34.

39.   Coltman DW, Wilson K, Pilkington JG, Stear MJ, Pemberton JM. A microsatellite polymorphism in the gamma interferon gene is associated with resistance to gastrointestinal nematodes in a naturally-parasitized population of Soay sheep. Parasitology. 2001;122(Pt 5):571–82.

40.   Davies G, Stear MJ, Bishop SC, Road B, Glasgow G: Genetic relationships between indicator traits and nematode parasite infection levels in 6-month-old lambs. Vet Parasitol. 2005;80(02):143–150.

41.   Prada Jiménez de Cisneros J, Matthews L, Mair C, Stefan T, Stear MJ. The transfer of IgA from mucus to plasma and the implications for diagnosis and control of nematode infections. Parasitology. 2014;141:875–9.

42.   Stear MJ, Strain SAJ, Bishop SC. How lambs control infection with Ostertagia circumcincta. Vet Immunol Immunopathol. 1999;72:213–8.

43.   Mair C, Matthews L, De Cisneros JPJ, Stefan T, Stear MJ: Multitrait indices to predict worm length and number in sheep with natural, mixed predominantly Teladorsagia circumcincta infection. Parasitology 2015, FirstView:1–10.

12

MicroRNA profiling of dogs with transitional cell carcinoma of the bladder using blood and urine samples

Michael S. Kent[1], Allison Zwingenberger[1], Jodi L. Westropp[2], Laura E. Barrett[3], Blythe P. Durbin-Johnson[4], Paramita Ghosh[5,6,7*] and Ruth L. Vinall[5,6,8*] (iD)

Abstract

Background: Early signs of canine transitional cell carcinoma (TCC) are frequently assumed to be caused by other lower urinary tract diseases (LUTD) such as urinary tract infections, resulting in late diagnosis of TCC which could be fatal. The development of a non-invasive clinical test for TCC could dramatically reduce mortality. To determine whether microRNAs (miRNAs) can be used as non-invasive diagnostic biomarkers, we assessed miRNA expression in blood and/or urine from dogs with clinically normal bladders ($n = 28$), LUTD ($n = 25$), and TCC ($n = 17$). Expression levels of 5 miRNA associated with TCC pathophysiology (miR-34a, let-7c, miR-16, miR-103b, and miR-106b) were assessed by quantitative real-time PCR.

Results: Statistical analyses using ranked ANOVA identified significant differences in miR-103b and miR-16 levels between urine samples from LUTD and TCC patients (miR-103b, $p = 0.002$; and miR-16, $p = 0.016$). No statistically significant differences in miRNA levels were observed between blood samples from LUTD versus TCC patients. Expression levels of miR-34a trended with miR-16, let-7c, and miR-103b levels in individual normal urine samples, however, this coordination was completely lost in TCC urine samples. In contrast, co-ordination of miR-34a, miR-16, let-7c, and miR-103b expression levels was maintained in blood samples from TCC patients.

Conclusions: Our combined data indicate a potential role for miR-103b and miR-16 as diagnostic urine biomarkers for TCC, and that further investigation of miR-103b and miR-16 in the dysregulation of coordinated miRNA expression in bladder carcinogenesis is warranted.

Keywords: microRNA, Canine bladder cancer, Urine and blood analysis

Background

Transitional cell carcinoma (TCC) is the most common bladder tumor in dogs representing approximately 2% of all canine tumors [1–3]. Further, the prevalence of this disease is increasing [4, 5]. The recognized causes of TCC are varied with identified risk factors including use of topical insecticides, living in houses where the yards have been treated with insecticides, and living near marshes sprayed for mosquitoes or industrial areas [6, 7]. Female dogs and obese dogs appear to have an increased incidence of disease, in contrast to humans where the

disease is more prevalent among male patients [3, 7]. There are also several breed predilections for TCC, including Scottish terriers, beagles, Shetland sheep dogs, wire fox terriers and West Highland white terriers, suggesting a genetic component to this disease [4, 8].

The extent of tumor locally as well as locoregional and distant metastasis is staged using the Tumor, Lymph Node and Metastasis (TNM) staging system [9]. Most dogs are diagnosed with TCC later in the course of disease with higher stage tumors being most common [10]. It has also been shown that having a higher stage of disease can negatively affect response to treatment. Treatment for TCC involves the use of surgery, radiotherapy, nonsteroidal anti-inflammatory agents and chemotherapy. Even with aggressive therapy, most dogs

* Correspondence: paghosh@ucdavis.edu; rvinall@cnsu.edu
[5]Department of Urology, University of California, Davis, School of Medicine, Sacramento, CA, USA
Full list of author information is available at the end of the article

fail treatment and die from their disease [3, 11–17]. Some of the biggest gains in survival in human cancer medicine have occurred because of early detection of disease. This has proven true for prostate cancer, breast cancer and colon cancer as well as TCC. While ~80% of human patients present with superficial TCC, 10–30% of these patients will progress to invasive TCC and frequent screening has allowed for earlier detection of progression and has helped improve outcomes including survival [18–20]. Given this, early detection of TCC in dogs is likely to impact their response and survival.

Currently the diagnosis of TCC is most commonly made after dogs show advanced signs of disease, including hematuria, stranguria, and pollakiuria, all of which can mimic lower urinary tract disease (LUTD) [1]. Abdominal ultrasound may reveal structural changes to the urinary bladder, but lacks specificity and is also relatively expensive [4, 21]. Aspirates and open surgical biopsy of bladder tumors carry the risk of distant seeding of tumor cells [22, 23]. Other methods of definitive diagnosis, including traumatic catheterization and cystoscopically obtained biopsies, carry their own risks of complication and associated costs, making their use as a screening tool impractical [21]. The V-BTA rapid latex agglutination urine dipstick test to detect dogs with TCC proved not to be useful due to a low positive predictive value, resulting in only 3% of positive tests occurring in dogs with TCC [4, 24]. This indicates the need for an improved diagnostic screening test to detect dogs with TCC vs LUTD.

MicroRNAs (miRNAs) are small, highly stable, non-coding RNAs which facilitate post-transcriptional control of gene expression [25]. Multiple studies have demonstrated that dysregulation of miRNA expression levels can play a functional role in the initiation and progression of many cancers, and that miRNA can be used as diagnostic, prognostic, and predictive biomarkers [26]. Importantly, miRNA are relatively stable in most body fluids meaning they have the potential to be used clinically as non-invasive biomarkers [27–29]. The majority of miRNA biomarker discovery studies have focused on assessing miRNA levels in blood, and several blood-based miRNA biomarkers are currently in development. Assessment of miRNA levels in urine is possible but has proved much more challenging due to accelerated RNA degradation as a result of RNA being in an acidic environment [30–32]. As urine is in direct contact with the bladder (and bladder cancers, if present), urine samples are more likely than blood samples to contain miRNA which are derived from bladder cells and therefore any alterations in miRNA expression which are observed in urine samples are likely to reflect actual changes in miRNA expression which are occurring in bladder cells.

Altered expression of several miRNA has been observed in human bladder cancer progression [33–37].

We previously determined that assessment of miRNA in canine tissue specimens can be used to distinguish between inflammatory disease and TCC [38]; a statistically significant difference in expression levels of miR-34a, miR-16, miR-103b and miR-106b was observed between tissue specimens from canine LUTD and TCC patients. All of these miRNA have the ability to control expression of molecules which play a role in driving human bladder cancer initiation and progression, including components of the p53, Rb and/or Bcl-2 signaling pathways and likely play a role in driving bladder carcinogenesis in canines [39–45]. In addition, we recently demonstrated that the miRNA let-7c plays an important role in the response of human patients with bladder cancer to chemotherapy [46]. Based on these results, the goal of the current study was to determine whether assessment of these same miRNA is feasible in canine blood and urine samples, and whether these miRNA show potential for use as non-invasive biomarkers which can distinguish between non-neoplastic LUTD, such as urinary tract infections (UTI) and cystic calculi, and TCC, in canine patients.

The development of a non-invasive method versus an invasive method to distinguish between common inflammatory LUTD and TCC in canine patients is highly desirable for both economical and feasibility reasons and could have implications for human medicine [30–32, 47, 48].

Methods

Patient samples

Dogs with newly diagnosed, untreated transitional cell carcinoma of the urinary bladder and two control groups, clinically normal dogs and dogs with non-neoplastic lower urinary tract disease (such as dogs with UTI and cystic calculi), were entered into the study.

Definitions of disease

A clinically normal dog was defined as a dog with no lower urinary tract signs, a normal bladder on ultrasound examination done by a board certified veterinary radiologist, a normal urinalysis and a negative urine culture result. Dogs were only enrolled if they were not receiving any antibiotics, non-steroidal or steroidal medications. Dogs with inflammatory or infectious lower urinary tract disease were defined as dogs with a positive urine culture and/or urolithiasis and no bladder mass seen under ultrasound evaluation, during surgical exploration of the bladder or during cystoscopy. Dogs with TCC were defined as dogs having either a histopathological or cytological diagnosis of transitional cell carcinoma. Only dogs not receiving any treatment for this disease including chemotherapy, non-steroidal anti-inflammatory medications or antibiotics at the time of sampling could be enrolled. As part of the study design, the person performing the molecular analyses was blinded as to the group inclusion of the sample until after sample analyses were complete.

Analysis of canine blood

2.5 mls of whole blood was obtained from the jugular vein of each dog and placed in a PAXgene RNA Blood collection tube (Qiagen - Cat# 762165). PAXgene tubes were then inverted 8–10 times and stored at room temperature (20C) for 2 h before being transferred to -20C for 24 h. After 24 h, the tubes were transferred to -80C and stored until the time of analysis. The PAXgene blood miRNA kit (PreAnalytiX – Cat# 762165) was used to isolate RNA from blood samples per manufacturer's instructions. To allow for normalization during subsequent qPCR analysis, a synthetic RNA was added to RNA preps (5.6×10^8 copies of cel-miR-39 (Qiagen, Cat# 217184) per sample). This is a well accepted method for normalization [49].

Analysis of canine urine

10mls of urine was collected by ultrasound guided antepubic cystocentesis. 3 mls was submitted for urinalysis, 2 mls was used for urine culture, and 5 mls was stored in 1 ml aliquots at –80 °C until the time of analysis. Prior to RNA extraction, urine was thawed on ice then centrifuged at 250xG for 5 min to pellet exfoliated cells present in the urine. The Qiagen miRNeasy kit (Qiagen – Cat# 217004) was used to extract RNA from cell pellets.

miRNA analysis

RNA extracted from blood and urine extractions was quantified using a NanoDrop 2000 spectrophotometer. Relative expression levels of miR-34a, let-7c, miR-16, miR-103b, and miR-106b were assessed using predesigned TaqMan primer/probes sets (Applied Biosystems) in combination with the TaqMan MicroRNA Reverse Transcription and Universal PCR Master Mix (no AmpErase UNG) kit (Applied Biosystems, Cat# 4324018) per manufacturer's protocol. Three replicates were included for each sample. Twenty nanograms of total RNA was used for each RT reaction. Cel-miR-39 expression levels were assessed to allow for normalization of miRNA expression in blood samples. To allow for normalization of miRNA expression in urine samples, RNU6 expression levels were assessed using predesigned TaqMan primer/probes sets (Applied Biosystems)). RNU6 is frequently used as an endogenous control gene for miRNA expression studies [50]. Expression values of miR-34a, let-7c, miR-16, miR-103b, and miR-106b are expressed relative to these normalization controls using the 2(–delta delta cycle threshold) method.

Statistical analysis

We determined that inclusion of 20 normal, 20 LUTD, and 17 TCC patients would provide a power of 0.8 for our study (28 normal, 25 LUTD, and 17 TCC patients were included in the actual study). Data from each of the groups were graphed and parametric and/or nonparametric analyses performed to generate descriptive and inferential statistical data using a commercially available software program (GraphPad Prism, GraphPad Software, La Jolla, CA). The following variables were assessed in this study; age (continuous variable), weight (continuous variable), miRNA levels (miR-34a, let-7c, miR-16, miR-103b, miR-106b, continuous variable), gender (categorical variable (male/female)), presence of cystic calculi (categorical variable (yes/no)), presence of UTI (categorical variable (yes/no)). The Chi-squared test was used to determine whether differences in patient characteristics existed between groups for gender, while standard ANOVA was used to determine whether differences in age, weight, and amount of miRNA isolated from patient blood and urine specimens existed between groups. MiRNA expression levels were compared between groups using Kruskal-Wallis One Way ANOVA on Ranks (Ranked ANOVA), a method which is becoming common place in biomarker discovery studies because it is able to take into account the different levels of variation which are present in the groups being assessed [51–56]. It is of note that this type of analysis is considered exploratory in nature, i.e. is used for hypothesis-generation. Correlation between miRNA expression in the 3 patient groups was estimated by Pearson Product moments analysis. Statistical significance for all tests was set at $p < 0.05$.

Results

Patient characteristics

A total of 70 dogs, including 28 normal control dogs, 25 dogs with LUTD and 17 dogs with TCC were included in the study (Table 1). A statistically significant difference in mean age was observed between the groups (Table 1, $P < 0.0001$). Statistically significant differences in gender and weight were not observed (Table 1). In the normal control group there were 11 male castrated dogs and 17 female spayed dogs. In the LUTD control group there were 11 male castrated dogs, 1 intact male dog, 10 female spayed dogs and 3 intact female dogs. In the TCC group there were 9 male castrated dogs and 8 female spayed dogs. In the normal control group there were 15 mixed breed dogs, 3 Labrador retrievers, 2 border collies, 2 dachshunds and 1 each of 6 different pure bred dogs. All had negative urine cultures results and all had no evidence of LUTD on abdominal ultrasound. In the LUTD group there were 5 mixed breed

Table 1 Patient Characteristics

# Patients	Normal control	Dogs with LUTD	Dogs with TCC	p-value
	28	25	17	
Gender				
Male	11 (39.3%)	12 (48%)	9 (53%)	>0.5
Female	17 (60.7%)	13 (52%)	8 (47%)	>0.5
Characteristics				
Mean Age (Range) years	5.2 ± 2.98 (0.67–12.0)	7.5 ± 3.9 (0.5–14.0)	10.0 ± 2.4 (6–14)	<0.0001
Mean Weight (Range) Kg	17.85 ± 10.9 (3.4–40.0)	14.15 ± 12.16 (2.9–50.0)	20.97 ± 15.37 (5.1–69.0)	>0.5
Disease				
Cystic Calculi (CC)	0	11	0	
Urinary Tract infection (UTI)	0	2	3	
CC + UTI	0	11	0	
TCC based on biopsy	0	0	5	
TCC based on cytology	0	0	12	

dogs, 3 Bishon Frises, 2 pit bull terriers and 1 each of 14 different pure bred dogs. For the dogs with LUTD, 11 were diagnosed with cystic calculi, 11 were diagnosed with both cystic calculi and a urinary tract infection based on a positive aerobic bacterial urine culture, and 2 were diagnosed with chronic urinary tract infections. In the TCC group there were 4 mixed breed dogs, 2 Australian shepherds, 2 German shepherd dogs, 2 West Highland white terriers and 1 each of 7 different pure bred dogs. Five were diagnosed on biopsy and 12 were diagnosed on cytology. All dogs were assumed to have muscle invasive disease based on appearance on ultrasound examination but as not all dogs had biopsies taken this could not be fully evaluated. Three had a concurrent urinary tract infection based on results of aerobic bacterial urine cultures.

Extraction of miRNA from canine urine and blood samples

Based on recent publications comparing the levels of miRNA in blood and urine of bladder cancer patients [57–59], we assessed both blood and urine samples. Bladder cells are in direct contact with urine and as a number of the cells present in urine are of urothelial origin; the higher content of bladder cells in urine versus blood makes it more likely that observed changes in miRNA expression in urine samples are reflective of alterations that directly mediate bladder inflammation or TCC.

We chose to isolate RNA from cells present in urine samples rather than isolate RNA which is present 'free' in the urine because other studies have demonstrated isolating sufficient amounts of high quality 'free' RNA from urine is challenging due to low pH and high levels of nucleases [30–32]. The median quantities of RNA isolated from cells present in canine patient urine samples from the three groups were: 181.6 ng (Normal patients, range; 70.8 ng – 760.4 ng, $n = 28$), 938.6 ng (LUTD patients, range; 93.6 ng – 42,337.6, $n = 20$), 1192.4 ng (TCC patients, range; 117.6 ng – 55,468.8 ng, $n = 11$) (Fig. 1A). There was not a statistically significant difference in the quantity of RNA isolated from the 3 patient groups.

The Qiagen PAXGene kit was used to isolate RNA from canine blood samples. The median quantities of RNA isolated from canine patient blood samples from the three groups were: 1839.8 ng (Normal patients, range; 320 ng – 9510.8 ng, n = 28), 1999.2 ng (LUTD patients, range; 12.4 ng – 7279.6 ng, $n = 25$), 1887.2 ng (TCC patients, range; 146.4 ng – 8636.6 ng, $n = 17$) (Fig. 1B). There was not a statistically significant difference in the quantity of RNA isolated from the 3 groups.

A statistically significant difference in RNA yields from blood versus urine samples collected from normal patients was observed ($p = 0.0001$, 10-fold difference), however, there was not a statistically significant difference in RNA yield for LUTD or TCC patients (Fig. 1A, B).

Age-related differences in miR-34a expression in normal dogs and those with LUTD but not TCC

Expression of 5 miRNAs associated with TCC pathophysiology (miR-34a, let-7c, miR-16, miR-103b, and miR-106b) [38, 60], was assessed in RNA extracted from clinically normal, LUTD, and TCC canine blood and urine samples using quantitative real time PCR. Since a statistically significant difference in age was observed between dogs with normal bladder, LUTD and TCC (Table 1), we first investigated whether any age-related differences in miRNA expression were observed in the three patient groups (Fig. 2). There

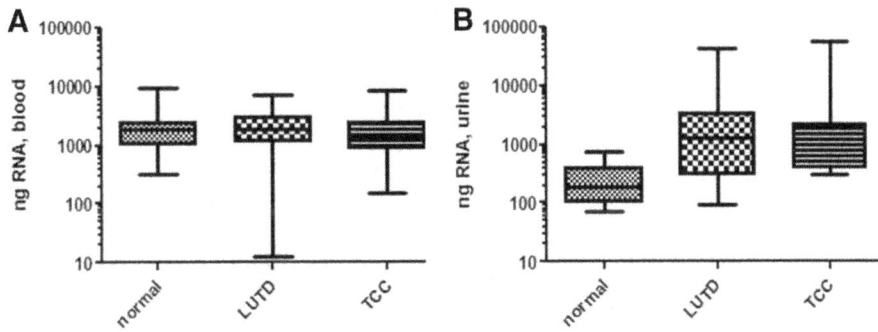

Fig. 1 Relative quantities of RNA extracted from blood and urine specimens from canine patients with normal bladder, lower urinary tract disease (LUTD), and transitional cell carcinoma (TCC) of the bladder. Statistically significant differences in the quantity of RNA isolated from blood specimens (**a**) or urine specimens (**b**) from the 3 patient groups were not observed. However, there was a statistically significant difference in the quantity of RNA isolated from blood versus urine from patients with normal bladders ($p = 0.0001$). No statistically significant difference was observed in quantity of RNA isolated from blood versus urine from patients with LUTD, or patients with TCC. Standard ANOVA was used for these comparisons

were no age-related differences observed in either let-7c, miR-16, miR-103b or miR-106b in urine or blood samples, however, urine miR-34a expression correlated strongly with age in both the normal group and the LUTD group, but not in the TCC group (Fig. 2). Correlation between age and miR-34a was not observed in blood samples. Neither gender nor body weight correlated with the expression of any of the miRNA tested (data not shown). It is possible that suppression of miR-34a expression may occur in aging TCC patients. Age-matched control studies will be necessary to confirm this.

Paired analysis of miRNA expression in patient urine samples demonstrate that miR-34a correlations with other miRNAs are disrupted in TCC

As several of the miRNAs analyzed in this study target the same molecules and/or same signaling pathways (miR-34a targets; Bcl-2, CCND1, CDK4/6, CREB, DLL1, E2F3, MET, c-MYC, SIRT-1, HMGA2, Notch1, Let-7c targets; LIN28, Ras, HMGA2, c-myc, Bcl-xL, miR-16 targets; BCL2, MCL1, CCND1, WNT3A; miR-103b targets; CCNE1, CDK2, CREB1, miR-106b targets; CCND1, E2F3, RBL1/2, WEE1, [24–30]), we rationalized that there may be a correlation between their relative expression levels in individual patient specimens. We used Pearson Product Moment Correlation to assess the correlation between individual miRNA in urine and blood (Additional file 1: Tables S1–S6). In blood specimens from normal, LUTD, and TCC patients, expression levels of all 5 miRNA analyzed trended together in individual patients. In urine samples from normal patients, expression of miR-34a trended with let-7c, miR-16, and miR-103b, but not miR-106b (Fig. 3A). In urine samples from LUTD patients, expression of miR-34a trended with let-7c and miR-103b but not miR-16 or miR-106b (Fig. 3B). In urine from TCC patients, miR-34a

expression was completely independent of let-7c, miR-16, miR-103b, and miR-106b (Fig. 3C). Thus, miR-34a correlation with the other miRNAs examined decreased from normal > LUTD > TCC. Conversely, miR-16 was *not* correlated with miR-103b or miR-106b in urine from normal canine but significant correlation was observed in the diseased states. These data indicate that alteration of coordinated expression of miRNAs occurs in patients with LUTD and TCC. It is noteworthy that no correlation between miRNA expression and RNA yield was observed in any of these settings.

MiRNA expression levels in normal, LUTD, and TCC blood and urine samples

Next, we investigated whether any of the miRNA tested were differentially expressed in blood and urine samples from normal dogs and those with LUTD or TCC. Kruskal-Wallis one-way ANOVA on ranks (ranked ANOVA), an exploratory non-parametric method that is frequently used in biomarker discovery studies [51–56], was used for these analyses. No significant differences in expression of miR-34, let-7c, miR-16, or miR-106b were observed in blood samples from the three groups (Fig. 4A-C, E, Table 2), however, one-way ANOVA on ranks identified statistically significant differences in the expression levels of miR-103b in the blood of normal vs LUTD ($p = 0.028$) and normal vs TCC patients ($p = 0.011$), but not LUTD vs TCC patients ($p > 0.05$) (Fig. 4D, Table 2).

We also examined the levels of miRNA in urine from these three groups of patients (Fig. 5, Table 2). As in blood samples, there was no significant difference in miR-34a levels in the urine of animals from the three groups (Fig. 5A). A statistically significant difference in miR-106b levels in the urine of normal vs TCC patients (Fig. 2E, p<0.001) was observed. Comparison of patients with LUTD and TCC determined that only miRNA-16

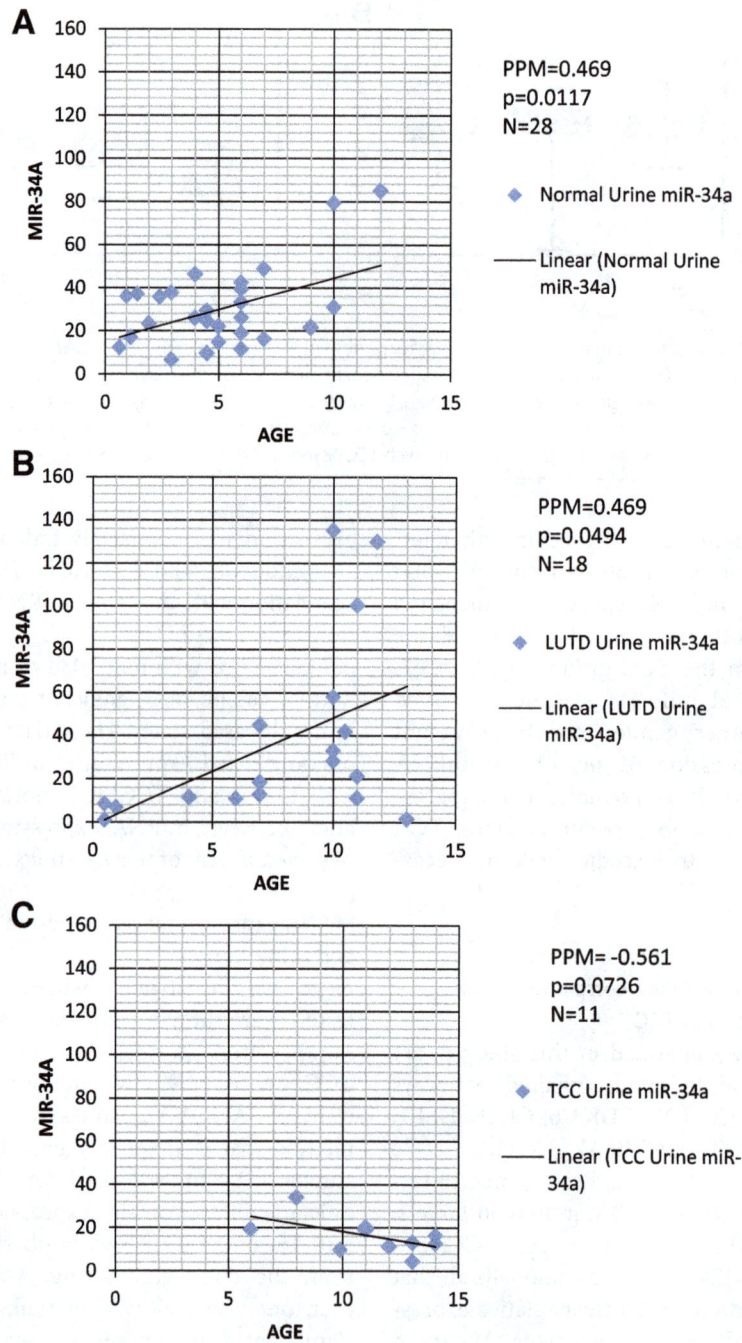

Fig. 2 Age-related differences in miR-34a expression exist in urine samples from normal dogs and those with lower urinary tract disease (LUTD) but not in urine samples from dogs with transitional cell carcinoma (TCC) of the bladder. Urine miR-34a expression correlated strongly with age in both the normal group (a) and the LUTD group (b), but not in the TCC group (c). There were no age-related differences observed in let-7c, miR-16, miR-103b, or miR-106b expression (data not shown). A correlation between age and miRNA expression was not observed in canine blood samples (data not shown). Pearson Product Moment Correlation was used to generate these data

($p = 0.016$) and miR-103b ($p = 0.002$) appeared to have any significant differences (Fig. 5C, D, Table 2). Thus, these two miRNAs are potential candidates for distinguishing biomarkers of TCC vs LUTD.

Discussion

There is a clinical need to develop non-invasive and inexpensive tests that have fast turnaround to distinguish between canine patients with non-neoplastic LUTD and

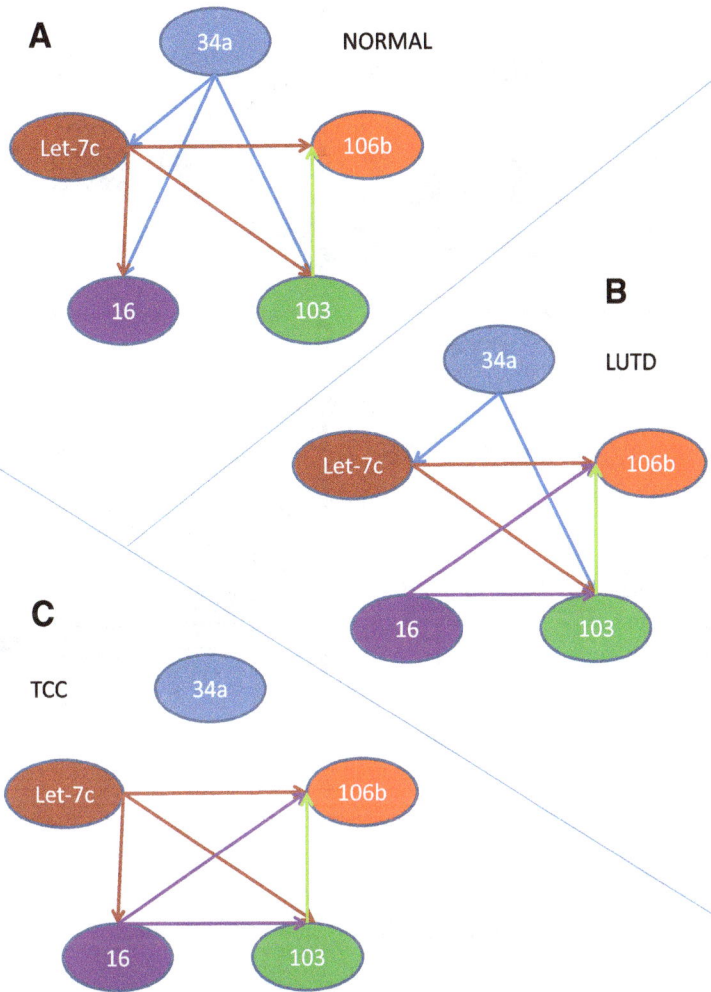

Fig. 3 The correlation of miR-34a expression with other miRNAs is disrupted in TCC. In urine samples from normal and LUTD patients, expression of miR-34a trended with other related miRNA: let-7c, miR-16, and miR-103b, but not miR-106b (**a**). MiR-34a expression was independent of miR-16 in LUTD patients (**b**), and completely independent of any other miRNA tested in TCC (**c**). Thus, miR-34a correlation with the related miRNAs examined decreased normal > LUTD > TCC. In blood specimens from normal, LUTD, and TCC patients, expression levels of all 5 miRNA analyzed trended together in individual patients (data not shown)

canine patients with TCC. The goal of this study was to determine whether assessment of miRNA expression in canine urine and blood samples is possible and could help address this need. We successfully assessed expression of five miRNA (miR-34a, let-7c, miR-16, miR-103b, and miR-106b) in canine urine and blood samples. Analysis of miRNA in canine urine has not previously been reported. Statistically significant differences in miR-103b (p = 0.002) and miR-16 (p = 0.016) expression levels were observed in canine urine specimens from LUTD versus TCC patients, however, no difference in miRNA expression levels was observed in canine blood specimens from these 2 groups. It should be noted that this study was exploratory in nature and a larger prospective study will be necessary to validate the association of miR-103b and miR-16 expression levels with canine TCC. It should also

be noted that while it has been shown that some dog breeds are predisposed to TCC [3] this study was not powered to detect whether miRNA expression contributes to these predispositions and there were too few of any one breed in the TCC and control groups to attempt meaningful analysis. Lastly, the study was not powered to determine whether these miRNA are expressed early in the course of disease or only after they progress to become muscle invasive. More work is need to determine if these miRNA are associated with earlier superficial forms of the disease.

To our knowledge, this is the first study to observe differential expression of miR-103b and miR-16 in body fluids from canine bladder cancer patients versus patients with LUTD. Jiang et al. very recently reported lower miR-103b expression levels predict worse outcome

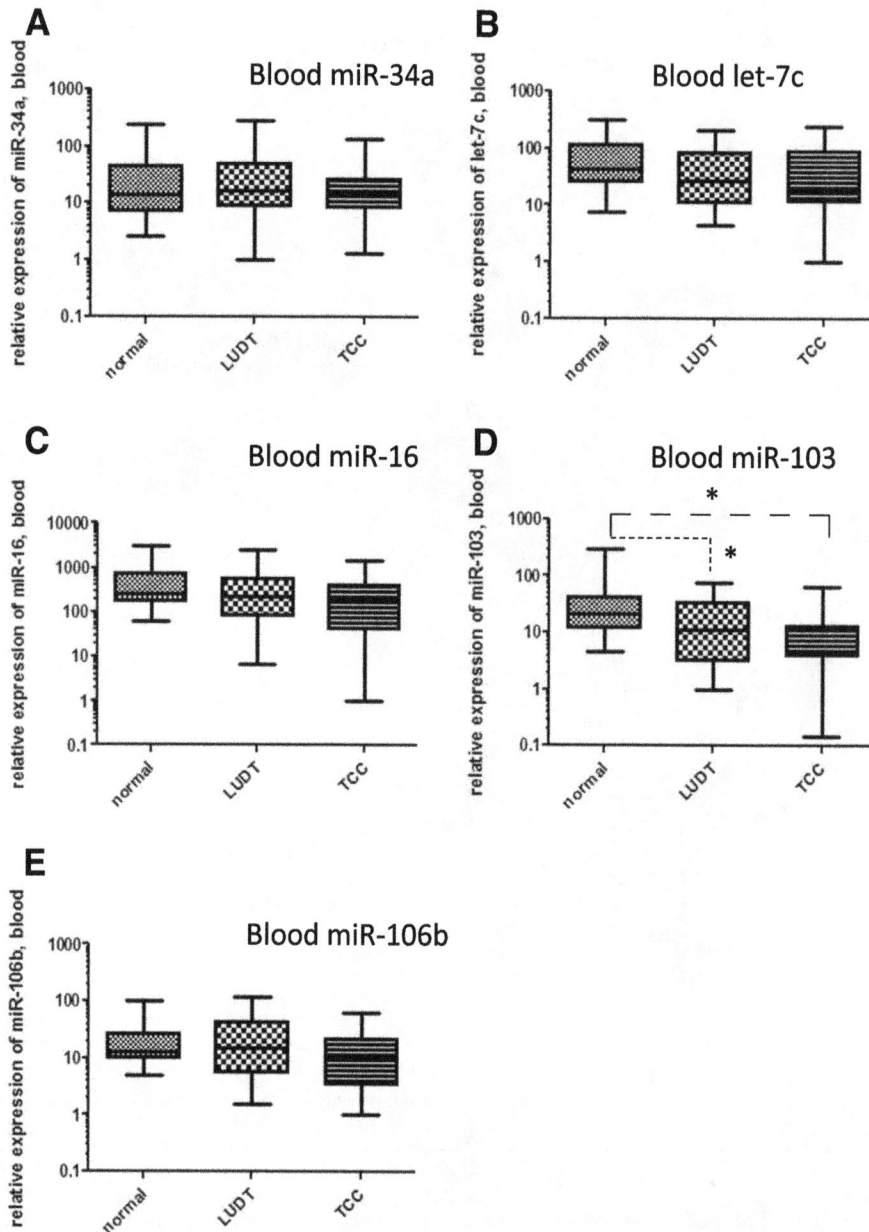

Fig. 4 Comparison of expression levels of miR-34a, let-7c, miR-16, miR-103b, and miR-106b in blood specimens from patients with normal bladders, lower urinary tract disease (LUTD), and transitional cell carcinoma (TCC) of the bladder. One-way ANOVA on ranks identified statistically significant differences in the expression levels of miR-103b in the blood of normal vs LUTD ($p = 0.028$) and normal vs TCC patients ($p = 0.011$), but not LUTD vs TCC patients ($p > 0.05$) (**d**). No statistically significant differences in expression levels were observed between the 3 patient groups for miR-34a, let-7c, miR-16, or miR-106b (**a**, **b**, **c**, and **e**)

for humans with muscle invasive bladder cancer [61]. This group assessed miR-103b expression in human blood but not urine samples. It is possible lack of statistical power is a reason why we did not observe differences of miR-103b in canine blood samples in addition to urine samples. In addition, the genetics of the human bladder may be different from that of canine bladder. MiR-103b has been shown to target several molecules which play a role in carcinogenesis in other cell types,

for example CCNE1, CDK2, CREB1, DICER, and PTEN [62] [44], and colorectal cancer cell line studies indicate dysregulation of miR-103b expression can drive cancer progression [62–64]. In addition to validating miR-103b as a non-invasive biomarker to distinguish between canine LUTD and TCC, our future studies will focus on identifying downstream targets of miR-103b in bladder cancer cells and the impact of miR-103b on bladder cancer cell growth and survival; it is possible that miR-103b

Table 2 Median values of miRNA from blood and urine of dogs with normal bladders, LUTD and TCC and one-way ANOVA on ranks analysis

Age	MEDIAN VALUES			p-values (one-way ANOVA on ranks)		
	NORMAL	LUTD	TCC	NORMAL vs LUTD	NORMAL vs TCC	LUTD vs TCC
	5	7	11	0.0371	<0.001	0.002
Blood miR-34a	13.882	16.393	15.047	>0.05	>0.05	>0.05
Blood Let-7c	41.478	26.022	19.420	>0.05	>0.05	>0.05
Blood miR-16	247.180	223.006	211.826	>0.05	>0.05	>0.05
Blood miR-103b	21.427	11.097	11.757	0.028	0.011	0.709
Blood miR-106b	12.663	14.910	10.452	>0.05	>0.05	>0.05
Urine miR-34a	26.152	19.947	16.305	>0.05	>0.05	>0.05
Urine Let-7c	36.801	5.603	1.788	<0.001	<0.001	0.092
Urine miR-16	37.730	64.643	21.398	0.066	0.095	0.016
Urine miR-103b	8.539	5.199	2.038	0.298	<0.001	0.002
Urine miR-106b	8.380	6.623	2.923	0.276	0.001	0.063

may have utility as a therapeutic target as well as a diagnostic biomarker. The targets of miR-16 in bladder cancer cells have not been determined and its impact on bladder cancer cell growth and survival remains unknown, however, studies in other cancer cell types, including chronic lymphocytic lymphoma (CLL) and prostate cancer, have demonstrated dysregulation of miR-16 expression is associated with cancer initiation and/or progression [65–67]. The loss of correlation of miR-34a expression with age in TCC patients as well as the loss of coordinated expression of miR-34a with let-7c, miR-103b, and miR-106b (a progressive loss of miR-34a coordination with these miRNA was observed from normal > LUTD > TCC patients), indicates miR-34a may also contribute to bladder carcinogenesis. Coordinated control of miRNA expression has been shown to be important in many biological systems to allow for the regulation of complex cellular processes and can occur through genomic clustering, epigenetic regulation, or regulation by a shared transcription factor [68, 69]. In vitro studies will be necessary to determine how dysregulation of coordinated miRNA expression occurs in bladder cancer cells and how this contributes to carcinogenesis.

Key differences were observed between our current study and a prior study in which we assessed expression of miR-106b, miR-34a, miR-16, and miR-103b, and let-7c in archival paraffin-embedded tissue samples which were collected at time of necropsy or biopsy from canine patients with LUTD versus TCC [38]. In archival tissue samples, expression of miR-106b, miR-34a, miR-16, and miR-103b was higher in canine LUTD versus TCC patients. In our current study, no difference in expression of miR-106b and miR-34a was observed in blood or urine samples and miR-103b and miR-16 expression levels were decreased in urine samples from LUTD

versus TCC patients. Greater variability in miRNA levels in body fluids versus tissue may account for why differences in miR-34a and miR-106b expression levels were not observed in the current study; within group variances were much higher for these miRNA in the urine and blood analyses described in the current manuscript compared to our previous archival tissue analyses. In case of miR-103b and miR-16, it is possible that the miRNA is produced in the LUTD affected tissue and is retained there, while in TCC, although produced in the tissue, they are then released into the circulation easily. In support of this, several groups have recently shown that some cancer cells can selectively export miRNA [70–72]. Hence selective export of miRNA by in TCC but not LUTD could explain why the levels of these miRNA are lower in the TCC tissue compared to LUTD, but higher in the released urine. Other studies have shown miRNA expression levels can be extremely variable in body fluid specimens [47, 48]. It is possible the difference in direction in trend of miR-16 and miR-103b in urine versus tissue samples is due, at least in part, to differences in the type of cells present in tissue versus urine samples and their relative proportion. For example, presence and/or proportion of immune cells in the urine samples from the three groups could be a factor. In the current study, 3 out of the 17 (17.6%) patients with TCC had urinary tract infections at the time of diagnosis. This rate is comparable to a recent study where 25% of dogs diagnoses with TCC had a positive urine culture prior to beginning chemotherapy [73]. It is likely the archival tissue samples contained a higher proportion of bladder cells compared to the blood and urine samples. Differences in collection and processing that urine and blood samples versus tissue samples went through may have also contributed to the observed differences. While a direct comparison of miRNA expression between

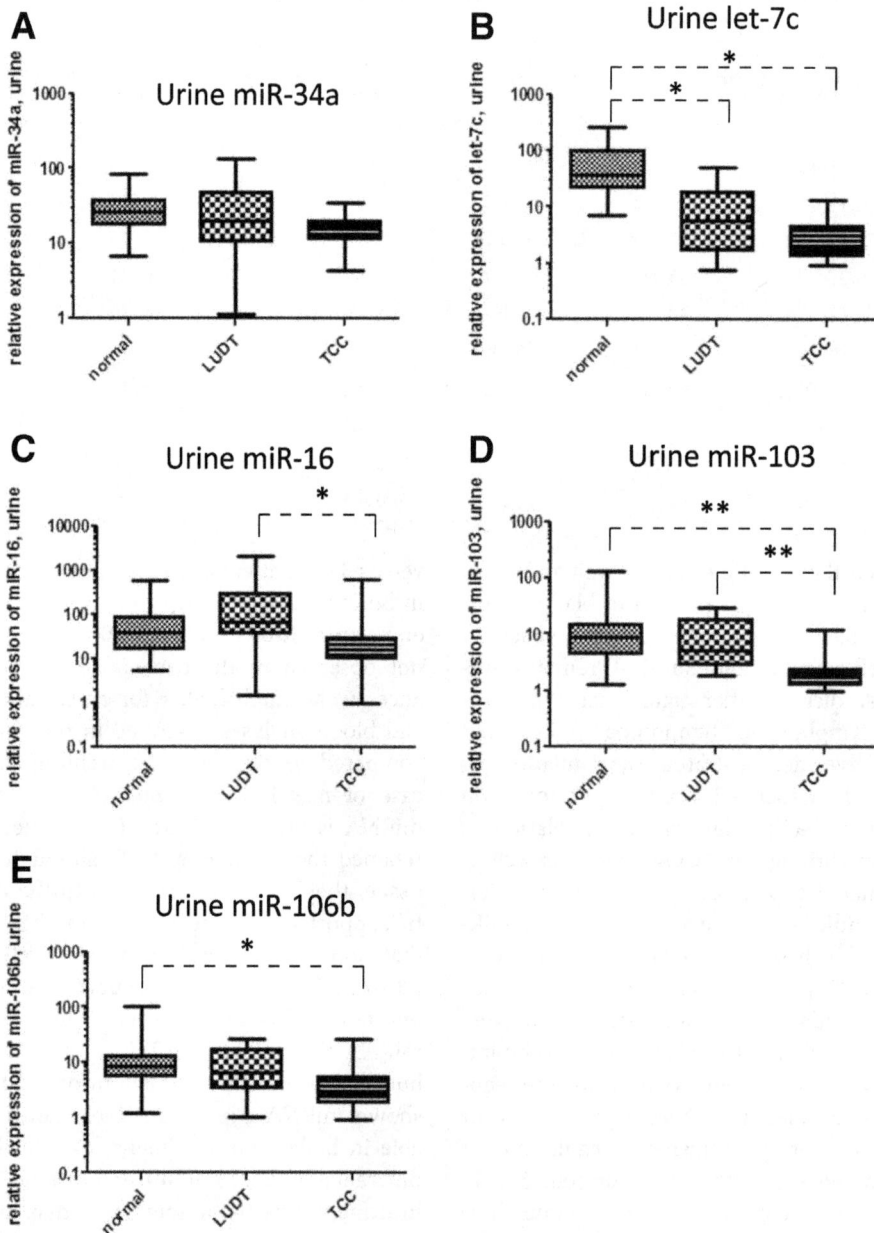

Fig. 5 Comparison of expression levels of miR-34a, let-7c, miR-16, miR-103b, and miR-106b in urine specimens from patients with normal bladders, lower urinary tract disease (LUTD), and transitional cell carcinoma (TCC) of the bladder. One-way ANOVA on ranks identified significant differences in the expression levels of miR-16 and miR-103b in the urine of LUTD vs TCC patients (**c** and **d**, $p < 0.05$ and $p < 0.005$, respectively), of let-7c levels in the urine of normal vs TCC and LUTD patients (**b**, $p < 0.05$ for both), and of miR-106b levels in the urine of normal vs TCC patients (**e**, $p < 0.05$). A statistically significant difference in miR-34a expression levels was not observed between the 3 patient groups (**a**)

matched tissue, blood, and urine samples is certainly warranted to address the observed discrepancies between the two studies it will likely prove challenging both financially and logistically as bladder biopsies are not routinely performed for canine patients and owners may not be willing to give consent for this procedure due to associated risks.

To our knowledge, extraction and assessment of miRNA from canine urine has not previously been performed, and only a limited number of studies have assessed miRNA expression using human urine samples [30–32]. Urine analysis is ideally suited to biomarker discovery studies for TCC and other urological diseases because urine is in direct contact with the bladder and it can easily be obtained from patients. The fact that we observed statistically significant differences in levels of 4 of the 5 miRNAs assessed in urine specimens (differential expression of miR-103b and miR-16 in LUTD versus

TCC patients, and differential expression of let-7c and miR-106b in clinically normal versus LUTD and/or TCC patients) versus only 1 in blood specimens (differential expression of miR-103b in clinically normal versus TCC patients) between the 3 patient groups, and also observed progressive loss of coordinated expression of miR-34a, supports the use of urine specimens rather than blood specimens for urological biomarker discovery studies.

Conclusions

In summary, our data demonstrate an association exists between miR-103b and miR-16 expression levels in urine and TCC, and show that miRNA can be isolated and quantified in canine urine as well as blood specimens. Our results indicate that further investigation of these miRNA as diagnostic non-invasive biomarkers for canine TCC is warranted.

Additional files

Additional file 1: Table S1. *P* values for correlation of miRNA expression in RNA extracted from blood samples from canine patients with normal bladders, **Table S2.** *P* values for correlation of miRNA expression in RNA extracted from urine samples from canine patients with normal bladders, **Table S3.** *P* values for correlation of miRNA expression in RNA extracted from blood samples from canine patients with LUTD, **Table S4.** *P* values for correlation of miRNA expression in RNA extracted from urine samples from canine patients with LUTD, **Table S5.** *P* values for correlation miRNA expression in RNA extracted from blood samples from canine patients with TCC, **Table S6.** *P* values for correlation of miRNA expression in RNA extracted from urine samples from canine patients with TCC. (DOCX 28 kb)

Additional file 2: Table S7. Demographic and miRNA expression data. (XLSX 25 kb)

Abbreviations

AUC: Area under the curve; IACUC: Institutional animal care and use committee; LUTD: Lower urinary tract disease; miRNA: MicroRNA; OR: Odds ratio; ROC: Receiver operating characteristic; SD: Standard deviation; TCC: Transitional cell carcinoma; TNM: Tumor, Lymph Node and Metastasis; UTI: Urinary tract infection

Acknowledgements

We would like to thank Ms. Teri Guerrero for her help in collecting and processing samples.

Funding

This study was supported by a grant from the Center for Companion Animal Health, School of Veterinary Medicine, University of California, Davis.

Author contributions

MSK: Study conception and design, data collection, data interpretation and analysis, drafting and revising manuscript, final approval of manuscript. AZ: Study design, data collection, data interpretation and analysis, drafting and revising manuscript, final approval of manuscript. JLW: Study design, data collection, data interpretation and analysis, drafting and revising manuscript, final approval of manuscript. LEB: Study design, data collection, data interpretation and analysis, drafting and revising manuscript, final approval of manuscript. BDJ: Statistical analyses, final approval of the manuscript. PMG: Study conception and design, data interpretation and analysis, drafting and revising manuscript, final approval of manuscript. RLV: Study conception and design, data collection, data interpretation and analysis, drafting and revising manuscript, final approval of manuscript

Competing interests

None.

Author details

[1]Department of Surgical and Radiological Sciences, School of Veterinary Medicine, University of California, Davis, CA, USA. [2]Department of Medicine and Epidemiology, School of Veterinary Medicine, University of California, Davis, CA, USA. [3]William R. Pritchard Veterinary Medical Teaching Hospital, School of Veterinary Medicine, University of California, Davis, CA, USA. [4]Department of Public Health Sciences, University of California Davis, Davis, California 95616, USA. [5]Department of Urology, University of California, Davis, School of Medicine, Sacramento, CA, USA. [6]Department of Biochemistry and Molecular Medicine, University of California, Davis, School of Medicine, Sacramento, CA, USA. [7]VA Northern California Health Care System, Sacramento, CA, USA. [8]Department of Pharmaceutical and Biomedical Sciences, California Northstate University College of Pharmacy, Elk Grove, CA, USA.

References

1. Norris AM, Laing EJ, Valli VE, Withrow SJ, Macy DW, Ogilvie GK, Tomlinson J, McCaw D, Pidgeon G, Jacobs RM. Canine bladder and urethral tumors: a retrospective study of 115 cases (1980-1985). J Vet Intern Med. 1992;6(3):145–53.
2. Priester WA, McKay FW. The occurrence of tumors in domestic animals. Natl Cancer Inst Monogr. 1980;54:1–210.
3. Fulkerson CM, Knapp DW. Management of transitional cell carcinoma of the urinary bladder in dogs: a review. Vet J. 2015;205(2):217–25.
4. Mutsaers AJ, Widmer WR, Knapp DW. Canine transitional cell carcinoma. J Vet Intern Med. 2003;17(2):136–44.
5. Knapp DW, Ramos-Vara JA, Moore GE, Dhawan D, Bonney PL, Young KE. Urinary bladder cancer in dogs, a naturally occurring model for cancer biology and drug development. ILAR J. 2014;55(1):100–18.
6. Glickman LT, Raghavan M, Knapp DW, Bonney PL, Dawson MH. Herbicide exposure and the risk of transitional cell carcinoma of the urinary bladder in Scottish terriers. J Am Vet Med Assoc. 2004;224(8):1290–7.
7. Glickman LT, Schofer FS, McKee LJ, Reif JS, Goldschmidt MH. Epidemiologic study of insecticide exposures, obesity, and risk of bladder cancer in household dogs. J Toxicol Environ Health. 1989;28(4):407–14.
8. Davis BW, Ostrander EA. Domestic dogs and cancer research: a breed-based genomics approach. ILAR J. 2014;55(1):59–68.
9. Owen LN. TNM classification of Tumours in domestic animals. 1st ed. Geneva: World health Organization; 1980.
10. Knapp DW, Glickman NW, Denicola DB, Bonney PL, Lin TL, Glickman LT. Naturally-occurring canine transitional cell carcinoma of the urinary bladder a relevant model of human invasive bladder cancer. Urol Oncol. 2000;5(2):47–59.
11. Chun R, Knapp DW, Widmer WR, Glickman NW, DeNicola DB, Bonney PL. Cisplatin treatment of transitional cell carcinoma of the urinary bladder in dogs: 18 cases (1983-1993). J Am Vet Med Assoc. 1996;209(9):1588–91.
12. Greene SN, Lucroy MD, Greenberg CB, Bonney PL, Knapp DW. Evaluation of cisplatin administered with piroxicam in dogs with transitional cell carcinoma of the urinary bladder. J Am Vet Med Assoc. 2007;231(7):1056–60.
13. Mohammed SI, Craig BA, Mutsaers AJ, Glickman NW, Snyder PW, deGortari AE, Schlittler DL, Coffman KT, Bonney PL, Knapp DW. Effects of the cyclooxygenase inhibitor, piroxicam, in combination with chemotherapy on tumor response, apoptosis, and angiogenesis in a canine model of human invasive urinary bladder cancer. Mol Cancer Ther. 2003;2(2):183–8.
14. Shapiro W, Kitchell BE, Fossum TW, Couto CG, Theilen G. Cisplatin for treatment of transitional cell and squamous cell carcinomas in dogs. J Am Vet Med Assoc. 1988;193(12):1530–3.

15. Poirier VJ, Forrest LJ, Adams WM, Vail DM. Piroxicam, mitoxantrone, and coarse fraction radiotherapy for the treatment of transitional cell carcinoma of the bladder in 10 dogs: a pilot study. J Am Anim Hosp Assoc. 2004;40(2):131–6.

16. Upton ML, Tangner CH, Payton ME. Evaluation of carbon dioxide laser ablation combined with mitoxantrone and piroxicam treatment in dogs with transitional cell carcinoma. J Am Vet Med Assoc. 2006;228(4):549–52.

17. Bilbrey SA, Withrow SJ, Klein MK, Bennett RA, Norris AM, Gofton N, DeHoff W. Vulvovaginectomy and perineal urethrostomy for neoplasms of the vulva and vagina. Vet Surg. 1989;18(6):450–3.

18. Kamat AM, Hahn NM, Efstathiou JA, Lerner SP, Malmstrom PU, Choi W, Guo CC, Lotan Y, Kassouf W. Bladder cancer. Lancet. 2016;388(10061):2796–810.

19. Bell MD, Yafi FA, Brimo F, Steinberg J, Aprikian AG, Tanguay S, Kassouf W. Prognostic value of urinary cytology and other biomarkers for recurrence and progression in bladder cancer: a prospective study. World J Urol. 2016;34(10):1405–9.

20. Kojima T, Kawai K, Miyazaki J, Nishiyama H. Biomarkers for precision medicine in bladder cancer. Int J Clin Oncol. 2016;

21. Henry CJ. Management of transitional cell carcinoma. Vet Clin North Am Small Anim Pract. 2003;33(3):597–613.

22. Anderson WI, Dunham BM, King JM, Scott DW. Presumptive subcutaneous surgical transplantation of a urinary bladder transitional cell carcinoma in a dog. Cornell Vet. 1989;79(3):263–6.

23. Vignoli M, Rossi F, Chierici C, Terragni R, De Lorenzi D, Stanga M, Olivero D. Needle tract implantation after fine needle aspiration biopsy (FNAB) of transitional cell carcinoma of the urinary bladder and adenocarcinoma of the lung. Schweiz Arch Tierheilkd. 2007;149(7):314–8.

24. Henry CJ, Tyler JW, McEntee MC, Stokol T, Rogers KS, Chun R, Garrett LD, McCaw DL, Higginbotham ML, Flessland KA, et al. Evaluation of a bladder tumor antigen test as a screening test for transitional cell carcinoma of the lower urinary tract in dogs. Am J Vet Res. 2003;64(8):1017–20.

25. Jonas S, Izaurralde E. Towards a molecular understanding of microRNA-mediated gene silencing. Nat Rev Genet. 2015;16(7):421–33.

26. Di Leva G, Garofalo M, Croce CM. MicroRNAs in cancer. Annu Rev Pathol. 9:287–314.

27. Mraz M, Malinova K, Mayer J, Pospisilova S. MicroRNA isolation and stability in stored RNA samples. Biochem Biophys Res Commun. 2009;390(1):1–4.

28. Kruhoffer M, Dyrskjot L, Voss T, Lindberg RL, Wyrich R, Thykjaer T, Orntoft TF. Isolation of microarray-grade total RNA, microRNA, and DNA from a single PAXgene blood RNA tube. J Mol Diagn. 2007;9(4):452–8.

29. Brase JC, Wuttig D, Kuner R, Sultmann H. Serum microRNAs as non-invasive biomarkers for cancer. Mol Cancer. 2010;9:306.

30. Puerta-Gil P, Garcia-Baquero R, Jia AY, Ocana S, Alvarez-Mugica M, Alvarez-Ossorio JL, Cordon-Cardo C, Cava F, Sanchez-Carbayo M. miR-143, miR-222, and miR-452 are useful as tumor stratification and noninvasive diagnostic biomarkers for bladder cancer. Am J Pathol. 180(5):1808–15.

31. Yun SJ, Jeong P, Kim WT, Kim TH, Lee YS, Song PH, Choi YH, Kim IY, Moon SK, Kim WJ. Cell-free microRNAs in urine as diagnostic and prognostic biomarkers of bladder cancer. Int J Oncol. 41(5):1871–8.

32. Yamada Y, Enokida H, Kojima S, Kawakami K, Chiyomaru T, Tatarano S, Yoshino H, Kawahara K, Nishiyama K, Seki N, et al. MiR-96 and miR-183 detection in urine serve as potential tumor markers of urothelial carcinoma: correlation with stage and grade, and comparison with urinary cytology. Cancer Sci. 102(3):522–9.

33. Rosenberg E, Baniel J, Spector Y, Faerman A, Meiri E, Aharonov R, Margel D, Goren Y, Nativ O. Predicting progression of bladder urothelial carcinoma using microRNA expression. BJU Int.

34. Han Y, Chen J, Zhao X, Liang C, Wang Y, Sun L, Jiang Z, Zhang Z, Yang R, Li Z, et al. MicroRNA expression signatures of bladder cancer revealed by deep sequencing. PLoS One. 6(3):e18286.

35. Pignot G, Cizeron-Clairac G, Vacher S, Susini A, Tozlu S, Vieillefond A, Zerbib M, Lidereau R, Debre B, Amsellem-Ouazana D, et al. microRNA expression profile in a large series of bladder tumors: identification of a 3-miRNA signature associated with aggressiveness of muscle-invasive bladder cancer. Int J Cancer, 132. (11):2479–91.

36. Kurozumi A, Goto Y, Okato A, Ichikawa T, Seki N. Aberrantly expressed microRNAs in bladder cancer and renal cell carcinoma. J Hum Genet. 2016;

37. Xu Z, YQ Y, Ge YZ, Zhu JG, Zhu M, Zhao YC, LW X, Yang XB, Geng LG, Dou QL, et al. MicroRNA expression profiles in muscle-invasive bladder cancer: identification of a four-microRNA signature associated with patient survival. Tumour Biol. 2015;36(10):8159–66.

38. Vinall RL, Kent MS, deVere White RW. Expression of microRNAs in urinary bladder samples obtained from dogs with grossly normal bladders, inflammatory bladder disease, or transitional cell carcinoma. Am J Vet Res. 73(10):1626–33.

39. Johnson SM, Grosshans H, Shingara J, Byrom M, Jarvis R, Cheng A, Labourier E, Reinert KL, Brown D, Slack FJ. RAS is regulated by the let-7 microRNA family. Cell. 2005;120(5):635–47.

40. He XY, Chen JX, Zhang Z, Li CL, Peng QL, Peng HM. The let-7a microRNA protects from growth of lung carcinoma by suppression of k-Ras and c-Myc in nude mice. J Cancer Res Clin Oncol. 136(7):1023–8.

41. Mayr C, Hemann MT, Bartel DP. Disrupting the pairing between let-7 and Hmga2 enhances oncogenic transformation. Science. 2007;315(5818):1576–9.

42. Shimizu S, Takehara T, Hikita H, Kodama T, Miyagi T, Hosui A, Tatsumi T, Ishida H, Noda T, Nagano H, et al. The let-7 family of microRNAs inhibits Bcl-xL expression and potentiates sorafenib-induced apoptosis in human hepatocellular carcinoma. J Hepatol. 52(5):698–704.

43. Hermeking H. The miR-34 family in cancer and apoptosis. Cell Death Differ. 17(2):193–9.

44. Liao Y, Lonnerdal B. Global microRNA characterization reveals that miR-103 is involved in IGF-1 stimulated mouse intestinal cell proliferation. PLoS One. 5(9):e12976.

45. Aqeilan RI, Calin GA, Croce CM. miR-15a and miR-16-1 in cancer: discovery, function and future perspectives. Cell Death Differ. 17(2):215–20.

46. Vinall RL, Tepper CG, Ripoll AA, Gandour-Edwards RF, Durbin-Johnson BP, Yap SA, Ghosh PM, deVere White RW. Decreased expression of let-7c is associated with non-response of muscle-invasive bladder cancer patients to neoadjuvant chemotherapy. Genes Cancer. 2016;7(3–4):86–97.

47. Huang X, Liang M, Dittmar R, Wang L. Extracellular microRNAs in urologic malignancies: chances and challenges. Int J Mol Sci. 14(7):14785–99.

48. De Guire V, Robitaille R, Tetreault N, Guerin R, Menard C, Bambace N, Sapieha P. Circulating miRNAs as sensitive and specific biomarkers for the diagnosis and monitoring of human diseases: promises and challenges. Clin Biochem. 46(10–11):846–60.

49. Roberts TC, Coenen-Stass AM, Wood MJ. Assessment of RT-qPCR normalization strategies for accurate quantification of extracellular microRNAs in murine serum. PLoS One. 9(2):e89237.

50. Galiveti CR, Rozhdestvensky TS, Brosius J, Lehrach H, Konthur Z. Application of housekeeping npcRNAs for quantitative expression analysis of human transcriptome by real-time PCR. RNA. 2010;16(2):450–61.

51. Jung Y, Huang JZ, Hu J. Biomarker detection in association studies: modeling SNPs simultaneously via logistic ANOVA. J Am Stat Assoc. 2014;109(508):1355–67.

52. Bartel J, Krumsiek J, Theis FJ. Statistical methods for the analysis of high-throughput metabolomics data. Computational and structural biotechnology journal. 2013;4:e201301009.

53. Lu S, Li J, Song C, Shen K, Tseng GC. Biomarker detection in the integration of multiple multi-class genomic studies. Bioinformatics. 2010;26(3):333–40.

54. Smilde AK, Jansen JJ, Hoefsloot HC, Lamers RJ, van der Greef J, Timmerman ME. ANOVA-simultaneous component analysis (ASCA): a new tool for analyzing designed metabolomics data. Bioinformatics. 2005;21(13):3043–8.

55. Bauer C, Kleinjung F, Smith CJ, Towers MW, Tiss A, Chadt A, Dreja T, Beule D, Al-Hasani H, Reinert K, et al. Biomarker discovery and redundancy reduction towards classification using a multi-factorial MALDI-TOF MS T2DM mouse model dataset. BMC bioinformatics. 2011;12:140.

56. Poon TC, Hui AY, Chan HL, Ang IL, Chow SM, Wong N, Sung JJ. Prediction of liver fibrosis and cirrhosis in chronic hepatitis B infection by serum proteomic fingerprinting: a pilot study. Clin Chem. 2005;51(2):328–35.

57. Xiao S, Wang J, Xiao N. MicroRNAs as noninvasive biomarkers in bladder cancer detection: a diagnostic meta-analysis based on qRT-PCR data. Int J Biol Markers. 2016;0

58. Armstrong DA, Green BB, Seigne JD, Schned AR, Marsit CJ. MicroRNA molecular profiling from matched tumor and bio-fluids in bladder cancer. Mol Cancer. 2015;14:194.

59. Ralla B, Stephan C, Meller S, Dietrich D, Kristiansen G, Jung K. Nucleic acid-based biomarkers in body fluids of patients with urologic malignancies. Crit Rev Clin Lab Sci. 2014;51(4):200–31.

60. Zhou H, Tang K, Xiao H, Zeng J, Guan W, Guo X, Xu H, Ye Z. A panel of eight-miRNA signature as a potential biomarker for predicting survival in bladder cancer. J Exp Clin Cancer Res. 2015;34:53.

61. Jiang X, Du L, Duan W, Wang R, Yan K, Wang L, Li J, Zheng G, Zhang X, Yang Y, et al. Serum microRNA expression signatures as novel noninvasive

biomarkers for prediction and prognosis of muscle-invasive bladder cancer. Oncotarget. 2016;

62. Geng L, Sun B, Gao B, Wang Z, Quan C, Wei F, Fang XD. MicroRNA-103 promotes colorectal cancer by targeting tumor suppressor DICER and PTEN. Int J Mol Sci. 2014;15(5):8458–72.

63. Hong Z, Feng Z, Sai Z, Tao S. PER3, a novel target of miR-103, plays a suppressive role in colorectal cancer in vitro. BMB Rep. 2014;47(9):500–5.

64. Chen HY, Lin YM, Chung HC, Lang YD, Lin CJ, Huang J, Wang WC, Lin FM, Chen Z, Huang HD, et al. miR-103/107 promote metastasis of colorectal cancer by targeting the metastasis suppressors DAPK and KLF4. Cancer Res. 2012;72(14):3631–41.

65. Nana-Sinkam SP, Croce CM. MicroRNA in chronic lymphocytic leukemia: transitioning from laboratory-based investigation to clinical application. Cancer Genet Cytogenet. 2010;203(2):127–33.

66. Aqeilan RI, Calin GA, Croce CM. miR-15a and miR-16-1 in cancer: discovery, function and future perspectives. Cell Death Differ. 2010;17(2):215–20.

67. Cho WC. OncomiRs: the discovery and progress of microRNAs in cancers. Mol Cancer. 2007;6:60.

68. Shalgi R, Lieber D, Oren M, Pilpel Y. Global and local architecture of the mammalian microRNA-transcription factor regulatory network. PLoS Comput Biol. 2007;3(7):e131.

69. Budd WT, Weaver DE, Anderson J, Zehner ZE. microRNA dysregulation in prostate cancer: network analysis reveals preferential regulation of highly connected nodes. Chem Biodivers. 2012;9(5):857–67.

70. Falcone G, Felsani A, D'Agnano I. Signaling by exosomal microRNAs in cancer. J Exp Clin Cancer Res. 2015;34:32.

71. Ohshima K, Inoue K, Fujiwara A, Hatakeyama K, Kanto K, Watanabe Y, Muramatsu K, Fukuda Y, Ogura S, Yamaguchi K, et al. Let-7 microRNA family is selectively secreted into the extracellular environment via exosomes in a metastatic gastric cancer cell line. PLoS One. 2010;5(10):e13247.

72. Ostenfeld MS, Jeppesen DK, Laurberg JR, Boysen AT, Bramsen JB, Primdal-Bengtson B, Hendrix A, Lamy P, Dagnaes-Hansen F, Rasmussen MH, et al. Cellular disposal of miR23b by RAB27-dependent exosome release is linked to acquisition of metastatic properties. Cancer Res. 2014;74(20):5758–71.

73. Budreckis DM, Byrne BA, Pollard RE, Rebhun RB, Rodriguez CO, Jr., Skorupski KA: Bacterial urinary tract infections associated with transitional cell carcinoma in dogs. Journal of veterinary internal medicine / American College of Veterinary Internal Medicine 2015, 29(3):828–833.

13

Risk factors of different hemoplasma species infections in cats

Michèle Bergmann[1*], Theresa Englert[1], Bianca Stuetzer[1], Jennifer R. Hawley[2], Michael R. Lappin[2] and Katrin Hartmann[1]

Abstract

Background: Hemoplasma species (spp.) commonly cause infections in cats worldwide. However, data on risk factors for infections are limited. The aim of this study was to determine the prevalence of hemoplasma spp. infections in cats in Southern Germany and to assess risk factors associated with infection.

Results: DNA was extracted from blood samples of 479 cats presented to different veterinary hospitals for various reasons. DNA of feline hemoplasmas was amplified by use of a previously reported PCR assay. Direct sequencing was used to confirm all purified amplicons and compared to hemoplasma sequences reported in GenBank. Results were evaluated in relation to the age, sex, housing conditions, feline leukemia virus (FeLV) and feline immunodeficiency virus (FIV) status of the cats.

The overall hemoplasma prevalence rate was 9.4% (45/479; 95% CI: 7.08–12.36). 'Candidatus Mycoplasma (M.) haemominutum' (Mhm) DNA was amplified from 42 samples, M. haemofelis from 2, and M. haemocanis from 1 sample. There was a significantly higher risk of hemoplasma infection in cats from multi-cat households, in outdoor cats, as well as in cats with FIVinfection and in cats with abortive FeLV infection, but not in cats with progressive or regressive FeLV infection.

Conclusions: Mhm infection is common in cats in Southern Germany. Higher prevalence in multi-cat households and associations with FeLV infection likely reflect the potential for direct transmission amongst cats. Outdoor access, male gender, and FIV infection are additional risk factors that might relate to aggressive interactions and exposure to vectors.

Keywords: Feline, Hemoplasmosis, *Mycoplasma* spp, PCR, Vector-borne, FeLV, FIV

Background

Hemoplasma species (spp.) (or hemotrophic *Mycoplasma* spp.) are bacteria without cell walls that can cause hemolytic anemia in different species. At least 3 hemoplasma spp. have been described in cats, *Mycoplasma (M.) haemofelis* (Mhf), 'Candidatus (Ca.) M. haemominutum' (Mhm), and 'Ca. M. turicensis' (Mtc). Hemoplasma spp. attach to the external surface of red blood cells. Besides transmission through arthropod vectors, there is evidence of horizontal transmission (e.g., blood transmission during aggressive interactions between cats, blood transfusion) between cats [17].

Hemoplasma strains that occur in cats differ in their size and pathogenicity. Mhf and Mtc seem to have a higher pathogenicity and are more often associated with anemia than Mhm [2]. However, clinical relevance of hemoplasmas as a cause of anemia is not fully understood. Many authors believe them to be an important primary cause of anemia [20, 21, 25]; others regard hemoplasmas more as opportunistic pathogens [5, 12].

Natural hemoplasma infection is mostly subclinical. Clinical signs can occur after a longer latency under immunosuppressed conditions. Feline immunodeficiency virus (FIV) and feline leukemia virus (FeLV) infection can be associated with the development of clinical signs in some cats [4, 5, 24]. After developing clinical signs, alternating periods with anemia and subclinical phases can occur [2, 25].

Worldwide, cats are commonly infected by hemoplasma spp. [11, 12, 14, 21, 26, 27] and prevalence was found to be 9.9% in Switzerland [27] and 38.5% in Africa [14]. In Southern Germany, two studies investigated the

* Correspondence: n.bergmann@medizinische-kleintierklinik.de
[1]Clinic of Small Animal Medicine, Centre for Clinical Veterinary Medicine, LMU Munich, Veterinaerstrasse 13, 80539 Munich, Germany
Full list of author information is available at the end of the article

prevalence of hemoplasma spp. infection in 135 cats [11] and in 296 cats [12] so far. These studies only evaluated preselected cats with anemia. Current data in a non-selected cat population are missing. Thus, the aim of the present study was to determine the prevalence of hemoplasma spp. by investigating blood samples of 479 cats by PCR. In addition, associations between hemoplasma spp. infections with the age, sex, housing conditions, and FIV and FeLV infection status of the cats were evaluated.

Methods
Animals
The 479 cats evaluated in this study were presented to different veterinary clinics in Southern Germany for various reasons. Health status of the cats was evaluated by physical examination. In each cat, a complete blood count (CBC) was performed and the FIV and FeLV status was examined. FIV antibodies were detected using a commercial enzyme-linked immunosorbent assay (ELISA) (SNAP Kombi Plus FeLV/FIV antibody test®, IDEXX GmbH, Ludwigsburg, Germany). FeLV infection status was investigated by performing tests for free FeLV p27 antigen using a commercial ELISA (SNAP Kombi Plus FeLV/FIV antibody test; IDEXX GmbH, Ludwigsburg, Germany), FeLV provirus using polymerase chain reaction (PCR) as well as anti-FeLV-p45

antibodies using an indirect ELISA, both as previously described [1]. Progressively FeLV- infected cats are persistently viremic and thus, FeLV antigen- and provirus-positive [9]. Regressively FeLV-infected cats are antigen-negative and provirus-positive; they are considered FeLV carriers. Cats with abortive FeLV infection never become viremic; they are antigen-, and provirus-negative but have FeLV-specific antibodies [9].

A total of 298 cats were male (62.2%) and 181 cats were female (37.8%) (Table 1). The cats´ ages ranged from 3 months to 19 years. Median age was 7.4 years (age of 40 cats was unknown). Of the 468 cats, 106 (22.6%) were purebred cats and 362 (77.4%) were Domestic Shorthair (DSH). Breed was unknown in 11 (2.3%) cats. Nine of 479 cats (1.9%) were progressively FeLV-infected, 7 of 479 cats (1.5%) were regressively FeLV-infected, and 22 of 479 cats (4.5%) were abortively FeLV-infected. A total of 7 cats were FIV antibody-positive (1.5%); two of these 7 FIV-infected cats were also progressively FeLV-infected.

Hemoplasma spp. PCR
Total DNA had previously been extracted from whole blood of the 479 cats using the MagNA Pure LC Total Nucleic Acid Isolation Kit (Roche Diagnostics AG, Rotkreuz, Switzerland) and stored at −80 °C until assayed in this study. The samples were thawed at room temperature and

Table 1 Cats with and without hemoplasma species (spp.) infection, and analysis of the risk factors housing conditions, feline immunodeficiency virus (FIV), and feline leukemia virus (FeLV) infection status

		n	Hemoplasma spp.-positive[a]	Hemoplasma spp.-negative[a]	p	Mhm[a]	Mhf[a]	Mhc[a]
Total		479	45 (9.4)	434 (90.6)	-	42 (93.3)	2 (4.5)	1 (2.2)
Age (median)		439	9.0 years	7.2 years	-	9.3	17	2
Gender	male	298	38 (12.8)	260 (87.2)	0.001	37 (97.4)	0 (0.0)	1 (2.6)
(n = 470)	female	181	7 (3.9)	174 (96.1)		5 (71.4)	2 (28.6)	0 (0.0)
Origin	shelter	56	10 (17.9)	56 (82.1)	0.104	10 (100.0)	0 (0.0)	0 (0.0)
(n = 479)	private	423	35 (8.3)	388 (91.7)		32(91.4)	2 (5.7)	1 (2.9)
Household	multi-cat	378	44 (11.6)	334 (88.4)	0.007	41 (93.2)	2 (4.5)	1 (2.3)
(n = 445)	single-cat	67	1 (1.5)	66 (98.5)		1 (100.0)	0 (0.0)	0 (0.0)
Access	outdoor	229	37 (16.2)	192 (83.8)	<0.0001	39 (95.1)	2 (4.9)	0 (0.0)
(n = 432)	indoor	203	4 (2.0)	199 (98.0)		3 (75.0)	0 (0.0)	1 (25.0)
FIV infection	positive	7	5 (71.4)	2 (28.6)	<0.0001	5 (100.0)	0 (0.0)	0 (0.0)
(n = 477)	negative	470	40 (8.5)	430 (91.5)		37 (92.5)	2 (5.0)	1 (2.5)
Progressive FeLV infection	positive	9	1 (11.1)	8 (88.9)	ns	1 (100.0)	0 (0.0)	0 (0.0)
(n = 479)	negative	470	44 (9.4)	426 (91.5)	ns	41 (93.2)	2 (4.5)	1 (2.3)
Regressive FeLV infection	positive	7	2 (28.6)	5 (71.4)	ns	2 (100.0)	0 (0.0)	0 (0.0)
(n = 479)	negative	472	43 (9.1)	429 (90.9)	ns	40 (93.0)	2 (4.7)	1 (2.3)
Abortive FeLV infection	positive	22	12 (54.5)	10 (45.5)	<0.0001	12 (100.0)	0 (0.0)	0 (0.0)
(n = 459)	negative	437	28 (6.4)	409 (93.6)		23 (82.2)	2 (7.2)	1 (3.6)

n numbers of cats in every group, p p-value, ns not significant, Mhm 'Candidatus Mycoplasma (M.) haemominutum', Mhf M. haemofelis, Mhc M. haemocanis; [a]the percentages are presented in parenthesis prepared for the amplification of hemotropic *Mycoplasma* spp. DNA in a previously reported conventional polymerase chain reaction (PCR) assay [10]. Briefly, each 2.5 µl DNA sample was added to the PCR master mix (10 mM Tris, pH 8.3, 50 mM KCl, 3.5 mM MgCl2, 200 µM each dNTP, 400 µM dUTP, 0.5 units uracil N-glycosylase (UNG) and 1.25 units Taq polymerase) with the final reaction volume of 25 µl.

PCR products were visualized on a 3% agarose gel using 6X EZVision One DNA Dye (Amersco; Solon, OH) according to manufacturer specifications.

Appropriate negative and positive controls were run with each sample. Positive PCR controls were obtained from diagnostic whole blood samples received by the Center for Companion Animal Studies (Department of Clinical Sciences, Colorado State University). Negative controls consisted of PCR (molecular grade) water being added in lieu of DNA template. Any positive sample was purified (QIAquick Gel Extraction Kit; Qiagen Germantown, MD) and sequenced to confirm genus and species (Colorado State University Proteomics and Metabolomics Facility; Fort Collins Colorado).

Statistical analysis

Statistical analysis was performed with Graph PadPrism 6.0. Confidence intervals were determined by an exact binomial test. The exact binomial test was one-tailed and was used to prove the alternative hypotheses that the prevalence of hemoplasma infection was within the 95% confidence interval (CI). A significance level of < 0.05 was chosen. Fisher´s exact test was used to assess associations between hemoplasma infection, cats´ age, gender, and housing conditions, as well as FIV and FeLV status.

Results

Prevalence of hemoplasma spp. infections

The overall hemoplasma prevalence rate was 9.4% (45/479; 95% CI: 7.08–12.36) (Table 1). Mhm DNA was amplified from 42 samples, Mhf from 2 samples, and *Mycoplasma hemocanis* (Mhc) from 1 sample (Table 1). All PCR-negative and extract-negative controls were always negative in all assays.

Hemoplasma-infected cats

Of the hemoplasma-positive cats, 84.5% (38/45) were male. Infected cats ages ranged from 9 months to 17 years (median 9 years). Most of the hemoplasma-infected cats were ≥ 9 years old (25/41); 8 cats were ≤ 3 years old (age of 4 cats was unknown).

Most of the infected cats were allowed to roam outside (90.2%; 37/41) and lived in multi-cat-households (97.8%; 44/45) (Table 1).

Ten of the infected cats were healthy and presented for neutering and/or routine health checks (22.2%; 10/

45); the remaining cats were presented with a history of illness (77.8%; 35/45). Six infected cats had anemia (13.4%; 6/45), whereas 67 (21.1%; 67/317) of the non-infected cats had anemia. The hematocrit of the 6 hemoplasma-infected anemic cats ranged from 0.22 to 0.29 l/l (reference range: 0.30–0.44 l/l). None of these cats showed signs of regenerative anemia, such as polychromasia, macrocytosis, and in none of these cats nucleated red blood cells were present.

Risk factors

Due to the low number of cats infected with the species Mhf or Mhc, all of the hemoplasma-infected cats were evaluated together for risk factor analysis. Male cats had a significantly higher risk of infection with a hemoplasma spp. than female cats ($p = 0.001$; odds-ratio (OR): 3.633; 95% CI: 1.586–8.322) (Table 1). In addition, cats with outdoor access ($p < 0.0001$; OR: 9.59; 95% CI: 3.35–27.42) and cats from multi-cat households ($p = 0.007$; OR: 8.66; 95% CI: 1.18–64.25) had a significantly higher risk of infection with a hemoplasma spp. Cats from shelters ($p = 0.104$; OR: 1.98; 95% CI: 92.8–421.9) had no significantly higher risk of hemoplasma-infection than cats from private homes.

Of the hemoplasma-positive cats, 5 cats were coinfected with FIV; 12 cats were abortively FeLV-coinfected, 2 cats were regressively and 1 cat was progressively coinfected with FeLV. Hemoplasma spp. bacteremia was significantly more often found in FIV-positive cats ($p < 0.0001$; OR: 26.88; 95% CI: 5.05–143.00) and in cats with abortive FeLV infection ($p = 0.019$; OR: 2.64; 95% CI: 1.26–5.51). Cats with progressive ($p = 0.592$) and regressive ($p = 0.134$) FeLV infections had no higher risk of being infected with hemoplasma spp..

Mhc-infected cat

The Mhc-infected cat was a 10 months old, female neutered British Shorthair. The cat lived in a multi-cat household. The cat had no access to outdoors, no contact to dogs, and no travelling history. The cat was presented for routine health care. Physical and laboratory examination were unremarkable.

Discussion

The present study revealed an overall prevalence rate of hemoplasma infections in cats of 9.4%. Worldwide, prevalence differs between about 10% in Switzerland [27] to over 30% in Africa [14]. Thus, prevalence of hemoplasma infection seems to be higher in countries with warmer climates. The infection rate in Southern Germany is similar to that in Switzerland, presumably due to the similar climate. An association between prevalence of potential vectors and prevalence of feline hemoplasma infections is likely [18, 23].

Similar to previous studies, Mhm was the most common hemoplasma spp. in the present study. None of the cats was positive for Mtc, although Mtc infections in cats from Southern Germany have been reported previously [11, 12]. Surprisingly, a 10 months old British Short Hair cat was infected with Mhc, the most prevalent hemoplasma spp. in dogs. Hemoplasmas are not necessarily strictly species-specific and there are reports stating that Mhc could infect cats and that cats might act as reservoir for Mhc [15, 16]. Mhc is most prevalent in dogs from Mediterranean countries; transmission is suspected *via Rhipicephalus sanguineus*, a tick that is not endemic in Germany [22, 28]. Source of Mhc infection in this cat of the present study is unclear. The cat was never allowed to go out and lived only indoors without any contact to dogs. Tick transmission therefore seemed unlikely; as this cat was still young, vertical transmission, which has been reported in cattle, might be the most likely source of infection [3].

Most of the Mhm- and Mhf-infected cats were older (≥9 years). Due to the subclinical nature of Mhm infection, this follows the presumption of becoming infected as a result of prolonged exposure during lifetime [23, 27].

As reported previously, infection was more prevalent in male cats and in cats with outdoor access [27]. This supports the hypotheses of horizontal transmission during aggressive interactions between cats and transmission through arthropod vectors [17]. In addition, cats from multicat-households were significantly more likely to be infected with hemoplasma spp., which could be due to a higher risk for aggressive interactions in multicat-environments.

Associations between hemoplasma spp. infection and clinical disease in naturally infected cats are not fully understood. Natural hemoplasma spp. infection is mainly subclinical in cats, but some cats develop severe anemia with fever, inappetence and lethargy [21]. It has been discussed whether retrovirus and hemoplasma infections are associated and whether immunosuppression could lead to enhanced pathogenicity of hemoplasma spp. [8, 23, 27].

A surprisingly strong association of FIV and hemoplasma spp. infection was found in the present study. Cats with hemoplasma infection were 26 times more likely to be FIV infected. This emphasizes, that hemoplasma spp. can be transmitted through similar routes as FIV, such as through biting. Similar to a recent study, FIV infection was predominantly associated with Mhm but not with Mhf and Mtc [23]. However, none of the hemoplasma FIV-coinfected cats showed signs of clinical manifestation of hemoplasmosis. It has been discussed that specific FIV strains might be the reason for more severe disease in coinfected cats [5], but this has never been proven so far.

In the present study, cats with hemoplasma infection were also more likely to be FeLV-infected. This is presumably attributable to outdoor access and multi-cat household, which increases the risk of FeLV infection through cat contact [7]. Only 3 of 28 FeLV hemoplasma-coinfected cats showed mild non-regenerative anemia which was likely caused by chronic kidney disease present in these 3 cats. In contrast, Harrus and colleagues found that Mhf-positive and cats positive for FeLV-p27 antigen were more often anemic than cats with Mhf infection alone [8]. However, most of the hemoplasma-positive cats in the present study were only abortively FeLV-infected (12/45), and cats with abortive FeLV infection never become viremic [9]. Abortive infections develop in immunocompetent cats. Due to effective immune response, these cats are able to terminate viral replication, and cats have no clinical signs [9]. Thus, immunocompetence is likely the reason for the missing enhanced pathogeniticity of hemoplasmas in the cats with abortive FeLV coinfections. In addition, all of the FeLV hemoplasma-coinfected cats were infected with Mhm, a strain that has an inherently low pathogenicity [2]. None of the progressively and regressively FeLV hemoplasma-coinfected cats showed clinical signs either. All this supports the hypothesis that the association of FIV and FeLV with hemoplasma spp. infection is likely the same mode of transmission and not necessarily an enhanced pathogenicity.

If hemoplasma spp. infection is clinically apparent, it usually results in regenerative hemolytic anemia [19]. In the present study, only 6 Mhm-infected of all 45 hemoplasma-infected cats had anemia. All of these cats had non-regenerative anemia, and other diseases that were likely responsible for the non-regenerative anemia (chronic kidney disease ($n = 3$), anemia of chronic disease caused by chronic respiratory tract disease ($n = 2$); tumor of the central nervous system ($n = 1$); chronic weight loss ($n = 1$)). Thus, other reasons than Mhm infection were presumably responsible for anemia in these cats. Although Mhf is thought to be more pathogenic, none of the Mhf-infected cats in the present study showed clinical signs. This could be due to a low hemoplasma load or infection with a less virulent strain. The Mhc-infected cat also showed no clinical signs of hemoplasmosis. Pathogenicity of this species in cats is unknown. Mhc can cause acute disease in immunosuppressed [6] or splenectomized dogs [13].

The major limitation of the study was the low number of cats with Mhf and Mhc infections and the fact that no cat in the present study was positive for Mtc. Thus, comparison between the different hemoplasma species was not possible. In addition, pretreatment of the cats in the present study was unknown, and treatment with antibiotics, e.g., doxycycline or enrofloxacin, prior to blood sampling could have led to termination of bacteremia and underestimation of hemoplasma prevalence [21].

Conclusions

Feline hemoplasma infection is relatively common in cats, and if cats are infected, they are usually infected with Mhm, a species with low pathogenicity. A higher risk exists for male sex, outdoor access, multi-cat environment, and FIV- and FeLV-infected cats which seems to be related to similar mechanisms for transmission during aggressive interactions and through arthropod vectors.

Abbreviations

Ca.: Candidatus; CBC: Complete blood count; DSH: Domestic Shorthair; ELISA: Enzyme-linked immunosorbent assay; FeLV: Feline leukemia virus; FIV: Feline immunodeficiency virus; M.: Mycoplasma; Mhc: Mycoplasma haemocanis; Mhf: Mycoplasma haemofelis; Mhm: 'Candidatus Mycoplasma haemominutum'; Mtc: 'Candidatus Mycoplasma turicensis'; n: Numbers of cats in every group; ns: Not significant; p: P-value; PCR: Polymerase chain reaction; spp.: Species

Acknowledgements

The authors would like to thank Prof. Dr. Ralf S. Mueller, Clinic of Small Animal Medicine, for his assistance in the statistical examination.
Parts of the results were presented as a poster at the ACVIM Symposium in San Francisco, USA, 2014.

Funding

This research received no grant from any funding agency in the public or commercial sectors but was supported in part by the Center for Companion Animal Studies, a non-profit organization, at Colorado State University.

Authors' contributions

KH chaired the research group. Acquisition of data was performed by TE under the supervision of KH. PCR was performed by BS and JH under the supervision of ML at the Veterinary Diagnostic Laboratories, Colorado State University. MB did the data analysis and wrote the paper. All authors read, commented, and approved the final manuscript.

Competing interests

The authors declare that they have no competing interests.

Consent for publication

Not applicable.

Author details

[1]Clinic of Small Animal Medicine, Centre for Clinical Veterinary Medicine, LMU Munich, Veterinaerstrasse 13, 80539 Munich, Germany. [2]Center for Companion Animal Studies, Department of Clinical Sciences, College of Veterinary Medicine and Biomedical Sciences, Colorado State University, Fort Collins, CO, USA.

References

1. Englert T, Lutz H, Sauter-Louis C, Hartmann K. Survey of the feline leukemia virus infection status of cats in Southern Germany. J Feline Med Surg. 2012;14:392–8.

2. Foley JE, Harrus S, Poland A, Chomel B, Pedersen NC. Molecular, clinical, and pathologic comparison of two distinct strains of Haemobartonella felis in domestic cats. Am J Vet Res. 1998;59:1581–8.

3. Fujihara Y, Sasaoka F, Suzuki J, Watanabe Y, Fujihara M, Ooshita K, Ano H, Harasawa R. Prevalence of hemoplasma infection among cattle in the western part of Japan. J Vet Med Sci. 2011;73:1653–5.

4. Gentilini F, Novacco M, Turba ME, Willi B, Bacci ML, Hofmann-Lehmann R. Use of combined conventional and real-time PCR to determine the epidemiology of feline haemoplasma infections in northern Italy. J Feline Med Surg. 2009;11:277–85.

5. George JW, Rideout BA, Griffey SM, Pedersen NC. Effect of pre-existing FeLV infection or FeLV and feline immunodeficiency virus coinfection on pathogenicity of the small variant of Haemobartonella felis in cats. Am J Vet Res. 2002;63:1172–8.

6. Handcock WJ. Clinical haemobartonellosis associated with use of corticosteroid. Vet Rec. 1989;125:585.

7. Hardy Jr WD, Hirshaut Y, Hess P. Detection of the feline leukemia virus and other mammalian oncornaviruses by immunofluorescence. Bibl Haematol. 1973;39:778–99.

8. Harrus S, Klement E, Aroch I, Stein T, Bark H, Lavy E, Mazaki-Tovi M, Baneth G. Retrospective study of 46 cases of feline haemobartonellosis in Israel and their relationships with FeLV and FIV infections. Vet Rec. 2002;151:82–5.

9. Hartmann K. Clinical aspects of feline retroviruses: a review. Viruses. 2012;4:2684–710.

10. Jensen WA, Lappin MR, Kamkar S, Reagan W. Use of a polymerase chain reaction assay to detect and differentiate two strains of Haemobartonella felis in naturally infected cats. Am J Vet Res. 2001;62:604–8.

11. Just F, Pfister K. Detection frequency of haemoplasma infections of the domestic cat in Germany. Berl Munch Tierarztl Wochenschr. 2007;120:197–201.

12. Laberke S, Just F, Pfister K, Hartmann K. Prevalence of feline haemoplasma infection in cats in Southern Bavaria, Germany, and infection risk factor analysis. Berl Munch Tierarztl Wochenschr. 2010;123:42–8.

13. Lester SJ, Hume JB, Phipps B. Haemobartonella canis infection following splenectomy and transfusion. Can Vet J. 1995;36:444–5.

14. Lobetti RG, Tasker S. Diagnosis of feline haemoplasma infection using a real-time PCR assay. J S Afr Vet Assoc. 2004;75:94–9.

15. Lumb WV. Canine haemobartonellosis and its feline counterpart. Calif Vet. 1961;14:24–5.

16. Luria BJ, Levy JK, Lappin MR, Breitschwerdt EB, Legendre AM, Hernandez JA, Gorman SP, Lee IT. Prevalence of infectious diseases in feral cats in Northern Florida. J Feline Med Surg. 2004;6:287–96.

17. Museux K, Boretti FS, Willi B, Riond B, Hoelzle K, Hoelzle LE, Wittenbrink MM, Tasker S, Wengi N, Reusch CE, Lutz H, Hofmann-Lehmann R. In vivo transmission studies of 'Candidatus Mycoplasma turicensis' in the domestic cat. Vet Res. 2009;40:45.

18. Novacco M, Meli ML, Gentilini F, Marsilio F, Ceci C, Pennisi MG, Lombardo G, Lloret A, Santos L, Carrapico T, Willi B, Wolf G, Lutz H, Hofmann-Lehmann R. Prevalence and geographical distribution of canine hemotropic mycoplasma infections in Mediterranean countries and analysis of risk factors for infection. Vet Microbiol. 2009;142:276–84.

19. Pennisi MG, Hartmann K, Addie DD. Blood transfusion in cats ABCD guidelines for minimizing risk of infectious iatrogen complications. J Feline Med Surg. 2015;17:588–93.

20. Piros des Santes A, de Oliveira Conrado F, Messick JB, Biondo AW, Tostes de Oliviera S, Sa Guimarares AM, Cannes do Nascimento N, Pedralli V, Lasta CS, Doiaz Gonzales FH. Hemplasma prevalence and hematological abnormalities associated with infection in three different cat populations from Southern Brazil. Braz J Vet Parasitol. 2014;23:428–34.

21. Reynolds CA, Lappin MR. "Candidatus Mycoplasma haemominutum" infections in 21 client-owned cats. J Am Anim Hosp Assoc. 2007;43:249–57.

22. Seneviratna P, Weerasinghe N, Ariyadasa S. Transmission of Haemobartonella canis by the dog tick, Rhipicephalus sanguineus. Res Vet Sci. 1973;14:112–4.

23. Sykes JE, Drazenovich NL, Ball LM, Leutenegger CM. Use of conventional and real-time polymerase chain reaction to determine the epidemiology of hemoplasma infections in anemic and nonanemic cats. J Vet Intern Med. 2007;21:685–93.

24. Sykes JE, Terry JC, Lindsay LL, Owens SD. Prevalences of various hemoplasma species among cats in the United States with possible hemoplasmosis. J Am Vet Med Assoc. 2008;232:372–9.

25. Weingart C, Tasker S, Kohn B. Infection with haemoplasma species in 22 cats with anemia. J Feline Med Surg. 2016;18:129–36.

26. Willi B, Tasker S, Boretti FS, Doherr MG, Cattori V, Meli ML, Lobetti RG, Malik R, Reusch CE, Lutz H, Hofmann-Lehmann R. Phylogenetic analysis of *Candidatus* Mycoplasma turicensis" isolates from pet cats in the United Kingdom, Australia, and South Africa, with analysis of risk factors for infection. J Clin Microbiol. 2006;44:4430–5.
27. Willi B, Boretti FS, Baumgartner C, Tasker S, Wenger B, Cattori V, Meli ML, Reusch CE, Lutz H, Hofmann-Lehmann R. Prevalence, risk factor analysis, and follow-up of infections caused by three feline hemoplasma species in cats in Switzerland. J Clin Microbiol. 2006;44:961–9.
28. Willi B, Novacco M, Meli M, Wolf-Jäckel G, Boretti F, Wengi N, Lutz H, Hofmann-Lehmann R. Haemotropic mycoplasmas of cats and dogs: transmission, diagnosis, prevalence and importance in Europe. Schweiz Arch Tierheilkd. 2010;152:237–44.

14

Sarcoptic mange in the Scandinavian wolf *Canis lupus* population

Boris Fuchs[1]* (iD), Barbara Zimmermann[1], Petter Wabakken[1], Set Bornstein[2], Johan Månsson[3], Alina L. Evans[1], Olof Liberg[3], Håkan Sand[3], Jonas Kindberg[4], Erik O. Ågren[5] and Jon M. Arnemo[1,4]

Abstract

Background: Sarcoptic mange, a parasitic disease caused by the mite *Sarcoptes scabiei*, is regularly reported on wolves *Canis lupus* in Scandinavia. We describe the distribution and transmission of this parasite within the small but recovering wolf population by analysing 269 necropsy reports and performing a serological survey on 198 serum samples collected from free-ranging wolves between 1998 and 2013.

Results: The serological survey among 145 individual captured Scandinavian wolves (53 recaptures) shows a consistent presence of antibodies against sarcoptic mange. Seropositivity among all captured wolves was 10.1 % (*CI.* 6.4 %–15.1 %). Sarcoptic mange-related mortality reported at necropsy was 5.6 % and due to secondary causes, predominantly starvation. In the southern range of the population, seroprevalence was higher, consistent with higher red fox densities. Female wolves had a lower probability of being seropositive than males, but for both sexes the probability increased with pack size. Recaptured individuals changing from seropositive to seronegative suggest recovery from sarcoptic mange. The lack of seropositive pups (8–10 months, $N = 56$) and the occurrence of seropositive and seronegative individuals in the same pack indicates interspecific transmission of *S. scabiei* into this wolf population.

Conclusions: We consider sarcoptic mange to have little effect on the recovery of the Scandinavian wolf population. Heterogenic infection patterns on the pack level in combination with the importance of individual-based factors (sex, pack size) and the north–south gradient for seroprevalence suggests low probability of wolf-to-wolf transmission of *S. scabiei* in Scandinavia.

Keywords: *Canis lupus*, Grey wolf, *Sarcoptes scabiei*, Sarcoptic mange, Ectoparasites, ELISA, Red fox, *Vulpes vulpes*, Wildlife disease

Background

Sarcoptic mange is an epizootic skin disease caused by the mite *Sarcoptes scabiei* worldwide infesting over 100 mammalian hosts including wild and domestic canids [1, 2]. The mite, burrowing through the stratum corneum, causes the host to mount a humoral immunological response [3–5]. Wolves *Canis lupus* infested by *S. scabiei*, develop alopecia due to intense scratching and biting triggered by a hypersensitive response and may become debilitated and emaciated due to secondary bacterial infections and difficulties in catching the natural prey [1, 2, 6]. *S. scabiei* infections can reduce pack size, annual pack growth rate and cause additive mortality [7, 8]. However, recovery from even severe sarcoptic mange on wolves is reported from northern Spain and Yellowstone National Park [7, 9].

S. scabiei actively seek olfactory and thermal stimuli and are able to survive, in suitable environments, for up to 19 days off the host. All life stages remain infective for at least one-half to two-thirds of their survival time [10]. Transmission normally occurs through close contact between hosts and is assumed to be host-density dependent [1] but also fomites in the host environment can be a source of transmission [10]. In Yellowstone National Park, the spatio-temporal patterns of *S. scabiei* infestation on wolves are related to distance to the next infested pack, indicating wolf-to-wolf transmission [7]. In Scandinavia interspecific transmission of *S. scabiei* var. *vulpes* from red fox *Vulpes vulpes* is the most likely

* Correspondence: boris.fuchs@hihm.no
[1]Faculty of Applied Ecology and Agricultural Sciences, Hedmark University College, Campus Evenstad, N-2480 Koppang, Norway
Full list of author information is available at the end of the article

origin for mange in wolves, domestic dog *Canis lupus familiaris*, arctic fox *Alopex lagopus*, lynx *Lynx lynx* and domestic cat *Felis catus* [11, 12]. In northern Spain, wolves are infested with *S. scabiei* originated from both red foxes and ungulates, emphasising the prey-to-predator transmission [13].

The wolf was regarded as functionally extinct in Scandinavia during the late 1960's. In 1983, two immigrant wolves from the Finnish-Russian wolf population reproduced for the first time and became the founders of the present Scandinavian wolf population, [14–16]. During the following 30 years, the population increased from less than 10 individuals to an estimated size of approximately 400 wolves [17]. By 2013, only five Finnish-Russian founders had genetically contributed to this population, and severe inbreeding depression has been confirmed [15]. Although mortality of Scandinavian wolves is mainly human-caused [18], sarcoptic mange may be an important cause of natural mortality [11]. Sarcoptic mange arrived in Scandinavia in the mid-1970's with devastating effects on the red fox population, [19, 20]. A previous study focusing on immunoglobulin E (IgE) levels found 14/57 Scandinavian wolves seropositive for sarcoptic mange [21]. Effects of sarcoptic mange on the demography of the Scandinavian wolf population remain unclear but have the potential to influence this small, inbred population. Here we analyse and present an overview of the distribution of sarcoptic mange in the Scandinavian wolf population.

Between 1998 and 2013 a total of 198 serum samples from live wolves were collected and analysed by two different enzyme-linked immunosorbent assays (ELISA) and complemented by Western Blot. In addition, we evaluated necropsy reports of 269 dead wolves collected in Sweden between 2003 and 2013.

The aim of our study is to describe the occurrence of sarcoptic mange in the Scandinavian wolf population and to identify demographic and environmental factors that relate to the probability of finding seropositive samples. Based on the literature and personal observations we expected sarcoptic mange to be a minor threat to the Scandinavian wolf population. We predicted the probability of sarcoptic mange occurrence to depend on population level factors including red fox and wolf territory density rather than on individual-based factors such as age and sex of wolves.

Results

Seropositivity on captured wolves

In total 178 of the 198 samples (89.9 %) (Tables 1 and 2) were tested seronegative and 20 samples (10.1 %, Wilson 95 % CI 6.4 %–15.1 %) were tested seropositive. Mean annual proportion of seropositive samples was 11.3 % (SE 2.5 %), ranging from 40.0 % in 1999 ($N = 5$) to zero

Table 1 Demographic distribution of the serum samples and observed lesions indicating sarcoptic mange among the captured individuals

		Total number of serum samples	Seropositive serum samples
Pups	Pups total	56	0
	Females	28	0
	Males	28	0
	Single/Dispersing	0	0
	Pair	0	0
	Pack	56	0
	Unclear pack structure	0	0
	Alopecia reported	0	0
Adults	Adults total	142	20
	Females	66	6
	Males	76	14
	Single/Dispersing	11	1
	Pair	54	6
	Pack	71	13
	Unclear pack structure	6	1
	Alopecia reported	9	7

Pups are < 1 year old, adults > 1 year old. Single/Dispersing wolves are outside the parental territory and have no territory established yet. Pairs are a male and a female in an established territory. Packs are one or two reproducing wolves with their < 2 year old offspring. Alopecia reported on the capture form

in 2008 ($N = 7$) and 2010 ($N = 15$) (Fig. 1a). The annual proportion of the wolf population that was sampled decreased during the study period ($\chi_{1,13} = 18.82$; $p < 0.01$) (Fig. 1b). The annual sample size did not allow for further temporal analysis.

Among the 38 recaptured individuals, eight were tested seropositive at least once. Six were seropositive at first capture and four seronegative at recapture 1 year later. Two individuals were seropositive both at first capture and at recapture 2 years later (Table 2).

In 61 of 95 territory sampling events, multiple wolves were captured within the same territory. In 13 of these 61 sampling events, at least one individual was seropositive and there were always also seronegative wolves in the same sampling event. In two family groups, both the adult male and female tested seropositive but their captured pups (two each) were seronegative at time of capture. In eight territories, seropositive individuals were recaptured and six tested seronegative at recapture. In one territory, both the adult male and female were captured in two consecutive years, the male tested seropositive twice and the female seronegative twice.

Sarcoptic mange from wolves at necropsy

The average annual prevalence of sarcoptic mange among dead wolves collected in Sweden between 2003

Table 2 Results from ELISA and Western Blot analysis

ID Wolf	Sampling date	Sex	Age class	OD MSA – 1	OD Crude	Result ELISAs	Western Blots
9802	15.12.1998	Male	Adult	0.71	0.83	++	++
9803	15.12.1998	Female	Adult	0.73	0.91	++	+
9808	27.01.2000	Male	Adult	0.11	0.32	−+	−
0001	28.01.2000	Male	Adult	1.54	2.18	++	++
0002	28.01.2000	Female	Adult	0.11	0.09	−	-
0003	28.01.2000	Female	Juvenile	0.05	0.07	−	-
0104	10.02.2001	Female	Adult	1.14	1.20	++	++
0105	10.02.2001	Male	Adult	1.66	1.96	++	++
0105	05.02.2003	Male	Adult	0.76	0.73	++	+
0109	12.02.2001	Male	Adult	0.63	0.11	+−	-
0109	08.12.2001	Male	Adult	0.34	0.13	−	-
0106	12.02.2001	Female	Juvenile	0.11	0.14	−	-
0111	21.12.2001	Female	Adult	0.20	0.30	-?	+
0203	13.01.2002	Female	Adult	0.17	0.24	-?	-
0208	26.01.2002	Male	Adult	0.41	0.15	?-	-
0208	06.03.2003	Male	Adult	1.32	1.30	++	+
0215	01.02.2002	Male	Adult	0.20	0.25	-?	-
0214	05.03.2003	Male	Adult	0.70	0.92	++	+
0214	21.01.2004	Male	Adult	0.41	0.65	?+	+
0307	06.03.2003	Female	Adult	0.15	0.23	-?	-
0009	23.01.2004	Male	Adult	0.36	0.13	?-	-
0504	14.03.2005	Male	Adult	0.40	0.42	?+	+
0506	16.03.2005	Male	Adult	0.56	0.19	+−	?+
0506	09.03.2007	Male	Adult	0.43	0.07	?-	-
0507	16.03.2005	Female	Juvenile	0.26	0.15	−	-
0507	08.02.2008	Female	Adult	0.65	0.13	+−	-
0601	27.01.2006	Female	Adult	0.44	0.37	?+	-
0606	01.02.2006	Male	Adult	0.22	0.36	−+	+
0606	08.03.2007	Male	Adult	0.12	0.20	−	
0611	13.02.2006	Male	Adult	0.22	0.25	-?	+
0611	11.03.2007	Male	Adult	0.43	0.21	??	-
0704	07.03.2007	Female	Adult	0.67	0.70	++	+
0913	30.01.2009	Male	Juvenile	0.10	0.35	−+	-
0916	11.02.2009	Male	Adult	1.50	0.40	++	+
0918	12.02.2009	Male	Adult	1.01	0.80	++	+
0918	11.02.2010	Male	Adult	0.23	0.19	−	
1004	10.02.2010	Female	Juvenile	0.18	0.22	-?	-
1114	21.03.2011	Female	Adult	0.73	0.39	++	+
1114	11.12.2011	Female	Adult	0.98	0.37	++	-
1114	06.02.2012	Female	Adult	0.81	0.35	++	?-
1114	14.03.2013	Female	Adult	1.19	0.37	++	+
1202	16.12.2011	Male	Adult	1.54	0.98	++	+

OD MSA-1: Relative optical densities using the MSA-1 antigen in the ELISA, cut off are 0.35 (doubtful) and 0.499 (seropositive) respectively. OD Crude: Relative optical densities using the crude antigen in the ELISA, cut off 0.2 (doubtful) and 0.299 (seropositive). Result ELISAs are corresponding to the OD values and decide between: + (positive), − (negative) and ? (doubtful). Shown are all samples with either positive or doubtful results from one of the ELISA and five random selected with negative results

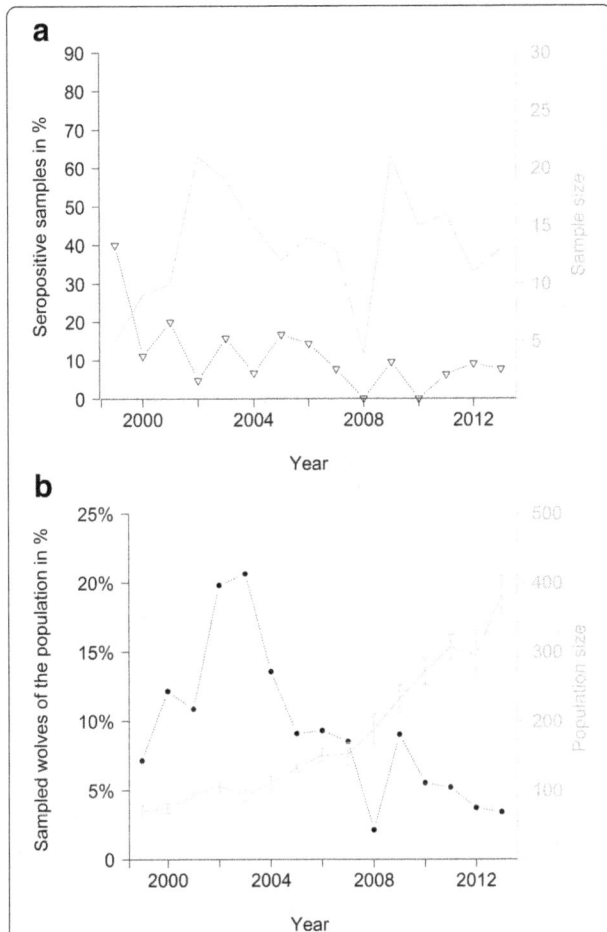

Fig. 1 The proportion of seropositive samples (**a**) and the sample size as the percentage of the Scandinavian wolf population (**b**). Triangles (**a**) show the proportion of seropositive samples to the sampled number of wolves each year (grey line). Solid dots (**b**) show the percentage of sampled wolves. The grey line (**b**) represents the mean number of individual wolves reported in Scandinavia with error bars representing minimum and maximum estimations [17]

it was not possible to include the necropsy data in to the statistical analysis.

The age distribution of the 19 wolves with known age and lesions of mange at necropsy was nine pups (5 to 12 months old; 47.3 %), seven juveniles (1 and 2 years old 36.8 %), and three adults (2 to 6 years old 15.8 %). The majority (9 and 7 respectively) of these wolves came from two different wolf territories. In one territory the adult pair and two 9 months old pups were captured. At capture, the adults were seropositive, while the pups were seronegative. However, the pups were euthanized at the age of 15 and 19 months due to lesions from sarcoptic mange [22]. One of them was seropositive at necropsy, while the serum of the other was not tested.

Probability of seropositive samples

All 56 pups captured within their parental territories, were seronegative and did not show any lesions of sarcoptic mange. They were therefore excluded from the statistical analysis. Annual mean seroprevalence of the adult population was 19.9 % (SE 6.5 %).

The model combining the population-level predictor latitude and the individual-based interaction of sex and pack size was the most parsimonious (Table 3). According to the relative AICc weight ratio, it had 1.5 higher evidence than the next-best model, which included the wolf territory density. Both models passed model validation with $r_s > 0.8$ (Table 3), but r_s is not penalized for additional variables. By adding body condition or removing pack size, the models decreased in evidence but remained within the AICc cut off value (Table 3). Latitude correlated negatively with the likelihood of finding seropositive adult wolves for all combinations of sex and pack size except for females in pairs (Fig. 2a, Table 4). The probability of finding seropositive adult wolves was 6.1 to 8.2 times higher in the southern part (eg UTM 6 600 000, seroprevalence males 36.5 %, females 10.5 %) in packs with 6 wolves (mean size of reproducing packs), as compared to the northern edge of the wolf distribution. The probability of finding seropositive adult males increased linearly with pack size, from 6.6 % seroprevalence in pairs to 38.9 % seroprevalence in packs of eight wolves in the southern part of the study area. For adult females in the same area, the model predicted a seroprevalence of 37.1 % for packs of eight wolves. No adult female from a pair without pups was seropositive, the model predicts a seroprevalence < 1 %.

Red fox harvest data was available for 49 Swedish territory centre points throughout the study period. There was no difference in red fox densities between territories with seropositive wolves (harvested red fox per 1000 ha ± SE = 1.6 ± 0.5) and territories with only seronegative wolves (harvested red fox per 1000 ha ± SE = 1.4 ± 0.2) (t = −0.31, df = 9.4; $p = 0.77$). However, the fox harvest

and 2013 was 4.5 % (SE = 1.3 %, N = 269). In the same period, seropositivity rate of sarcoptic mange among captured wolves in Sweden was 7.6 % (SE = 2.5 %, N = 112). Of the total 21 wolves considered to have sarcoptic mange at necropsy, ten were euthanized due to mange-caused emaciated status (starvation and alopecia), two were illegally shot, two were shot during licence hunt, one was culled to prevent predation on livestock, one was euthanized after a traffic accident and five were found dead. Of the five wolves found dead, four died due to mange-related starvation and one after a traffic accident. In summary, 15 (5.6 %) of the known wolf mortalities reported by the Swedish National Veterinary Institute (SVA) in Sweden between 2003 and 2013 were either euthanized or died because of sarcoptic mange. A systematic serological survey was not carried out on the necropsied wolves, thus

Table 3 Model selection for predictors of seroprevalence of sarcoptic mange in adult wolves captured in Scandinavia

Model	Parameters	K	AIC$_c$	ΔAIC$_c$	ω$_i$	r$_s$(SE)
Combined	Lat + Sex * Pack Size	5	78.16	0	0.38	0.86(0.02)
+ Density	Lat + Sex * Pack Size + Territory Density	6	79.00	0.84	0.24	0.86(0.03)
+ Body Condition	Lat + Sex * Pack Size + Body Condition	6	79.04	0.88	0.24	0.59(0.03)
– Pack Size	Lat + Sex	3	80.57	2.41	0.12	0.62(0.03)
Submodel intrinsic	Sex * Pack Size	4	83.36	5.20	0.01	-
Submodel density	Lat + Pack Size	3	84.83	6.67	0.01	-
Density	Lat + Long + Pack Size + Territory Density	4	88.47	10.31	0	-
Intrinsic	Sex * Pack Size + Body Condition + Age + Repro	6	90.41	12.25	0	-
Null model	1	1	92.00	13.84	0	-

Top models are validated by k-fold cross validation (r$_s$). Lat / Long: Latitude and longitude of the territory centre point, Repro: Reproducing or non-reproducing pair, Pack Size: Number of wolves within the territory, Territory Density: Mean Euclidian distance to the next three territory centre points, Body Condition: Individual residual distance to the linear regression line of log body weight and log body length. Presented are the two main models (Intrinsic, Density), the top models for each variable group, the model combining the top submodels, the combined model with variables ranking within the cut off in the variable group model selection and the null model

decreased along the geographical gradient from the southern to the northern most territories (Fig. 3; r^2 = – 0.59, df = 43, $p < 0.001$).

Discussion

The higher probability to find Scandinavian wolves seropositive to sarcoptic mange in their southern population range is consistent with a higher red fox density and higher habitat productivity resulting in smaller wolf territory size as described by J Mattisson, et al. [23] in these southern latitudes. The positive association between habitat productivity and frequency of mange on wolves is also reported from Yellowstone National Park [7]. In northern Spain reported seroprevalence (20 %, $N = 17/88$) is two times higher than the seropositivity rate in Scandinavia. This difference may be related to higher wildlife densities and more contact to livestock and domestic dogs in Spain [9, 24]. However, we could not find a direct relationship between red fox density and the occurrence of seropositive individual wolves. Reasons for this could be that red fox bag statistics do not represent the density of

infectious red foxes especially after a regional mange outbreak [25], and the occurrence of infected wolves after a mange peak in the red fox might be delayed [9]. Bag statistics in general have been shown to be an appropriate index to estimate population densities [25, 26].

Consistent with previous reports [7, 9], we found wolves that had recovered from sarcoptic mange and also cases of coexistence of seropositive wolves, both with and without clinical symptoms, with seronegative and healthy wolves within the territory. But we also had other cases with high mortality on the pack scale. Coinfection with other diseases in this population such as canine distemper virus (CDV), causing immune depression, could lead to increased mortality [27, 28]. The risk for a host to get infected may relate to the initial mite load. Possibly a threshold needs to be reached to overwhelm the host's immune system, resulting in a high total mite load and increased probability to spread the disease. In humans, *S. scabiei* transmission usually occurs in close body contact and patients carrying >100 adult female mites are much more likely to spread

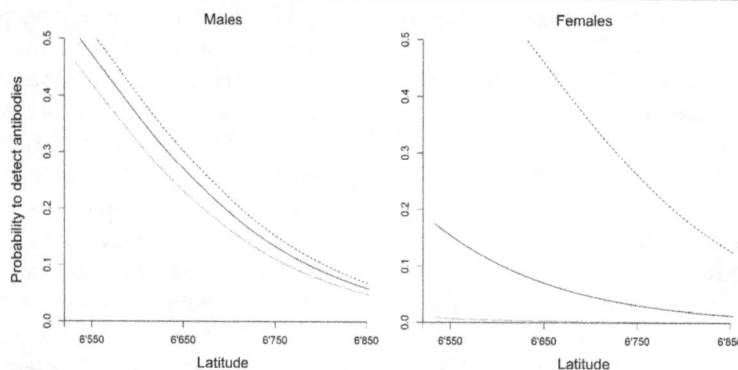

Fig. 2 Probability of seropositive serum samples from captured wolves depending on sex, pack size and latitude. Dotted line for pairs, solid line for a pack of six wolves and dashed for a pack with eight wolves. Both figures show the back transformed and averaged predictions of the combined model with e$^{(Combined/(1+Combined))}$

Table 4 Top model estimates explaining seroprevalence of sarcoptic mange in adult wolves captured in Scandinavia

Factors	Estimate	SE	Lower CI	Upper CI
Intercept	−57.16	26.3	5.56	108.76
Lat	- 0.88	0.39	- 1.64	- 0.11
Sex _female_	- 6.12	3.67	- 13.31	1.07
Pack Size	0.05	0.15	- 0.24	0.34
Sex _female_ * Pack Size	0.76	0.46	- 0.15	1.66
Territory Density	0.02	0.02	- 0.01	0.05
Body Condition	−4.09	3.53	- 11.01	2.82

Estimates are averaged among the four top models. Lat: Latitude of the territory centre point, Pack Size: Number of wolves within the territory, Territory Density: Mean Euclidian distance to the next three territory centre points, Body Condition: Individual residual distance to the linear regression line of log body weight and log body length

the disease than patients with lower mite rates [29]. Á Oleaga, et al. [9] reported mite rates of <100 isolated mites on wolves and a negative relation of isolated mites to the area of alopecic skin, suggesting a certain ability to control the mite development. The hypersensitive reaction leading to pruritus and alopecia might be present even if the mite rate is low [6]. In Yellowstone National Park, within-pack transmission occurs. Almberg et al. [30] reported a 61 % increased risk of individual infection with a 10 % increased prevalence within packs and that mortality hazards increased with the proportion of infected pack members or ambient temperatures above average but decreased with increasing prey availability.

The large proportion of young wolves among the infested individuals at necropsy demonstrates their sensitivity once infested with sarcoptic mange. In several North American wolf populations, sarcoptic mange

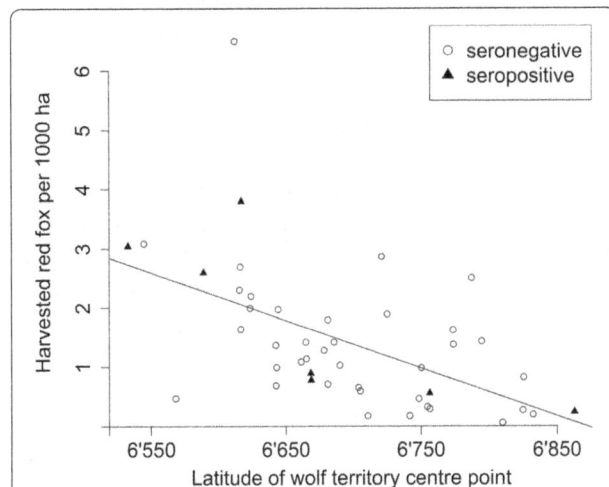

Fig. 3 Harvested red fox per 1000 ha for each sampled Swedish wolf territory along the latitudinal gradient (N = 49). Circles indicate territories with only seronegative samples, and triangles indicate territories with at least one seropositive sample in the respective years

decreased pup survival [8, 31, 32]. In Scandinavia, a large part of the mange-infested subadult wolves at necropsy came from only two territories and among the captured individuals, none of the pups were seropositive. We cannot rule out low detectability of infested pups due to high mortality before sampling during winter. In this case we would expect some seropositive survivors and, a negative relation between seroprevalence in adults and pack size. This is not supported by our findings. A seasonal cycle on wolves with lesions of mange has been observed in the Yellowstone National Park with peaks in November on population scale and in January on pack scale [30]. Our samples are collected between December and March.

During winter, Scandinavian wolf pups may be separated from their parents for a large part of the time even though they do not leave the territory until dispersal and do not generally contribute to the food acquirement of the family group [33]. For these wolf pups, exposure to live or recently-killed mange-infested red fox is likely to be very low. Experimentally measured seroconversion in domestic dogs and red foxes takes up to 1–5 weeks post-infection and 1–3 weeks from onset of clinical signs [3, 34] and persists for 1 to > 4.5 months after successful treatment in domestic dogs [35]. Infected pups, 7 to 10 months old at capture, would likely be detected by the ELISA. We suggest that wolf pups in Scandinavia are less exposed to S. scabiei than adults.

In contrast to other studies on sarcoptic mange and wolves [24, 30, 31], we found a lower probability of seroprevalence in adult females of small packs. Sex differences in the humoral response to sarcoptic mange are found in Iberian ibex Capra pyrenaica hispanica infested with S. scabiei and higher Immunoglobulin G (IgG) levels in females than males [36]. Higher IgG levels in females could lead to a longer duration of measurable antibody response potentially resulting, in contrast to our findings, in a higher detectability. Considering the observed recoveries, if higher antibody titres would lead to a faster clearance of the mite, detectability could be lower. IgG levels are currently not available for this data set and IgE or IgA levels measured on a subset of the wolf samples did not differ between males and females nor between mange seropositive and seronegative sera [21, 37] The observed positive correlation of mange prevalence in adult female wolves with pack size may be related to increased susceptibility to parasites during parturition and lactation [6].

Due to the high sociality and the monogamous mating system, sex differences in behaviour of breeding wolves are expected to be small, except during the early stage of nursing the pups [38]. Wolves display sexual dimorphism as male wolves are 20–30 % heavier than females [16, 39] and have a higher food intake [33, 40]. Exposure might be higher for males if they spend more time on carcasses shared with infested red foxes. The breeding wolf pairs in Scandinavia move together and use their territory equally during most of the year [23, 41]. However, we do not know if individual male and female wolves have different predation patterns on red fox or domestic dogs. Considering the assumption of restricted mite development on wolves and the heterogenic patterns on pack scale, individual variation regarding infection paths and immunological response might play an important role. Our small sample size, not allowing us to control for individual variation, might bias model based estimates on individual factors such as sex. Individuals to be captured where chosen according to the research- or management questions and sampling was opportunistic. However, to our knowledge this is the largest serological survey for sarcoptic mange on free-ranging wolves. This is a retrospective study, clinical evaluation of the captured animals was not standardized, did not classify mange lesions, or reports were incomplete. For seven of the 20 seropositive wolves, lesion consistent with sarcoptic mange (alopecia) was noted at capture. For five seropositive wolves normal fur was noted at capture and for eight seropositive wolves information was missing. Two wolves with seropositive test results had clinical signs (alopecia) at capture. No skin biopsies or skin scrapings have been conducted. We therefore were not able to define a nominal reference gold standard and do not report sensitivity and specificity of the ELISA. We confirmed the diagnosis using two ELISAs with different antigens in parallel and Western Blot in addition. Previous studies reported sensitivity and specificity of 92 and 96 % respectively, on domestic dogs with acute sarcoptic mange and 95 and 98 % in chronic cases applying the crude antigen [42]. For the same ELISA, sensitivity and specificity of 95 and 83 % respectively are reported on wild Norwegian red fox [43]. We assume similar values for the wolves, considering the close phylogenetic relation of the domestic dog and the red fox to the wolf. The ELISA using the MSA-1 along with the crude antigen is today used by SVA to diagnose sarcoptic mange on domestic dogs but not validated yet. We consider the three analyses to complement each other and assume sensitivity and specificity at least as high as in the validation studies.

Conclusions

Although continuously present, we do not consider sarcoptic mange as a significant factor of the sustainability and recovery of the Scandinavian wolf population. Wolf pups are less exposed to the parasite and mange dynamics in the wolf population are not related to the local density of wolf territories. Heterogenic seroprevalence distribution within the packs and repeated observed

recovery suggest an effective host - parasite response and a restricted wolf-to-wolf transmission. This disease cannot be regarded as a potential factor controlling population growth at this stage of population development. However, devastating mortality may occur on individual pack scale as a result of this parasite. The higher probability of sarcoptic mange in the southern part of the wolf distribution is probably related to landscape factors and red fox population dynamics. Sarcoptic mange could potentially become more important along with a southern expansion of the Scandinavian wolf population. Future research should address the individual humoral response of wolves and other canids to *S. scabiei*. In Scandinavia, the scale of research should include the entire carnivore guild for a more complete view on the dynamics and effects of this important disease.

Methods
Study area
The Scandinavian wolf population is located in central Sweden and south-eastern Norway (between 59 and 62°N, and 10–15°E) (Fig. 4) [17]. The area is primarily covered by managed forest stands of Norway spruce *Picea abies* and Scots pine *Pinus sylvestris* and wet lands, agricultural areas and settlements covering minor areas, primarily in the southern part of the wolf range [23]. The human population density is less than $1/km^2$ in large areas of the main wolf range [16]. The climate is continental with average temperatures of 15 °C in June and –7 °C in January and the area is snow covered from December to March with an average depth of 30–60 cm [41]. The main prey species are moose *Alces alces* and roe deer *Capreolus capreolus*, the latter mainly in the southern range of the wolf area. Other prey species represent a minor proportion of the diet [33, 44].

Serum collection and analysis
A total of 198 serum samples from 145 individual free-ranging wolves of 54 different packs in Sweden and Norway were analysed. All wolves were immobilized by darting from a helicopter during winter (December-March) between 1998 and 2013 as part of a long term joint Scandinavian research project or by national management, both following standard capture procedures [45] and in accordance with the NC3Rs ARRIVE guidelines for reporting animal research [46]. Captured animals were tagged with VHF or GPS collars and ear tags or microchips and the identity further confirmed by DNA- and pedigree analysis [15]. To change radio collars or for translocations 38 individuals were recaptured 1–3 times (Table 5). A sampling event per territory was defined as one or more wolves captured per winter within a pack, including recaptures. Sampled animals

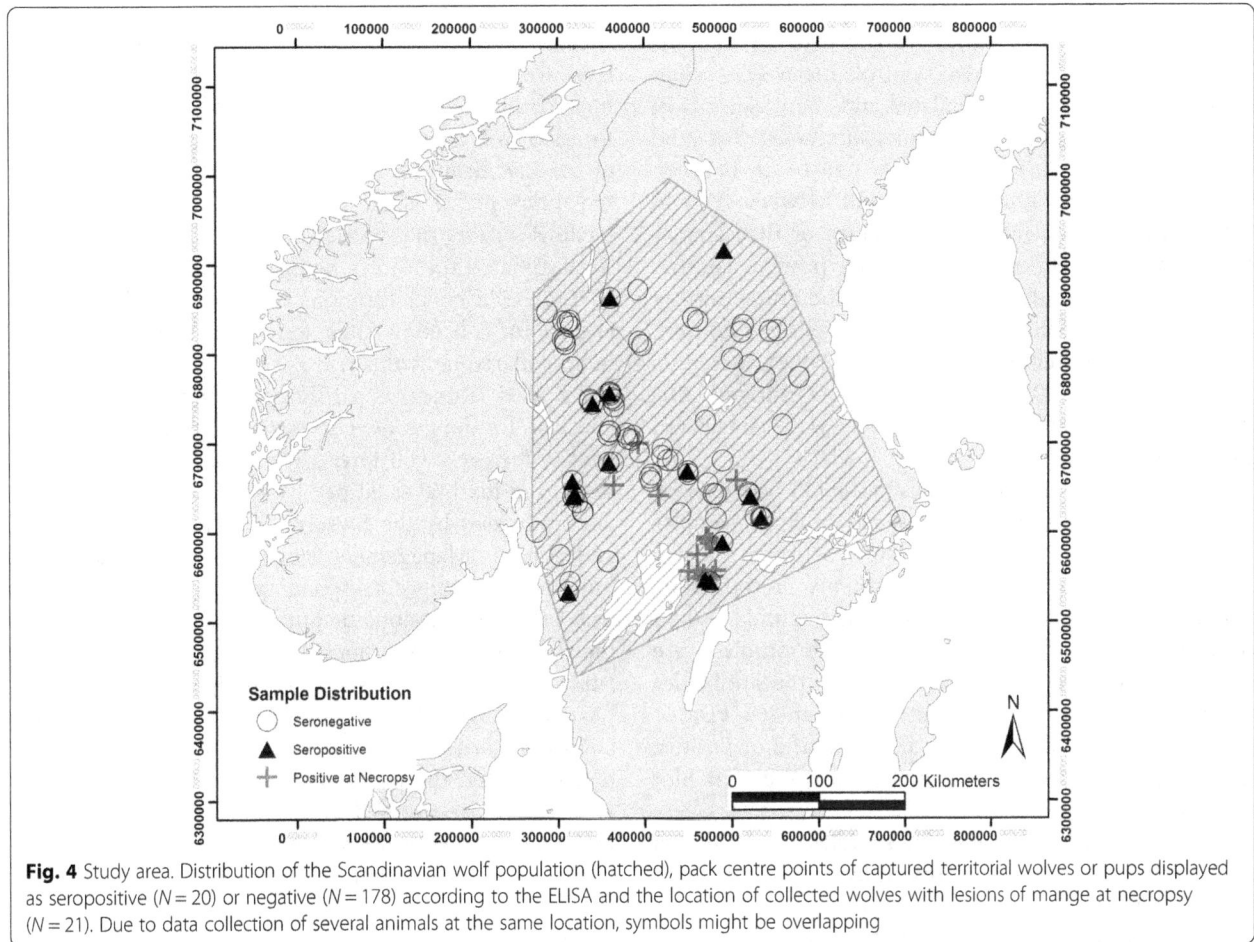

Fig. 4 Study area. Distribution of the Scandinavian wolf population (hatched), pack centre points of captured territorial wolves or pups displayed as seropositive (*N* = 20) or negative (*N* = 178) according to the ELISA and the location of collected wolves with lesions of mange at necropsy (*N* = 21). Due to data collection of several animals at the same location, symbols might be overlapping

were sexed (104 males, 94 females), weighed and measured. As a proxy for body condition, we used the residual distance from each individual to the linear regression line of log body weight and log body length (nose to base of the tail) estimated from all individuals in the data set [47]. This residual index was no longer correlated to body length ($r = -0.01$, df = 104, $p = 0.94$). The animals were grouped into pups (<1 year old) and adults. The age was estimated from tooth wear in adults and pups were identified by the growth zone on the radius and ulna [48]. Based on movement data from GPS-collared wolves, pups were assumed to be born in early

May [49]. The age of the sampled wolves ranged from 7 to 10 months for pups and over 10 years for adults. Age was adjusted if pedigree analysis could prove the year of birth. Clinical evaluation of the captured wolves was not standardized but anomalies, such as previous injuries, broken teeth or mange lesion, are mentioned on the capture form. Blood was collected from the cephalic vein using 8 ml sterile, evacuated serum-separator tubes with gel and clot activator (Venosafe™, Terumo Europe N.V, Leuven, Belgium). Serum was separated by centrifugation at 1500 rpm for 15 min the same day and kept frozen until shipment to the laboratory (Department of Virology, Immunobiology and Parasitology, SVA Uppsala, Sweden).

Serum samples were analysed by running two parallel ELISAs using a crude (*S. scabiei* var. *vulpes* extract) antigen according to Bornstein et al. 1993 [34], modified by a change of the substrate from 5-amino-2-hydroxybenzoic to 3-3-5 tetramethylebenzidin (TBM) and a recombinant major *S. scabiei* var. *vulpes* antigen (MSA-1) respectively [50]. In each series, samples were tested in duplicates and positive and negative control samples from dogs were included. Optical density (OD) was

Table 5 Age and recaptures among the captured individuals

| | Captured individuals | Recaptures | | | Total samples |
		1	2	3	
Pups	56				56
Pups, recaptured as adults		13	5	1	19
Adults	89	25	6	3	123
Total	145	38	11	4	198

Pups are < 1 year old, adults > 1 year old

measured at 450 nm with a multiscan EX (Thermo Labsystems, Vantaa, Finland). In order to get an OD value relative to the positive control, mean OD values for each duplicate were calculated and the mean OD of a blank (PBS-T instead of a sample) subtracted. For valid results, positive control OD values had to be between 0.8 and 1.6 for the crude antigen and between 0.7 and 2.0 for the MSA-1 antigen. OD values of the samples were divided by the OD value of the positive control. Positive results should reach > 0.3 for the crude antigen and > 0.5 for the MSA-1, relative to the positive control. Doubtful results were defined as 0.2–0.299 by the crude antigen and 0.35–0.499 by the MSA-1 antigen, OD values below 0.2 and 0.35 respectively were considered to be negative.

Western Blot as previously described [3], was used to confirm all seropositive samples, all doubtful samples and all samples with different results between the two ELISAs. In brief, the sarcoptes proteins in the crude antigen extract were separated by their atomic weight (kDa) on a nitrocellulose membrane. The samples were exposed to the proteins. When positive, the antibodies in the samples bound with the protein at 164 kDa or 147 kDa and 105 kDa. Samples with doubtful or positive ELISA values but confirmed positive by Western Blot were considered as seropositive.

The proportion of seropositive samples are presented with confidence intervals estimated by the Wilson score method [51].

Necropsy reports
After 2002, all dead wolves found in Sweden have been delivered for standard necropsy at SVA. Serology as described above (N = 15), microscopy (N = 4) or both (N = 2) were part of the standard necropsy if clinical signs of sarcoptic mange were detected. We compared observed seropositivity from captured Swedish wolves from 2003 to 2013 with the necropsy data.

Population data
The annual monitoring of the Scandinavian wolf population for the entire study area was based on snow tracking, DNA-analyses of scats and radio/GPS collar data [52]. This monitoring provided, for each winter, the total number and geographical distribution of established pairs and packs and estimates of pack- and population size. We expressed wolf density at two spatial scales. Within wolf territories, pack size represented the number of wolves per territory and ranged from one to ten wolves. The samples were classified as from single wolves, from pairs (two scent marking animals of opposite sex) or packs (one or two scent marking animals and pups or yearlings). Wolves older than two years within the parental territory and both parents present have

until the end of the study period not been detected by the monitoring in Scandinavia [17]. At the landscape level, we used distance to neighbouring packs as a proxy for territory density. We estimated the territory densitiy for each wolf territory and for each winter as the average of the Euclidean distances between its centre point and the centre points of the three nearest neighbouring wolf territories using the spatstat package [53] in R 3.0.3 [54]. We estimated the centre point coordinates by averaging VHF or GPS collar locations of territorial adult wolves, and DNA collection sites for wolf territories without radio-collared individuals.

We used latitude as a habitat productivity proxy and checked for longitude effects. As a proxy of red fox density for each wolf territory, we used the yearly number of red fox harvested per 10 km^2. These bag statistics were provided by the Swedish Association for Hunting and Wildlife Management on the hunting management unit level (mainly corresponding to a municipality) in Sweden. Mange lesions or other qualitative measures of the shot red fox were not reported. Using a two sample t-test, we tested if occurrence of seropositive wolves was related to high red fox densities. We used the red fox harvest record from those hunting management units that contained the centre points of the wolf territories. Accordingly, we tested if the latitude of the centre points was related to the red fox harvest record in the respective hunting management units.

Modelling seroprevalence
According to our hypothesis we formulated two full models à priori: 1) The individual-based model correlated the probability to find a seropositive serum sample to individual-based intrinsic factors; reproductive state, age, body condition, and the interaction of sex and pack size, assuming more physical contact of reproducing females with their pups, as well as a potential negative effect on pup survival with seropositive females. 2) The population-based model correlated the probability to find a positive serum sample to territory density, and to the projected, metric latitude and longitude of the wolf territory. Territory size of Scandinavian wolves increases with latitude, independently of available moose biomass but related to landscape structure and climate [23]. We did not include red fox density in this model because of missing values for the Norwegian territories. The response variable in both models was a binary term with 1 for seropositive and 0 for seronegative wolves, and models were statistically estimated using logistic regression. Due to a low number of events (seropositive) the risk of over-fitted models increases rapidly with every included variable [55]. We formulated sub models with fewer variables and included them in the selection.

Within both variable groups sub-models performed better than the full models (Table 3).

All analyses were done using statistical extensions available in R 3.0.3 [54]. Despite the inclusion recaptured individuals we did not include nested random factors to the models. This decision was based on the lack of the among-individual variance to the binary response variable resulting in a negligible effect when included as a random factor [56]. A large proportion of the individuals (107 of 145, Table 5) were sampled only once. In addition, the time interval between capture events was long enough for individuals to change from seropositive and seronegative and vice versa [34, 36]. The variance inflation factor of any continuous variable was <1 indicating no multicollinearity [57] and models did not show outliers (Cook's distance) [58].

We selected by parsimony for each full model the best sub-model (lowest AICc using the R-package AICcmodvag, no cut off). Then we used a cut-off point of delta AICc = 4 to find the best combination of predictors from both sub-models. Further, we used model-averaging to present the effect sizes of the predictors of the models within the cut-off [59]. Observations with lacking data were omitted before model selection ($N = 36$). Robustness of the selected models was verified by k-fold cross validation. The models were run 100 times on a training set including randomly selected 90 % of the data. Using the estimates of the training set, probabilities of being seropositive were predicted for the remaining 10 %. The predicted values were sorted and grouped into 10 equal-sized, ranked bins. For each bin, the frequency of seropositive individuals was correlated with the rank of the bin using a Spearman rank correlation (r_s). This process was repeated 10 times and the mean values of r_s are presented.

For the modelling process we omitted 36 out of the 198 samples either because data on body condition were missing ($N = 21$), the wolves were dispersing ($N = 4$) or were immigrants from the Finnish-Russian population resident but captured for translocation ($N = 2$). Four samples from one individual were excluded due to unclear results from both ELISA and Western Blot. On average, 9.3 % (SE 1.4 %) of the estimated mean Scandinavian wolf population was sampled each winter (Fig. 1a).

Acknowledgments
This paper is based on a Master thesis at Hedmark University College [60]. We are grateful to Per Ahlqvist, Thomas H. Strømseth and pilot Ulf Grinde, who captured and handled the wolves, together with Jon M. Arnemo. The SKANDULV project have been funded primarily by the Norwegian Research Council, Norwegian Environment Agency, Hedmark University of Applied Sciences, Norwegian Institute for Nature Research, County Governor of Hedmark, Swedish Research Council Formas, Swedish Environmental Protection Agency, Swedish University of Agricultural Sciences, Swedish Association for Hunting and Wildlife Management, and Worldwide Fund for Nature (Sweden). We thank A. Söderberg and K. Näslund for technical assistance and C. Milleret for R support. We also thank two anonymous reviewers for valuable comments on earlier versions of the manuscript.

Funding
This study was funded by Hedmark University College and the Scandinavian Wolf Research Network, SKANDULV.

Authors' contributions
BF, BZ, JMA, ALE and PW designed the study. JMA, ALE, PW and HS collected samples and data from live wolves, EOÅ and OL collected the data from the dead wolves and JK collected and organized the red fox data. BF and ALE organized and combined the data. BF participated in the laboratory analysis. BF and BZ performed the statistical analysis. BF drafted the manuscript. BZ, PW, JM, SB, JMA, ALE, HS, EOÅ and OL critically and substantially revised the manuscript. All authors approved the manuscript.

Competing interests
The authors declare that they have no competing interests.

Consent for publication
Not applicable.

Author details
[1]Faculty of Applied Ecology and Agricultural Sciences, Hedmark University College, Campus Evenstad, N-2480 Koppang, Norway. [2]Department of Virology, Immunobiology and Parasitology, National Veterinary Institute, SE-75189 Uppsala, Sweden. [3]Department of Ecology, Grimsö Wildlife Research Station, Swedish University of Agricultural Sciences, SE-73091 Riddarhyttan, Sweden. [4]Department of Wildlife, Fish and Environmental Studies, Swedish University of Agricultural Sciences, SE-90183 Umeå, Sweden. [5]Department of Pathology and Wildlife Disease, National Veterinary Institute, SE-75189 Uppsala, Sweden.

References
1. Pence DB, Ueckermann E. Sarcoptic mange in wildlife. Rev Sci Tech. 2002;21(2):385–98.
2. Bornstein S, Mörner T, Samuel WM. Sarcoptes scabiei and sarcoptic mange. In: Samuel WM, Pybus MJ, Kocan AA, editors. Parasitic diseases of wild mammals. 2nd ed. Ames: Iowa State University Press; 2001. p. 107–19.
3. Bornstein S, Zakrisson G, Thebo P. Clinical picture and antibody response to experimental Sarcoptes scabiei var. vulpes infection in red foxes (Vulpes vulpes). Acta Vet Scand. 1995;36(4):509–19.
4. Arlian LG, Morgan MS, Vyszenskimoher DL, Stemmer BL. Sarcoptes scabiei: The circulating antibody response and induced immunity to scabies. Exp Parasitol. 1994;78(1):37–50.
5. Falk ES. Serum immunoglobulin values in patients with scabies. Br J Dermatol. 1980;102(1):57–61.
6. Wobeser GA. Essentials of disease in wild animals. 1st ed. Ames: Blackwell Publishing Professional; 2006.
7. Almberg ES, Cross PC, Dobson AP, Smith DW, Hudson PJ. Parasite invasion following host reintroduction: A case study of Yellowstone's wolves. Phil Trans R Soc B. 2012;367(1604):2840–51.
8. Jimenez MD, Bangs EE, Sime C, Asher VJ. Sarcoptic mange found in wolves in the Rocky Mountains in western United States. J Wildl Dis. 2010;46(4):1120–5.
9. Oleaga Á, Casais R, Balseiro A, Espí A, Llaneza L, Hartasánchez A, Gortázar C. New techniques for an old disease: Sarcoptic mange in the Iberian wolf. Vet Parasitol. 2011;181(2–4):255–66.

10. Arlian LG. Biology, host relations, and epidemiology of Sarcoptes scabiei. Annu Rev Entomol. 1989;34(1):139–59.

11. Mörner T, Eriksson H, Bröjer C, Nilsson K, Uhlhorn H, Ågren E, Segerstad CH, Jansson DS, Gavier-Widén D. Diseases and mortality in free-ranging brown bear (Ursus arctos), gray wolf (Canis lupus), and wolverine (Gulo gulo) in Sweden. J Wildl Dis. 2005;41(2):298–303.

12. Ryser-Degiorgis MP, Hofmann-Lehmann R, Leutenegger CM, Segerstad CH, Mörner T, Mattsson R, Lutz H. Epizootiologic investigations of selected infectious disease agents in free-ranging eurasian lynx from Sweden. J Wildl Dis. 2005;41(1):58–66.

13. Oleaga A, Casais R, Prieto JM, Gortázar C, Balseiro A. Comparative pathological and immunohistochemical features of sarcoptic mange in five sympatric wildlife species in Northern Spain. Eur J Wildl Res. 2012;58(6):997–1000.

14. Vilà C, Sundqvist AK, Flagstad Ø, Seddon J, Björnerfeldt SB, Kojola I, Casulli A, Sand H, Wabakken P, Ellegren H. Rescue of a severely bottlenecked wolf (Canis lupus) population by a single immigrant. Proc R Soc Lond Ser B Biol Sci. 2003;270(1510):91–7.

15. Liberg O, Andrén H, Pedersen HC, Sand H, Sejberg D, Wabakken P, Åkesson M, Bensch S. Severe inbreeding depression in a wild wolf Canis lupus population. Biol Lett. 2005;1(1):17–20.

16. Wabakken P, Sand H, Liberg O, Bjärvall A. The recovery, distribution, and population dynamics of wolves on the Scandinavian peninsula, 1978–1998. Can J Zool. 2001;79(4):710–25.

17. Wabakken P, Svensson L, Kojola I, Maartmann E, Strømseth TH, Flagstad O, Akesson M, Zetterberg A. Ulv i Skandinavia og Finland: Sluttrapport for bestandsovervåking av ulv vinteren 2012–2013, vol. nr. 5–2013. Elverum: Høgskolen i Hedmark; 2013.

18. Liberg O, Chapron G, Wabakken P, Pedersen HC, Hobbs NT, Sand H. Shoot, shovel and shut up: Cryptic poaching slows restoration of a large carnivore in Europe. Proc R Soc Lond Ser B Biol Sci. 2012;279(1730):910–5.

19. Mörner T. Sarcoptic mange in Swedish wildlife. Rev Sci Tech. 1992;11(4): 1115–21.

20. Lindström ER, Andrén H, Angelstam P, Cederlund G, Hörnfeldt B, Jäderberg L, Lemnell PA, Martinsson B, Sköld K, Swenson JE. Disease reveals the predator: Sarcoptic mange, red fox predation, and prey populations. Ecology. 1994;75(4):1042–9.

21. Ledin A, Arnemo JM, Liberg O, Hellman L. High plasma IgE levels within the Scandinavian wolf population, and its implications for mammalian IgE homeostasis. Mol Immunol. 2008;45(7):1976–80.

22. Wabakken P, Aronson A, Sand H, Steinset OK, Kojola I. Ulv i Skandinavia: Statusrapport for vinteren 2001–2002, vol. 2–2002. Elverum: Høgskolen i Hedmark; 2002.

23. Mattsson J, Sand H, Wabakken P, Gervasi V, Liberg O, Linnell JDC, Rauset GR, Pedersen HC. Home range size variation in a recovering wolf population: Evaluating the effect of environmental, demographic, and social factors. Oecologia. 2013;173(3):813–25.

24. Oleaga A, Vicente J, Ferroglio E, Pegoraro de Macedo MR, Casais R, del Cerro A, Espí A, García EJ, Gortázar C. Concomitance and interactions of pathogens in the Iberian wolf (Canis lupus). Res Vet Sci. 2015;101:22–7.

25. Elmhagen B, Hellström P, Angerbjörn A, Kindberg J. Changes in vole and lemming fluctuations in northern Sweden 1960–2008 revealed by fox dynamics. Ann Zool Fenn. 2011;48(3):167–79.

26. Ueno M, Solberg EJ, Iijima H, Rolandsen CM, Gangsei LE. Performance of hunting statistics as spatiotemporal density indices of moose (Alces alces) in Norway. Ecosphere. 2014;5(2):art13.

27. Sykes JE. Immunodeficiencies caused by infectious diseases. Vet Clin N Am Small Anim Pract. 2010;40(3):409–23.

28. Åkerstedt J, Lillehaug A, Larsen IL, Eide NE, Arnemo JM, Handeland K. Serosurvey for canine distemper virus, canine adenovirus, Leptospira interrogans, and Toxoplasma gondii in free-ranging canids in Scandinavia and Svalbard. J Wildl Dis. 2010;46(2):474–80.

29. Mellanby K. The development of symptoms, parasitic infection and immunity in human scabies. Parasitology. 1944;35(04):197–206.

30. Almberg ES, Cross PC, Dobson AP, Smith DW, Metz MC, Stahler DR, Hudson PJ. Social living mitigates the costs of a chronic illness in a cooperative carnivore. Ecol Lett. 2015;18(7):660–67.

31. Todd AW, Gunson JR, Samuel WM. Sarcoptic mange: An important disease of coyotes and wolves in Alberta, Canada. In: Worldwide Furbearer Conference Proceedings: 3–11 August 1980; Frostburg: MD. Ed. J.A. Chapman D. and Pursley; 1980: 706–729.

32. Kreeger TJ. The internal wolf: Physiology, pathology, and pharmacology. In: Mech LD, Boitani L, editors. Wolves: Behavior, Ecology and Conservation. Chicago: The University of Chicago Press; 2003. p. 192–217.

33. Zimmermann B, Sand H, Wabakken P, Liberg O, Andreassen HP. Predator-dependent functional response in wolves: From food limitation to surplus killing. J Anim Ecol. 2015;84(1):102–12.

34. Bornstein S, Zakrisson G. Humoral antibody response to experimental Sarcoptes scabiei var. vulpes infection in the dog. Vet Dermatol. 1993;4(3):107–10.

35. Lower KS, Medleau LM, Hnilica K, Bigler B. Evaluation of an enzyme-linked immunosorbant assay (ELISA) for the serological diagnosis of sarcoptic mange in dogs. Vet Dermatol. 2001;12(6):315–20.

36. Sarasa M, Rambozzi L, Rossi L, Meneguz PG, Serrano E, Granados JE, González FJ, Fandos P, Soriguer RC, Gonzalez G, et al. Sarcoptes scabiei: Specific immune response to sarcoptic mange in the Iberian ibex Capra pyrenaica depends on previous exposure and sex. Exp Parasitol. 2010;124(3):265–71.

37. Frankowiack M, Olsson M, Cluff HD, Evans AL, Hellman L, Månsson J, Arnemo JM, Hammarström L. IgA deficiency in wolves from Canada and Scandinavia. Dev Comp Immunol. 2014;1:26–8.

38. Packard JM. Wolf behavior: Reproductive, social, and intelligent. In: Mech LD, Boitani L, editors. Wolves: Behavior, ecology, and conservation. Chicago: University of Chicago Press; 2003. p. 35–65.

39. Mech LD, Peterson RO. Wolf-prey relations. In: Mech LD, Boitani L, editors. Wolves: Behavior, ecology, and conservation. Chicago: University of Chicago Press; 2003. p. 131–60.

40. Peterson RO, Ciucci P. The wolf as a carnivore. In: Mech LD, Boitani L, editors. Wolves: Behavior, ecology, and conservation. Chicago: University of Chicago Press; 2003. p. 104–30.

41. Zimmermann B, Nelson L, Wabakken P, Sand H, Liberg O. Behavioral responses of wolves to roads: Scale-dependent ambivalence. Behav Ecol. 2014;25(6):1353–64.

42. Bornstein S, Thebo P, Zakrisson G. Evaluation of an enzyme-linked immunosorbent assay (ELISA) for the serological diagnosis of canine sarcoptic mange. Vet Dermatol. 1996;7(1):21–8.

43. Davidson RK, Bornstein S, Handeland K. Long-term study of Sarcoptes scabiei infection in Norwegian red foxes (Vulpes vulpes) indicating host/parasite adaptation. Vet Parasitol. 2008;156(3–4):277–83.

44. Sand H, Wabakken P, Zimmermann B, Johansson Ö, Pedersen HC, Olof L. Summer kill rates and predation pattern in a wolf-moose system: Can we rely on winter estimates? Oecologia. 2008;156(1):53–64.

45. Arnemo JM, Evans AL, Fahlman Å. Biomedical protocols for free-ranging brown bears, gray wolves, wolverines and lynx. Evenstad: Hedmark University College; 2012.

46. Kilkenny C, Browne WJ, Cuthill IC, Emerson M, Altman DG. Improving bioscience research reporting: the ARRIVE guidelines for reporting animal research. PLoS Biol. 2010;8(6):e1000412.

47. Jakob EM, Marshall SD, Uetz GW. Estimating fitness: A comparison of body condition indices. Oikos. 1996;77(1):61–7.

48. Gipson PS, Ballard WB, Nowak RM, Mech LD. Accuracy and precision of estimating age of gray wolves by tooth wear. J Wildl Manage. 2000;64(3):752–8.

49. Alfredéen A-C. Denning behaviour and movement pattern during summer of wolves Canis lupus on the Scandinavian Peninsula. In: Department of Conservation Biology, Swedish University of Agricultural Sciences. 2006.

50. Ljunggren EL, Bergström K, Morrison DA, Mattsson JG. Characterization of an atypical antigen from Sarcoptes scabiei containing an MADF domain. Parasitology. 2006;132(01):117–26.

51. Harrell FE, Charles D. Hmisc: Harrell Miscellaneous. R-package version 3.15-0. 2015.

52. Liberg O, Aronson Å, Sand H, Wabakken P, Maartmann E, Svensson L, Åkesson M. Monitoring of wolves in Scandinavia. Hystrix. 2011;23(1):29–34.

53. Baddeley A, Turner R. {spatstat}: An {R} package for analyzing spatial point patterns. J stat soft. 2005;12:1–42.

54. R Core Team. R: A language and environment for statistical computing. In: Warm Puppy, vol. 3.0.3. Vienna: R Foundation for Statistical Computing; 2014.

55. Babyak MA. What you see may not be what you get: A brief, nontechnical introduction to overfitting in regression-type models. Psychosom Med. 2004;66(3):411–21.

56. Pasch B, Bolker BM, Phelps SM. Interspecific dominance via vocal interactions mediates altitudinal zonation in neotropical singing mice. Am Nat. 2013;182(5):E161–73.

15

The use of primary murine fibroblasts to ascertain if *Spirocerca lupi* secretory/excretory protein products are mitogenic ex vivo

Kgomotso Sako[1], Ilse jv Rensburg[2], Sarah Clift[3] and Vinny Naidoo[1,2*]

Abstract

Background: *Spirocerca lupi* is a nematode that parasitizes vertebrates in particular canids, by forming nodules in the thoracic cavity specifically in the oesophagus. In 25% of *Spirocerca* infections of the domestic dog, nodules progress from inflammatory to pre-neoplastic to sarcomatous neoplasia. With the mechanism of neoplastic transformation being incompletely understood, this study investigates if *S. lupi* parasite proteinaceous secretory/ excretory products (ESPs) play a role in the neoplastic transformation.

Methods: To facilitate collection of ESPs, we maintained naturally harvested adult parasites in the laboratory under artificial conditions. Media in which the parasites were grown was subsequently evaluated for the presence of proteinaceous compounds using a mass spectroscopy library as well as for their ability to be mitogenic in primary murine fibroblastic cells.

Results: Chromatrography of the ethyl acetate extracted incubation media showed the presence of 9 protein compounds, of which three were identified as non-specific proteins isolated from *Nematostella vectensis*, *Caenorhabditis brenneri* and *Sus scrofa*, with the rest being unknown. Acetone, methanol, hexane and ethylacetate extracted culture media were unable to induce a mitogenic change in primary murine fibroblasts in comparison to the controls.

Conclusion: While no mitogenic effect was evident, further studies are required to understand the role of worm excretory/secretory products on clastogenesis under chronic exposure. In addition, while not of primary importance for this study, the observed duration of parasite survival indicates that ex vivo studies on *S. lupi* are possible. For the latter we believe that the worm culture method can be further optimized if longer survival times are required.

Keywords: *Spirocerca lupi*, Ex vivo culture, Viability, Mitogenic, Murine fibroblasts

Background

Spirocerca lupi is a nematode parasite with higher prevalence in both tropical and subtropical countries, despite its global distribution [1]. The life cycle of the parasite is well understood and includes intermediate hosts (coprophagous beetles), paratenic hosts (wild birds, lizards,

* Correspondence: vinny.naidoo@up.ac.za
[1]Section of Pharmacology and Toxicology, Department of Paraclinical Sciences, Faculty of Veterinary Science, University of Pretoria, Private Bag X04, Onderstepoort 0110, South Africa
[2]University of Pretoria Biomedical Research Centre, Faculty of Veterinary Science, Private Bag X04, Onderstepoort 0110, South Africa
Full list of author information is available at the end of the article

rodents, hedgehogs, rabbits and poultry) and the definitive host (dogs). *S. lupi* eggs containing stage 1 larvae (L1) are shed in the faeces or with the vomit of the canine definitive host. Coprophagous beetles of the Scarabaeidae family feed on the vomit or faeces, ingesting the larvated eggs. The emerging larvae (L1) then encyst in the tissues of the beetles and develop to stage 3 larvae (L3) within approximately 2 months. Paratenic hosts or the definitive host feeds on the coprophagous beetles, ingesting the L3 larvae. Following ingestion of L3 larvae by the definitive host, the larvae get released in the gastric lumen, then migrate within the gastric mucosa,

57. Fox J, Weisberg S. An {R} companion to applied regression. 2nd ed. Thousend Oaks: Sage; 2011.
58. Zuur A, Ieno EN, Walker N, Saveliev AA, Smith GM. Mixed effects models and extensions in ecology with R. 1st ed. New York: Springer; 2009.
59. Mazerolle MJ. AICcmodavg: Model selection and multimodel inference based on (Q)AIC(c). *R package version* 2014.
60. Fuchs B. Sarcoptic mange in the Scandinavian wolf population. Evenstad: Høgskolen i Hedmark; 2014.

serosa and gastric/coeliac arteries, reaching the caudal thoracic aorta, where they develop to stage 4 larvae (L4) and then to young adults. Thereafter, they migrate to the caudal thoracic oesophagus, where they settle and form nodule(s) in the serosa and submucosa [1–3].

Once a dog is infected with, the clinical signs most often seen include regurgitation, weight loss and/or dysphagia [4, 5]. The pathognomonic diagnostic lesions for spirocercosis include scarring of the caudal thoracic aorta with osseous metaplasia and/or aneurysm formation, caudal thoracic ventral vertebral body spondylitis and the formation of nodule(s) in the caudal thoracic esophagus [4]. In up to 25% of S. lupi-infested dogs, the esophageal nodules progress from inflammatory esophageal nodules to pre-neoplastic fibroblastic nodules and eventually to sarcoma [6]. S.lupi-induced sarcomatous neoplasia has been further classified histologically as osteosarcoma (the predominant S. lupi-induced sarcoma), fibrosarcoma and anaplastic (undifferentiated) sarcoma [2].

While the progression of the S. lupi nodule to neoplasia is well documented and described, the mechanism underlying the progression to neoplasia is poorly understood with current hypotheses linking neoplastic transformation to chronic inflammation [3, 7–9]. According to this supposition, it is believed that chronic irritation induces cellular metaplasia which eventually results in neoplastic transformation. In support of this, various studies have demonstrated that the initial esophageal inflammatory lesion induced by the parasites and its subsequent progression to neoplasia is associated with changes in C-reactive protein, vascular endothelial growth factor (VEGF), fibroblast growth factor (FGF), platelet-derived growth factor (PDGF) and interleukin 8 concentrations [3, 7–9]. However, these studies did not conclusively demonstrate that the inflammation seen was the cause of the progression to neoplasia, as opposed to being the expected response to the presence of a parasite.

Whilst inflammation is known to underpin carcinogenesis in some cases, very little attention has been given to the possibility that the worm could be secreting/excreting a mitogenic substance that might be responsible for the nodule formation and later neoplastic change. The human medical literature, to date, has reported numerous cases of infectious agents inciting direct neoplastic change. Clonorchis sinensis, a liver fluke, induces clonorchiosis and subsequent cholangiocarcinoma, and has been found to cause an increase in cyclins E and B, which play an important role in the regulation of the cell cycle, in the induction of mitosis, and in the behavior of neoplastic cells [10]. Opisthorchis viverrini, another liver fluke, known to induce cholangiocarcinoma in humans is also suspected to induce

oncogenesis via changes in the release of cyclin proteins [11]. As a result we believe it is important to evaluate the environment surrounding the parasite for the presence of oncogenic protein substances. The following study attempts to evaluate the secretory/excretory protein products (ESPs) of the Spirocerca adult worm collected from an ex vivo environment for their mitogenic effect using murine fibroblasts. In addition, since S. lupi worms have never been maintained in the laboratory to our knowledge, the other aim of this study was to establish if it was possible to maintain the parasite under laboratory conditions for ex vivo investigation, even if for limited periods.

Methods
Collection and maintenance of worms
Adult worms were collected from domestic dogs ($n = 4$) as soon as possible following euthanasia, and in all cases collection was opportunistic following euthanasia on humane grounds. Harvesting was approved by the Animal Use and Care Committee of the University of Pretoria (V063/12). Following esophageal nodule incision and careful removal of adult worms, they were placed into pre-warmed saline, Iscove's Modified Dulbecco's Medium (Iscove's), Dulbecco's Modified Eagle's Medium (DMEM), Ham's F12 Medium (Ham's) or Roswell Park Memorial Institute (RPMI) 1640 medium (RPMI) prior to transportation to the laboratory. All media was purchased from Highveld Biologicals (South Africa) and contained phenol red as a pH indicator. Prior to plating, parasites were rinsed three times using sterile phosphate buffered saline (PBS) to remove the detritus on the parasite's cuticle. The parasites were thereafter immersed in 2 ml of one of the four mentioned media or in prewarmed saline ($n = 6$ for RPMI and $n = 9$ for all other media) under serum free conditions. Plates were maintained in a humidified environment of 5% CO_2 in oxygen (Carbogen) at 37 °C. Culture media or saline was replaced at 48 h intervals. Following every media change, the removed media was frozen at –80 °C for future use. Worm survival (viability) was ascertained by parasite motility, the integrity of the esophagus and the color of the cuticle when non-motile.

Liquid chromatography
The supernatant (culture media or saline) was concentrated by removing the water using a Lyoquest freeze dryer (Telstar®) at a temperature of –77 °C and vacuum of 0.046 m-bar. Thereafter, samples were diluted in a mixture of water and acetonitrile (1:1). At least 20 µl of each of the samples was injected into an ultimate 3000 ultra-high performance liquid chromatography (U-HPLC) (Thermo Scientific and Dionex) fitted with an Acclaim™ 120 C18 column (Dionex) with a particle size of 3 µm, 2.1 mm × 100 mm

diameter and average pore diameter of 120 Å. The mobile phase (0.1% formic acid and water, 0.1% formic acid and acetonitrile) containing formic acid as an ion pairing agent was added to the column at a flow-rate of 0.3 ml/min. The U-HPLC was connected to a MicroTOF-QII (Bruker™) high resolution mass spectrophotometer (MS). Peaks were identified by use of an attached library.

Mitogenic assay
Preparation of the supernatant
Frozen media collected during the first incubation was thawed and mixed 1:1 with acetone, hexane or methanol. Mixed samples were subsequently centrifuged at 3500 rpm for 3 min (Allegra®, Beckman Coulter), at room temperature. Samples were rapidly frozen in a dry ice/methanol mixture to potentially remove the aqueous phase. After the ice-bath, the supernatant was dried using pressurized nitrogen (15 psi) at 60 °C for 60 min. The dried samples were preserved at 4 °C in a fridge until assessed. Prior to use the extracts were reconstituted at 750ul of their respective extraction solvent to 250ul of media, 500ul of solvent to 500ul of media or 250ul of solvent to 750ul of media.

Establishment of cell cultures
Skin samples were harvested from the pinnae of Balb/c mice (either sex ±3 months old) supplied by the UPBRC (University of Pretoria, Biomedical Research Centre). Sample collection was purely opportunistic following scheduled terminations from another approved study. Samples were cleaned using Bioscrub (Chlorhexidine gluconate), sterile water and 70% alcohol, digested in pre-warmed collagenase and hyaluronidase (Sigma Aldrich) solution at 37 °C in a humidified 5% CO_2 incubator for 24 h. After digestion, samples were centrifuged at 42 g, at 500 rpm for 5 min and the supernatant discarded. Pellets were suspended in DMEM HI (Sigma) and 40% heat inactivated fetal bovine serum (FBS-Scientific group) growth medium and gently agitated using the serological pipette tip and transferred into 50 ml TC flasks (Nunc, Thermo ScientificTM) with 5% antibiotic (Streptomycin, Neomycin and Penicillin). Cultures were maintained at 37 °C in 5% CO_2 in growth media for a week. After the first week of incubation, the culture medium was replaced with 10% FBS in DMEM in TC flasks and these were changed twice a week. Once cultures reached confluence of approximately 80–90%, they were rinsed twice with trypsin-versene solution and trypsinized. Cells were counted using the trypan blue exclusion method.

Exposure studies
The extracted Iscove's media were filter-sterilized (0.25 μm filters, Millipore corp.). Fibroblasts in suspension

(400 μl) were dispensed into each well of 8-well chambered slides (Lab-Tek, USA) and incubated for 24 h. After incubation, the culture medium was changed and fibroblasts were treated with 40 μl of one of the three concentrations of solvent-extracted secretory/excretory product for 48 h (final extract exposure of 10, 20 and 30 μl before dilution in the media was taken into consideration). The experiment was carried out in triplicates and in all cases compared to their respective solvent control. After the prerequisite exposure period, the slides were air dried, fixed in 100% methanol, and stained with Lily Mayer's haematoxylin and eosin using a laboratory optimized method. Detailed cytological evaluation was performed on digital photographs (4140 × 3096 pixel) obtained using an Olympus DP72 digital camera attached to an Olympus light microscope (Olympus, Japan). The photographs were downloaded onto a computer and adjusted to 50% (1360 × 1024 pixels) of their initial size in Paint (Microsoft Windows 7). A grid was superimposed over the photographs. Fibroblasts ($n = 100$), both normal and mitotic, were counted in an anticlockwise manner for each photograph.

Establishment of the cause of contamination
Prior to culture, the pH of thawed culture media or saline was measured using a standard pH meter. Samples were plated on MacConkey agar, sheep's blood agar (BAP), colistin-nalidixic acid agar (CNA) and broth containing methyl-umbellinferyl-β-glucuronide (MUG) and incubated at 35 °C in an aerobic atmosphere in an incubator for 24 h. Thereafter, growth of colonies and lactose consumption in samples plated on MacConkey agar was monitored. The recovered colonies of BAP and CNA were tested for biochemical reaction using catalase (–), lancefield group D (+) and pyrrolidonyl arylamidase [12].

Results
At the time of harvesting from the nodules the worms were curled-up and showed resistance to gentle pulling force. On placement in the warmed media the worms showed variable movement with time to harvest appearing to affect motility i.e. worms collected immediately after euthanasia of the host appeared to be more active and retained their pink-colored cuticle (Fig. 1a). After approximately 30 min within the warmed culture media, worms once again showed movement. Irrespective of the culture media, the worms all died by 96 h after harvest (Fig. 1b). Viability was longer in the plain saline, with only half of the parasites dying by 96 h, with the rest surviving to 144 h.

In all cases the death of the worms were associated with change in colour of the phenol red to yellow and an unpleasant smell of the media, with concurrent pH change of 7.38 ± 0.45; 7.67 ± 0.14; 7.24 ± 0.51 and

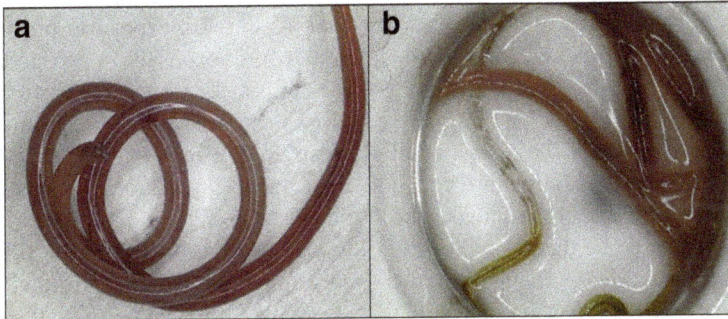

Fig. 1 Healthy adult *Spirocerca lupi* worm (**a**) and a dead parasite (**b**). The healthy worm is pink in colour while the dead worm has lost it colour

7.53 ± 0.26 for the Iscove's, DMEM, Ham's, RPMI media from a pH of 7.4. The pH of the saline control remained fairly constant at 6.00 ± 1.09 and remained unchanged from the pre-treatment pH of 6. Culture of the media and saline both revealed the presence of *Escherichia coli*, *Enterococcus faecalis*, *Pseudomonas aeruginosa* and *Serratia marcescens*.

Liquid chromatography revealed the presence of nine peaks, indicating the existence of nine different protein compounds of various sizes with mass to charge ratios of 166.0868 to 928.4730 m/z (Fig. 2) in the Iscoves and RPMI media. No peaks were present in the other media or the saline. Despite nine peaks being present, comparison with the molecular ion masses published from the protein library allowed for the characterization of only three of these proteins (same as the non-specific proteins produced by *Nematostella vectensis*, Caebren (*Caenorhabditis brenneri*) and *Sus scrofa*, with no information being available on their potential carcinogenic effects. None of the other chemicals were identifiable.

Following the exposure of fibroblasts to adult *S. lupi* ESPs (at various dilutions, 10, 20 and 30 µl), HE-stained cytological preparations were assessed for an increase in mitotic rate which would have been indicative of clastogenesis (Fig. 3). An increase in fibroblast proliferation was evident in both the adult *S. lupi* ESPs extracts and in the organic solvent groups, with a clear concentration-response relationship for the latter (Fig. 4).

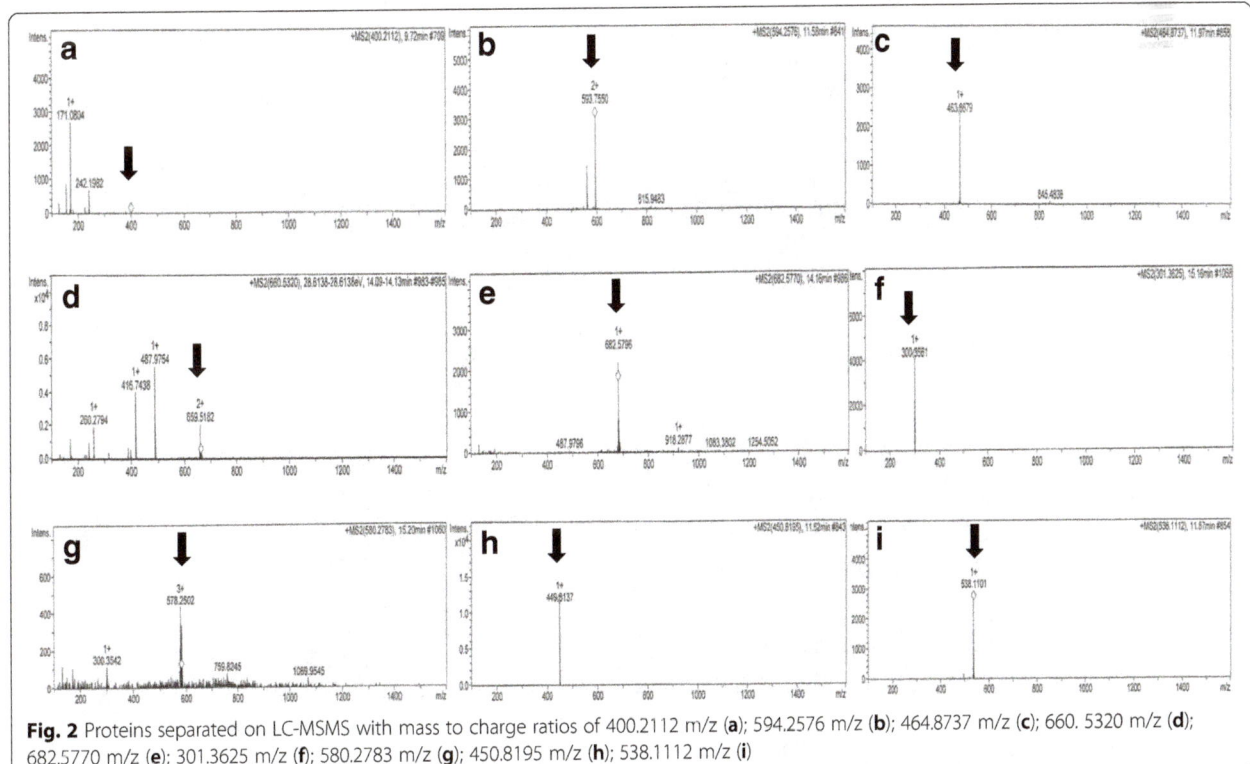

Fig. 2 Proteins separated on LC-MSMS with mass to charge ratios of 400.2112 m/z (**a**); 594.2576 m/z (**b**); 464.8737 m/z (**c**); 660. 5320 m/z (**d**); 682.5770 m/z (**e**); 301.3625 m/z (**f**); 580.2783 m/z (**g**); 450.8195 m/z (**h**); 538.1112 m/z (**i**)

Based on the similar results, it was evident that the *S. lupi* ESPs had no additional mitogenic effect over and above that of the solvents alone under experimental conditions.

Discussion

The aim of this study was to ascertain if the *S. lupi* adult parasite changed its surrounding environment through the release of secretory/excretory protein products, and whether any of these products could be the reason for the parasites ability to induce carcinogenic changes in the host. The latter was undertaken by placing live adult worms into specific media/saline for a limited period. Only the Iscoves's and RPMI media showed a difference in their protein content in comparison to the said media prior to culture. Of the two, the Iscove's media was selected for further analysis for the presence of a mitogenic effect, as preliminary TLC separation demonstrated the most intense staining bands (results not shown). In all cases the proteins identified were above 160 m/z. While in total nine additional proteins were identified on the spectra through LC-MSMS, only three of these were previously identified from other organisms. The three proteins have, however, thus far not been subjected to any further testing for the purpose of this study, nor could any published studies on the function or significance of these proteins be found. Another important question that should be answered is whether these proteins were from parasite or bacterial origin.

In an attempt to establish if these proteins could be mitogenic a cell culture assay was used. Following the exposure of fibroblasts to adult *S. lupi* ESPs (at various dilutions, 10, 20 and 30 μl), the in vitro fibroblasts were investigated in cytological preparation for an increase in

mitotic rate, which would have been indicative of clastogenesis. For the exposure, murine fibroblasts were harvested and exposed to extracts of excretory/secretory substances for a period of 48 h. The principle of the assay was based on use of primary fibroblast cultures to ascertain the mitogenic effect of environmental chemicals, under in vitro conditions [13]. As an increase in fibroblast proliferation was evident in both the adult *S. lupi* ESPs extracts and in the organic solvent groups, we concluded that *S. lupi* ESPs had no additional mitogenic effect over and above that of the solvents alone under the conditions of the study design. While the absence of a mitogenic effect tends to suggest that the parasite is not inducing its effect via the release of secretory/excretory proteinaceous substances, the time progression of infection to tumour development in vivo still needs to be taken into consideration. As such we believe that to conclusively rule out the effect of potentially mitogenic compounds, it may be necessary to undertake repeated exposure of the primary fibroblast cultures, in such a manner that with the periodical media change, the excretory/secretory products are replenished over a longer period of time.

While the main objective of the study was to ascertain if the parasites were releasing potentially mitogenic secretory/excretory products, to achieve this the parasite had to be maintained outside of its host for a period of time. To our knowledge this is the first description of an attempt to maintain adult *S. lupi* worms alive outside of the host animal, even for the short periods required for this study, and thus warrants some discussion. The worms in question were collected opportunistically from recently euthanized dogs through dissection of their

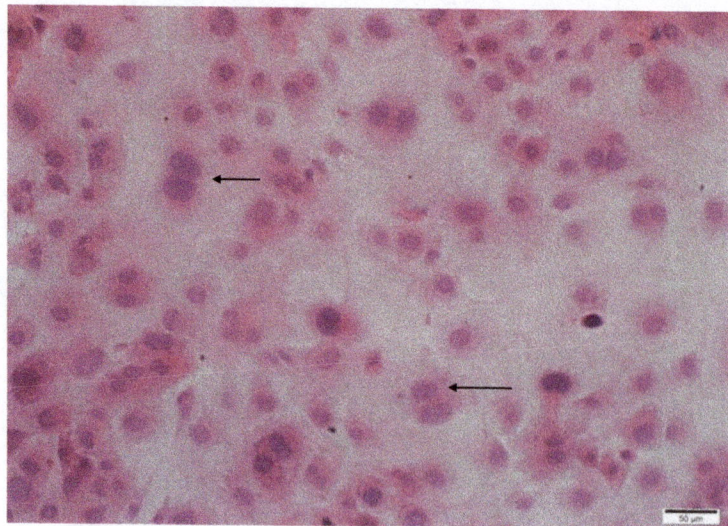

Fig. 3 Photograph of fibroblasts harvested from Balb/c mice, stained with HE, showing evidence of nuclear pleomorphism (bi-nucleates and karyomegaly) (arrows). Sample obtained from the acetone treated slides

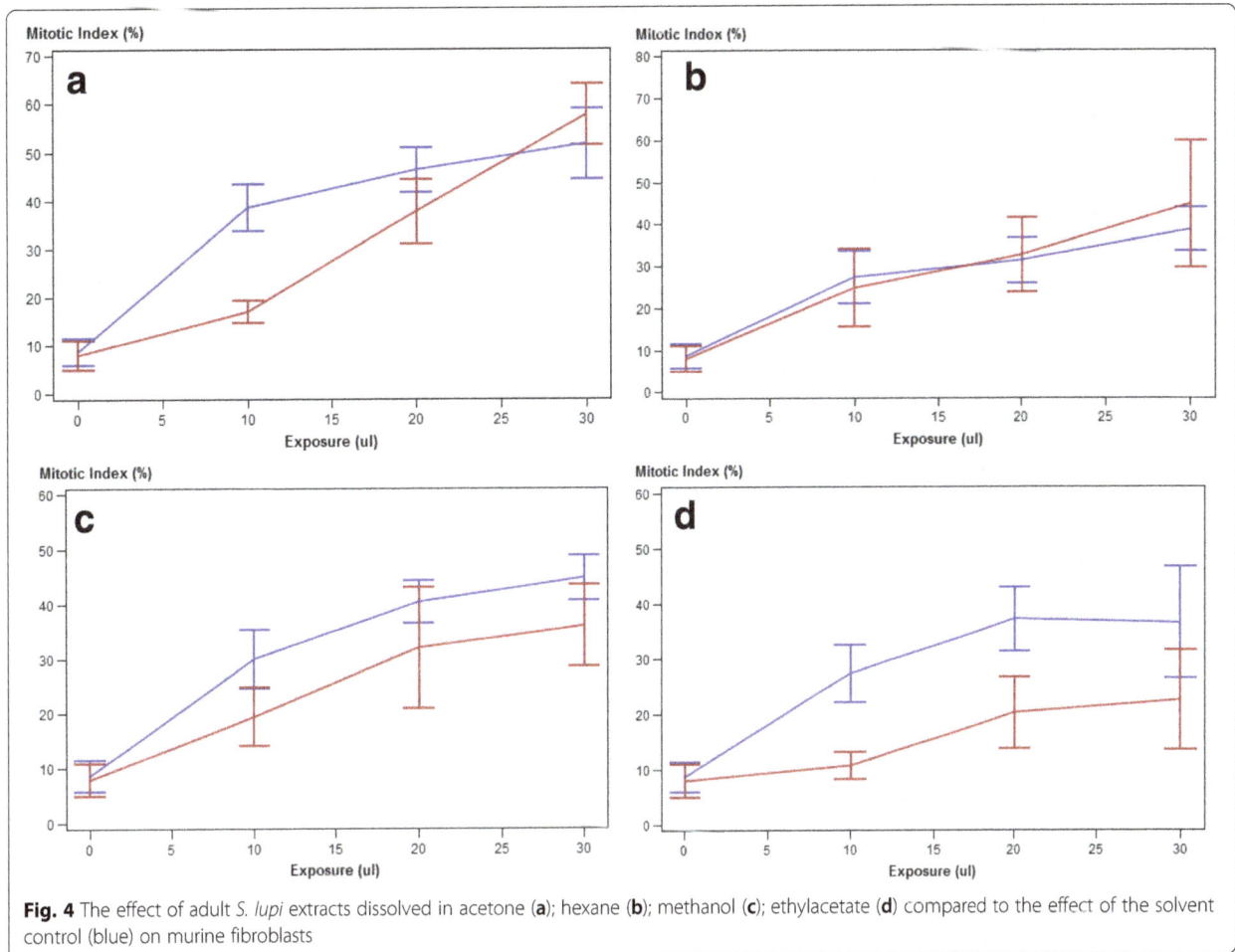

Fig. 4 The effect of adult *S. lupi* extracts dissolved in acetone (**a**); hexane (**b**); methanol (**c**); ethylacetate (**d**) compared to the effect of the solvent control (blue) on murine fibroblasts

esophageal nodules and the physical removal of the worms, without the necessity for collagenase digestion. Following nodule dissection, the harvested worms were deemed viable according to our established criteria of being pink in color, having an intact esophagus and showing some, albeit varied, motility. It would therefore appear that the physical harvesting of the worms had no adverse effect on parasite viability. A qualitative difference in movement was present between the worms, possibly due to the delay to time of nodule dissection and/or the pre-cooling that happens on placement of carcasses into a refrigerator at 4 °C, indicating that delays in harvesting should preferably be avoided.

Following harvest, the worms were placed in saline as the control or within Ham's F12 medium, DMEM, RPMI 1640 medium and / or Iscove's modification of DMEM for five to 7 days under serum free conditions. These media were selected based on prior reports of their use in in vitro culture of other parasites such as *Onchocerca* spp. and *Schistosoma* spp., and these media are also the most commonly used media in mammalian cell culture. The media differed from each other in their amino acid and glucose content and in their buffering systems. For

example, DMEM contained only sodium pyruvate and no buffer, RPMI 1640 medium contained only sodium bicarbonate as the buffer, Iscove's modification of DMEM contained lower concentrations of bicarbonate as HEPES was included as the buffer and Ham's F12 medium contained no buffer. In terms of their nutrient contents, the media contained different amino acids to support the growth of different cell types. Since *S. lupi* must survive off nutrients within their environment in esophageal nodules and with the selected cell media best representing the nutrient content within tissue fluid, it was speculated that these media would be able to meet the nutritional requirements of the parasite. Despite this, the parasites failed to thrive within the selected media with the worms progressively becoming weaker and more opaque until they died.

While we're uncertain as to the exact reason for the earlier death of the parasites in the various media, this was most likely an indication of the parasite's inability to utilise the nutrients within the media. This theory is supported by the measured change in pH of the media, as in all cases the parasites failed to modify the pH of the environment in which they were resident. From studies on *Ascaris suum* and *H. contortus*, one would have expected the parasite to modify their external environment to being a more acidic pH (circa pH 5 was reported for *A. suum*) [14, 15]. This pH modification is meant to arise from the excretion of the end-products of carbohydrate metabolism across the cuticle, in order to maintain the functionality of cuticle transporters. This would also explain why the parasites survived longer in the acidic saline, as the lower pH would have allowed for optimal functionality of the cuticle transporters for a longer period, with death probably eventually resulting from starvation as the incubation media was devoid of added nutrients. Support for the latter is evident by progressive increases in the parasite opaqueness, which from studies on *H. contortus* is an indication of glycogen stores depletion during starvation [16].

We propose some recommendations pertaining to future studies that potentially need the parasites to survive for a longer period of time. Firstly, the presence of *E. coli, E. faecalis, P. aeruginosa* and *S. marcescens*, indicates that the harvest of the parasites does result in the transfer of bacterial contaminants and that washing alone is not sufficient to remove them, warranting the need for antimicrobials in the media. Based on the organisms cultured, the aminoglycosides may a good antibiotic to include in the media. Nonetheless, we cannot at this stage associate the death of the parasite with the presence of the bacteria, as the four bacteria species were cultured equally well from all the media and the saline. The implication is that the bacteria cultured may be associated with the parasite, which is not uncommon as other nematode parasites have been reported to have bacteria attached to their cuticle e.g. urinary cysts caused by *Strongylus edentatus* are associated with genera such as *Escherichia, Enterobacter* and *Streptococcus* that are attached to the cuticle, while *E coli* and Pseudomonas have been associated with swine ascarids [17]. We also consider it unlikely that the bacteria were the cause of death of the parasites, especially since an intact cuticle purportedly protects nematode parasites against environmental insult [18]. Furthermore, living *S. lupi* parasites within esophageal nodules in infected dogs are routinely associated with purulent inflammation, necrotic cell debris and assorted bacteria in migratory tracts within these nodules. It may even be possible that the *S. lupi* parasite is the source of esophageal nodule contamination in a similar manner as described for *S. edentatus* cysts above.

A second consideration would be to lower the pH of the incubation media to 5 or 6, as the parasite may only be able to mobilise nutrients from the media at a lower pH, as seen with studies on Ascaris where it has been demonstrated that trans-cuticle transport is dependent on the pH of the surrounding environment [14]. Lastly perhaps the media should be supplemented with fetal

calf serum (FCS). For this study, with the attempt being the characterization of excretory/secretory protein products, we kept the additions of exogenous proteins to the media to a minimum. This is in contrast with other studies for which fetal calf serum is commonly added to mammalian and parasite cell cultures as a source of albumin and growth factors. For the parasite *Schistosoma spp.*, it has been shown that the parasite needs albumin for glycogen production, while supplementation with 10% FCS was vital for the prolonged viability of *Oesophagostomum gutturosa* adult parasites cultured in vitro using RPMI 1640 medium, Iscove's Modified Dulbecco's Medium and Minimum Essential Medium for 39 days [17]. The FCS is believed to provide parasites with necessary growth factors, e.g. platelet-derived growth factor (PDGF), epidermal growth factor (EGF), transforming growth factor-β (TGF-β) and insulin-like growth factor (IGF) [11].

Conclusion

The aim of this study was to culture adult *S. lupi* parasites in vitro using serum-free media to harvest the ESPs, for subsequent carcinogenic studies. While we were able to keep the parasite alive ex vivo for a short period of time, we were unable to demonstrate carcinogenic effects in cultured fibroblasts. We did, however, confirm that the ESPs are composed of proteins.

Acknowledgements

The authors wish to thank Sinoville Animal Clinic and the Onderstepoort Veterinary Academic Hospital for providing the worms; Ms. Naomi Timmerman for optimising the staining of the slides and Mintek for assisting with the LC-MSMS analysis at no cost. This project was sponsored by the National Research Foundation of South Africa and University of Pretoria (UP).

Author contributions

SC: Conceptualized the study and provided support for the cytological evaluation; VN: Conceptualized the study, participated in the chemical analysis and data analysis; IJvR: Responsible for maintaining the cell cultures and exposure assays; KS: undertook the laboratory studies, and participated in the data analysis; VN and SC were also student supervisors of KS. All authors participated in the preparation of the manuscript.

Competing interests

The authors declare that they have no competing interests.

Author details

[1]Section of Pharmacology and Toxicology, Department of Paraclinical Sciences, Faculty of Veterinary Science, University of Pretoria, Private Bag X04, Onderstepoort 0110, South Africa. [2]University of Pretoria Biomedical Research Centre, Faculty of Veterinary Science, Private Bag X04, Onderstepoort 0110, South Africa. [3]Section of Pathology, Department of Paraclinical Sciences, Faculty of Veterinary Science, University of Pretoria, Private Bag X04, Onderstepoort 0110, South Africa.

References
1. Bailey WS. *Spirocerca lupi:* A continuing inquiry. J Parasitol. 1972;58:3–22.
2. Van der Merwe L, Kirberger RM, Clift S, Williams M, Keller N, Naidoo V. *Spirocerca lupi* infection in the dog: a review. Vet J. 2008;176:294–309.
3. Dvir E, Clift SJ, Williams MC. Proposed histological progression of the *Spirocerca lupi*-induced oesophageal lesion in dogs. Vet Parasitol. 2010;168:71–7.
4. Mazaki-Tovi M, Baneth G, Aroch I, Harrus S, Kass PH, Ben-Ari T, Zur G, Aizenberg I, Bark H, Lavy E. Canine spirocercosis: clinical, diagnostic, pathologic, and epidemiologic characteristics. Vet Parasitol. 2002;107:235–50.
5. Ranen E, Lavy E, Aizenberg I, Perl S, Harrus S. Spirocercosis-associated esophageal sarcomas in dogs. A retrospective study of 17 cases (1997-2003). Vet Parasitol. 2004;119:209–21.
6. Dvir E, Kirberger RM, Malleczek D. Radiographic and computed tomographic changes and clinical presentation of spirocercosis in the dog. Vet Radiol Ultrasound. 2001;42:119–29.
7. Mukorera V, Dvir E, Van der Merwe LL, Goddard A. Serum C reactive protein concentration in benign and malignant canine spirocercosis. J Vet Intern Med. 2011;25:963–6.
8. Dvir E, Schoeman JP, Clift SJ, McNeilly TN, Mellanby RJ. Immunohistochemical characterization of lymphocyte and myeloid cell infiltrates in spirocercosis-induced oesophageal nodules. Parasite Immunol. 2011;33:545–53.
9. Dvir E, Mellanby RJ, Kjelgaard-Hansen M, Schoeman JP. Plasma IL-8 concentrations are increased in dogs with spirocercosis. Vet Parasitol. 2012;190:185.
10. Kim YJ, Choi MH, Hong ST, Bae YM. Resistance of cholangiocarcinoma cells to parthenolide-induced apoptosis by the excretory-secretory products of *Clonorchis sinensis*. Parasitol Res. 2009;104:1011–6.
11. Thuwajit C, Thuwajit P, Uchida K, Daorueang D, Kaewkes S, Wongkham S, Miwa M. Gene expression profiling defined pathways correlated with fibroblast cell proliferation induced by *Opisthorchis viverrini* excretory/secretory product. World J Gastroenterol. 2006;12:3585–92.
12. Kinzelman J, Ng C, Jackson E, Gradus S, Bagley R. Enterococci as indicators of lake Michigan recreational water quality: comparison of two methodologies and their impacts on public health regulatory events. Appl Environ Microbiol. 2003;69:92–6.
13. Grafstrom EF, Curren RD, Yang LL, Harris CC. Genotoxicity of formaldehyde in cultured human bronchial fibroblasts. Science. 1985;228:89–91.
14. Sims SM, Maga LT, Barsuhn CL, Ho NF, Geary TG, Thompson DP. Mechanisms of microenvironmental pH regulation in the cuticle of *Ascaris suum*. Mol Biochem Parasitol. 1992;53:135–48.
15. Sims SM, Ho NFH, Geary TG, Thomas EM, Day JS, Barsuhn CL, Thompson DP. Influence of organic acid excretion on cuticle pH and drug absorption by Haemonchus contortus. Int J Parasitol. 1996;26:25–35.
16. Beugnet F, Kerboeuf D, Nicolle J, Soubieux D. Use of free living stages to study the effects of thiabendazole, levamisole, pyrantel and ivermectin on the fine structure of *Haemonchus contortus* and *Heligmosomoides polygyrus*. Vet Parasitol. 1996;63:83–94.
17. Bird AL. The Namatode cuticle and its surface. In: Zuckerman B, editor. Nematodes as biological models, Volume 2. New York: Academic Press; 1980.
18. Page AP, Johnstone IL (2007) The cuticle. In The *C. elegans* Research Community (ed) WormBook, doi/10.1895/ wormbook.1.138.1, http://www.wormbook.org.

16

The prevalence of *Dirofilaria repens* in cats, healthy dogs and dogs with concurrent babesiosis in an expansion zone in central Europe

Anna Bajer[1*], Anna Rodo[2,3], Ewa J. Mierzejewska[1], Katarzyna Tołkacz[1] and Renata Welc-Faleciak[1]

Abstract

Background: *Dirofilaria repens* is a mosquito-transmitted, filarial nematode parasitizing dogs, cats and other carnivores. Recently, this parasite has spread in central Europe, including Poland. The aim of the present study was to estimate the prevalence of *D. repens* in cats and dogs in different regions of the country and to investigate the occurrence and consequences of co-infection with another fast-spreading vector-borne parasite, *Babesia canis*.

Results: In the period 2013–2015, 147 blood samples from cats from central Poland and 257 blood samples from dogs from central, northern, southern and western Poland were collected. Prevalence of *D. repens* was determined by amplification and sequencing of the *12S rDNA* gene fragment. Among dogs, 94 samples originated from clinically healthy dogs from central Poland (Masovia) and 58 samples originated from dogs that were infected with *B. canis*. Prevalence of *D. repens* was compared between these two groups of dogs.

For the first time *D. repens* was identified in a cat from central Europe (0.7 % [95 % CL: 0–4.1 %]). The DNA of the filarial endosymbiotic bacterium *Wolbachia* was detected in two cats (1.4 % [95 % CL: 0–5.5 %]). In dogs, the parasite was detected only in samples from central Poland (Masovia) (local prevalence = 38 % [95 % CL: 25.9–51.8 %]). Prevalence of *D. repens* was significantly higher in dogs with babesiosis (90 % [95 % CL: 81.6–94.5 %]). Co-infections of *D. repens* and *B. canis* were confirmed by sequencing in 30 dogs with babesiosis, but no co-infections were identified in healthy dogs from Masovia. Statistical analyses of blood parameters revealed that dogs with co-infections suffered more severe anemia and thrombocytopenia, but presented milder changes in biochemical parameters (i.e. less elevated concentration of alkaline phosphatase [ALP] and serum urea) suggesting lower risk of hepatic or renal failure in comparison to dogs infected only with *B. canis*.

Conclusions: These findings are important due to the spread of dirofilariosis and babesiosis in central Europe, as microfilaraemic dogs seem to be more prone to babesiosis. The possible protective effect of the nematode infection against hepatic or renal failure in canine babesiosis and its mechanisms require further investigations.

Keywords: *Dirofilaria repens*, *Babesia canis*, Co-infection, Dogs, Cats, Thrombocytopenia, Hepatic failure, Renal failure, Creatinine, Serum urea

Abbreviations: ALP, Alkaline phosphatase; ALT, Alanine aminotransferase; ANOVA, Analysis of variance; AST, Aspartate aminotransferase; CL, Confidence Interval; DNA, Deoxyribonucleic Acid; EDTA, Ethylene Diamine Tetra-acetic Acid; IBM, International Business Machines; MCHC, Mean Corpuscular Hemoglobin Concentration; MCV, Mean Corpuscular Volume; NS, Not significant; P, Probability values; PCR, Polymerase Chain Reaction; RBC, Red Blood Cell; RNA, Ribonucleic acids; SEM, Standard error of the mean; SPSS, Statistical Package for the Social Sciences

* Correspondence: anabena@biol.uw.edu.pl
[1]Department of Parasitology, Institute of Zoology, Faculty of Biology, University of Warsaw, 1 Miecznikowa Street, 02-096 Warsaw, Poland
Full list of author information is available at the end of the article

Background

Dirofilaria repens is a filarial species transmitted by more than 60 mosquito species acting as intermediate hosts of the parasite [1]. Dogs and other carnivores are its final hosts and humans are incidental hosts. *Dirofilaria repens* is a well-recognized parasite of dogs and humans in southern Europe [1–4] in the Ukraine [5, 6] and southern Russia [7]. Although cats appear to be competent hosts for *D. repens*, they are much more resistant to invasion and in endemic regions prevalence is considerably lower than in dogs [2].

Recently, the emergence of canine and human dirofilariosis due to *D. repens* has been reported in central European countries, a region that was previously considered to be non-endemic for this parasite species [2, 8–14]. Among the most probable reasons for this northward expansion of *D. repens* in Europe are climatic changes associated with global warming (facilitating the development of larval stages in the mosquito host) and translocation of infected dogs from southern to central Europe [15, 16]. The total number of human cases of dirofilariosis has changed dynamically, increasing from 1200 cases reported in 2009 [2] to over 4000 cases reported in 2015 [17], an increasing statistic that is likely also to be mainly attributable to a greater interest in the epidemiology of dirofilariosis in recent years. Thus dirofilariosis caused by *D. repens* is now considered to be an emerging zoonosis in Europe [1].

Dogs serve as the major source of infection of *D. repens* for mosquitoes which then transmit infection to humans. Therefore, the recognition, treatment and prevention of *D. repens* invasion in dogs is likely to help also the control of infection in humans [2]. Although there are new measures for the elimination of adult *D. repens* worms from dogs [18], a key problem is that neither the diagnosis nor the implementation of preventative/ control measures are common in newly established endemic regions in central Europe. Recent studies on the distribution of *D. repens* in Slovakia and Poland have detected high prevalence (34–60 %) of infection in clinically healthy working dogs [8, 19] and these asymptomatic infections are not usually recognized and treated. The presence of adult *D. repens* in dogs causes canine subcutaneous dirofilariosis, with a range of dermatological manifestations [20], but apparently may also be asymptomatic and chronic for several years [2, 8, 19]. The pathogenicity associated with accumulating high numbers of microfilariae in the circulating blood of infected dogs is also not well recognized but there are a few reports on possible acute and fatal outcomes of such infections associated with the presence of microfilariae in vital organs (heart, liver, kidney) [21].

Dirofilaria repens infections in dogs, humans and vectors have been reported often in recent years in countries in the vicinity of Poland [6, 13, 15, 17, 19]. In Germany at least two endemic regions have been recognized: between Stuttgart and Frankfurt/Men and in Branderburg federal state (near Berlin and possibly in the Oder River valley) [13, 15, 22, 23] In Slovakia, *D. repens* in dogs was recorded for the first time in 2005, and to date is widely spread and has been detected in *Aedes vexans* mosquitoes [11, 12, 19, 24]. In the Ukraine, dirofilariosis is a registerable zoonotic disease and about 91 new cases in humans are registered each year [6, 17].

To our knowledge, no data on the prevalence of *D. repens* in cats in central Europe is available.

In Poland, *D. repens* was recorded for the first time in a dog in 2009 [25] but already Central Poland is now well recognized as a recently established endemic region for this species, with a high prevalence having been reported in dogs, then in mosquitoes and as autochthonous zoonotic invasions in humans [5, 14, 26]. However, the distribution of the parasite in other regions of Poland is less well recognized.

The high prevalence of *D. repens* infections in dogs/ cats constitutes a new challenge for veterinarians due to the increasing probability of co-infection occurring with other blood parasites vectored by ticks [19]. Among the vector-borne diseases of greatest importance is canine babesiosis, caused by *Babesia canis* transmitted by *Dermacentor reticulatus* ticks [27–29]. In central and eastern regions of Poland canine babesiosis is endemic and hyper-endemic, causing thousands of life-threatening infections in dogs each year. As an example, over a period of 6 months (autumn 2013 to spring 2014) over 1200 canine babesiosis cases were treated in selected vet clinics in two districts in eastern Poland (Wysokie Mazowieckie and Semiatycze, Podlaskie voivodeship [large administrative region]) [30]. Prevalence of *B. canis* infections in *D. reticulatus* ticks may be as high as 8–16 % in central Poland [28] and this tick species dominates on dogs in this part of Poland [31]. To our knowledge, the impact of concurrent infections of *D. repens* with *B. canis* has not been investigated. Therefore we assessed the prevalence of *D. repens* and its effect on the host in dogs infected with *B. canis*, originating from the Mazovia region.

The aims of the present work were: (1) to estimate the prevalence of *D. repens* infection in cats and dogs from different regions of Poland (2) to compare the prevalence of *D. repens* in healthy dogs and dogs with babesiosis and finally (3) to analyze the influence of *D. repens* infections on the severity of canine babesiosis.

Methods

Sampling

Overall, 147 blood samples from cats were included in this study. These originated from pet cats that were regularly allowed to roam freely outside the house or

apartment of their owners, and were provided by the Lab-Wet diagnostic laboratory in the period 2013–2014.

In total, 257 individual blood samples were collected from dogs between October 2014 and November 2015, including samples from healthy dogs from central Poland, Warsaw area ($n = 94$; diverse group of dogs- pet dogs, sled dogs, dogs from shelters), samples from dogs from northern Poland (Gdańsk $n = 34$; Bydgoszcz $n = 5$); samples from southern Poland (Kraków $n = 30$; Katowice $n = 6$) and samples from western Poland (Wrocław $n = 30$). Samples from Gdańsk, Kraków and Wrocław were provided by Lab-Wet diagnostics laboratory, and originated from dogs referred for blood analysis because of a range of different medical reasons.

In addition to these 199 samples, the occurrence of *D. repens* was investigated among 58 dogs suspected for babesiosis. These samples originated from dogs presenting with a wide range of babesiosis symptoms, including fatal cases, originating from central Poland in the vicinity of Warsaw, a region that is known to be endemic both for canine babesiosis and dirofilariosis. Samples were enrolled into the study on the basis of a positive diagnosis of *B. canis* infection as detected by the Lab-Vet diagnostics laboratory.

To study the effect of concurrent infection with *D. repens* and *B. canis*, we analyzed standard data on blood cell concentrations (and related counts) available from 41 dogs and biochemistry parameters available from 37 dogs suffering from babesiosis. Blood parameters were compared between dogs with single (*B. canis*) and double (*B. canis* + *D. repens*) infections.

Molecular analysis

Infections with *D. repens* and *B. canis* in dogs were identified/confirmed based on specific PCR amplification and sequencing of reference genes [32–34]. Additionally, to detect *D. repens* invasions in cats, a fragment of the *ftsZ* gene of the filarial endosymbiotic bacterium, *Wolbachia*, was amplified and sequenced following Turba et al. (2012) [35]. Detection of *Wolbachia* in blood samples constitutes an indirect, but sensitive method for the assessment of the presence/absence of filarial infections.

Blood samples were collected into 0.001 M EDTA and frozen at a temperature of -20 °C until DNA extraction. DNA extractions were performed on whole blood using the AxyGen MiniPrep Blood kit (AxyGen, USA) or MO BIO Ultra Clean Blood Spin DNA Isolation kit (MO BIO Laboratories, USA). A combination of *D. repens* specific primers (12SF and 12SR2) extracted from a multiplex PCR developed by Gioia et al. (2010) [34] was used to amplify the *12S rRNA* gene fragment (327 bp) of *D. repens* [8]. Amplification of the *18S rRNA Babesia* gene fragment was performed using the previously described PCR protocol [32, 33]. Primers BAB GF2 (5′

GYYTTGTAA TTGGAATGATGG 3′) and BABGR2 (5′ CCAAAGACTTTGATTTCTCTC 3′) were used to produce a ~550 bp fragment. Positive controls were as follows: for *Babesia* detection- *B. microti* King's College strain genomic DNA [36]; for *D. repens*- *D. repens* genomic DNA from an adult nematode kindly provided by Dr. Aleksander Masny, National Institute of Health in Warsaw. Positive and negative (sterile H_2O as template) controls were included in each set of PCRs.

Amplicons were visualized with Midori Green stain (Nippon Genetics Europe GmbH, Germany) following the electrophoresis in 1.5 % agarose gels. Selected amplicons were purified and sequenced by a private company (Genomed S.A., Poland). DNA sequence alignments were conducted using MEGA version 6.0 [37]. The resulting sequences were compared with sequences deposited in GenBank NCBI.

Statistical methods

Prevalence of *D. repens* infection (% infected) in dogs with and without babesiosis was compared by Fisher exact test, INSTAT software. Comparison of mean blood parameter values between dogs with single (*B. canis*) and double (*B. canis* + *D. repens*) infections was carried out by Student's t-tests, implemented by the software package, IBM SPSS v. 21 (Table 1). An ANOVA was also used for the comparison of mean blood parameter values between dogs categorized in 3 classes of severity of babesiosis- to confirm correct categorization of scores (Table 2). The presence/absence of *D. repens* infection, fitted as a binary factor (infected =1, not infected =0) was included in a second ANOVA, incorporating also severity scores of babesiosis or scores for the severity of appropriate 'general' symptom as the dependent variables (anemia, hepatic or renal dysfunction, see below) (Table 3). These analyses were carried out to test our research hypothesis, that severity of babesiosis may be affected by concurrent *D. repens* infection through the negative impact of microfilariae on a range of blood parameters and the function of vital organs (liver, kidney) (as indicated in [19]). Thus, we performed a series of statistical comparisons with the presence/absence of *D. repens* as a factor associated with severity scores for three main 'general' symptoms and an overall severity score for babesiosis (explained below).

The severity of babesiosis was classified at 3 levels. As all dogs with babesiosis ($n = 58$) suffered from thrombocytopenia (only two dogs had thrombocytes count in the range 100–150, all the others had counts below 100 G/l) (Table 1), this parameter was not included in the classification. The three main groups of general symptoms (indicators of mortality in canine babesiosis) included: a. severity of anemia (severity score 0- RBC counts within normal range 5.5–8.0 T/l;

Table 1 Comparison of blood parameters between dogs co-infected with *B. canis* and *D. repens* and infected only with *B. canis*

Parameter	Mean parameter value ± SEM			Reference values	P
	Overall	Dogs with co-infection	Dogs with *B.canis*		
Counts (n = 41):		n = 36	n = 5		
Leukocytes (G/l)	5.850 ± 0.551	5.039 ± 0.320	7.50 ± 2.914	6.0–12.0	0.007
Erythrocytes (T/l)	4.885 ± 0.115	4.976 ± 0.191	4.18 ± 0.401	5.5–8.0	0.758NS
Hemoglobin (mmol/l)	7.238 ± 0.180	7.161 ± 0.254	7.404 ± 0.868	7.45–11.17	0.747 NS
Hematocrit (l/l)	0.332 ± 0.008	0.326 ± 0.012	0.342 ± 0.038	0.37–0.55	0.660 NS
MCV (fl)	67.26 ± 0.944	66.11 ± 0.778	70.44 ± 2.737	60–77	0.068 NS
MCHC (mmol/l)	21.86 ± 0.147	21.97 ± 0.109	21.58 ± 0.426	19.8–22.3	0.246 NS
Thrombocytes (G/l)	57.09 ± 5.007	45.40 ± 3.335	91.80 ± 26.79	200–580	0.001
Biochemical parameters (n = 37):		n = 32	n = 5		
AST (U/l)	120.66 ± 31.58	113.28 ± 18.83	249.40 ± 159.07	1–45	0.079 NS
ALT (U/l)	139.93 ± 39.63	126.25 ± 33.84	312.40 ± 156.41	3–60	0.081 NS
ALP (U/l)	203.98 ± 39.56	165.48 ± 20.71	432.80 ± 206.45	20–155	0.007
Serum glucose (mg/dl)	105.43 ± 7.066	100.33 ± 4.965	125.00 ± 30.33	70–120	0.151 NS
Creatinine (mg/dl)	1.541 ± 0.121	1.125 ± 0.134	1.780 ± 1.031	0.8–1.7	0.206 NS
Serum urea (mg/dl)	108.96 ± 8.376	61.50 ± 14.26	135.20 ± 98.20	20–45	0.158 NS
Total serum protein (g/l)	60.01 ± 1.177	59.59 ± 1.112	59.20 ± 2.437	55–75	0.896 NS

SEM standard error of the mean, *P* probability values from Student's t-tests, *MCV* mean corpuscular volume, *MCHC* mean corpuscular hemoglobin concentration, *AST* aspartate aminotransferase, *ALT* alanine aminotransferase, *ALP* alkaline phosphatase

severity score 1- RBC counts in a range 4.5–5.5 T/l; severity score 2- RBC below 4.5 T/l); b. hepatic dysfunction parameters (measures of enzymes activity [based on reference values for AST – aspartate aminotransferase and ALT- alanine aminotransferase; with accompanying ALP – alkaline phosphatase] within, above (up to 100 U/l) and profoundly above (>100 U/l) the normal range, representing scores of 0, 1 and 2, respectively, Table 2); c. renal dysfunction parameters (based on reference values for serum urea within, above (up to 100 mg/dl) and profoundly above (>100 mg/dl) the normal range, representing severity scores of 0, 1 and 2, respectively, Table 2).

Then all dogs with any of these three general symptoms classified as 'severity score 2' were assigned to

Table 2 Comparison of the selected parameters for the estimation of the severity of the three general symptoms, then used for classification of the severity of the babesiosis (classes 1–3)

Summarized symptom and parameters ± SEM	Severity class			P
	Class 0 (normal)	Class 1 (mild)	Class 2 (severe)	
1. Anemia:	n = 15	n = 14	n = 12	
Erythrocytes (T/l)	5.98 ± 0.183	5.02 ± 0.187	3.20 ± 0.235	0.000
Leukocytes (G/l)	4.89 ± 0.874	4.69 ± 0.896	9.06 ± 1.126	0.014
Hematocrit (l/l)	0.402 ± 0.013	0.347 ± 0.013	0.213 ± 0.017	0.000
Hemoglobin (mmol/l)	8.777 ± 0.286	7.558 ± 0.293	4.651 ± 0.368	0.000
Thrombocytes (G/l)	45.17 ± 7.945	59.83 ± 8.143	68.43 ± 10.234	0.103 NS
2. Hepatic dysfunction:	n = 5	n = 22	n = 10	
AST (U/l)	32.13 ± 77.238	78.20 ± 43.727	315.33 ± 47.672	0.029
ALT (U/l)	37.25 ± 96.948	66.58 ± 54.886	426.00 ± 59.838	0.011
ALP (U/l)	112.50 ± 96.599	141.69 ± 54.840	451.19 ± 59.622	0.026
3. Renal dysfunction:	n = 25	n = 7	n = 5	
Creatinine (mg/dl)	0.802 ± 0.151	0.983 ± 0.240	4.23 ± 0.304	0.000
Serum urea (mg/dl)	29.27 ± 10.459	55.92 ± 16.656	387.75 ± 21.116	0.000

P-probability values from ANOVA tests
Reference values for parameters and explanations as in legend to Table 1

Table 3 Comparison of blood parameters between dogs co-infected with *B. canis* and *D. repens* and infected only with *B. canis* in different severity classes

General symptom level	Parameter	Mean (± SEM) in dogs infected with *B.canis* + *D.repens*	Mean (± SEM) in dogs infected only with *B. canis*	F and P
I. Anemia				
Level 0:	Erythrocytes (T/l)	6.07 ± 0.181	6.00 ± 0.610	$F_{2,\,40} = 0.708$; $P = 0.408$
	Leucocytes (G/l)	5.12 ± 0.756	4.20 ± 2.661	$F_{2,\,40} = 2.734$; $P = 0.082$
	Thrombocytes (G/l)	52.56 ± 6.871	23.00 ± 24.188	$F_{2,\,40} = 6.866$; $P = 0.004$
	Hematocrit (l/l)	0.377 ± 0.014	0.450 ± 0.046	$F_{2,\,40} = 0.044$; $P = 0.835$
Level 1:	Erythrocytes (T/l)	4.80 ± 0.294	5.08 ± 0.431	
	Leucocytes (G/l)	4.39 ± 0.810	5.15 ± 1.881	
	Thrombocytes(G/l)	38.06 ± 7.360	92.50 ± 17.103	
	Hematocrit(l/l)	0.311 ± 0.022	0.365 ± 0.033	
Level 2:	Erythrocytes (T/l)	3.64 ± 0.249	3.95 ± 0.431	
	Leucocytes (G/l)	7.83 ± 1.402	11.50 ± 1.881	
	Thrombocytes (G/l)	39.89 ± 12.748	125.50 ± 17.103	
	Hematocrit (l/l)	0.247 ± 0.019	0.265 ± 0.033	
II. Hepatic dysfunction				
Level 0:	AST (U/l)	34.60 ± 24.153	nd	$F_{1,\,36} = 0.709$; $P = 0.407$
	ALT (U/l)	40.40 ± 51.35	nd	$F_{1,\,36} = 0.044$; $P = 0.835$
	ALP (U/l)	102.00 ± 48.093	nd	$F_{1,\,36} = 0.360$; $P = 0.554$
Level 1:	AST (U/l)	93.78 ± 15.868	81.00 ± 38.189	
	ALT (U/l)	60.33 ± 33.736	82.00 ± 81.192	
	ALP (U/l)	151.28 ± 31.726	119.50 ± 76.041	
Level 2:	AST (U/l)	307.67 ± 23.815	361.67 ± 31.181	
	ALT (U/l)	378.08 ± 50.632	466.00 ± 66.293	
	ALP (U/l)	259.00 ± 47.420	641.67 ± 62.087	
III. Renal dysfunction				
Level 0:	Creatinine (mg/dl)	0.87 ± 0.117	0.70 ± 0.334	$F_{2,\,36} = 11.68$; $P = 0.000$
	Serum urea (mg/dl)	28.94 ± 8.127	29.75 ± 23.131	$F_{2,\,36} = 16.16$; $P = 0.000$
Level 1:	Creatinine (mg/dl)	1.03 ± 0.236	0.90 ± 0.545	
	Serum urea (mg/dl)	52.88 ± 16.356	62.00 ± 37.773	
Level 2:	Creatinine (mg/dl)	2.55 ± 0.272	5.90 ± 0.545	
	Serum urea (mg/dl)	248.50 ± 18.886	527.00 ± 37.773	

P values derived from ANOVAs
D. repens presence x anemia level on erythrocytes count; *D. repens* presence x anemia level on leucocytes count; *D. repens* presence x anemia level on thrombocytes count
D. repens presence x hepatic dysfunction level on AST activity; *D. repens* presence x hepatic dysfunction level on ALT activity; *D. repens* presence x hepatic dysfunction level on ALP activity; *D. repens* presence x renal dysfunction level on serum creatinine; *D. repens* presence x renal dysfunction level on serum urea
Nd- not done, the lack of cases in this group

group 3 (severe babesiosis, severity level 3, $n = 20$); dogs presenting with more than one dysfunction (anemia, symptoms of hepatic or renal failure) at level 1 (abnormal) were assigned to group 2 (moderate babesiosis, severity level 2; $n = 11$) and finally dogs presenting only with one group of symptoms (mainly mild anemia and thrombocytopenia) were assigned to group 1 (mild babesiosis, severity level 1, $n = 10$). This final classification was carried out to assess the general impact of concurrent *D. repens* infection on the severity of babesiosis in dogs and

appropriate levels were implemented into multifactorial ANOVAs for each dog for each blood parameter (Table 2).

Finally, log-linear analyses of contingency tables were performed (SPSS v. 21) to compare prevalence of *D. repens* in dogs assigned to three severity classes (4 different classification: 1. anemia [0–2]; 2. symptoms of hepatic failure [0–2]; 3. symptoms of renal failure [0–2]; babesiosis severity [1–3]). This analysis was carried out to test our research hypothesis that the prevalence of *D. repens* infection should be higher in dogs suffering more severe symptoms (our scores 2 and 3 for 'general' symptoms or babesiosis, respectively). Again, this was done to seek evidence for an association between severity of the disease and presence of *D. repens*. We tested two models: anemia scale x babesiosis scale x *D. repens* presence (0, 1) and hepatic dysfunction class x renal dysfunction class x babesiosis scale x *D. repens* prevalence (0, 1).

Results
The occurrence of *Dirofilaria repens* and *Wolbachia* in cats
Dirofilaria repens
DNA was detected only in one blood sample, from one cat positive also for *Wolbachia* (0.7 % [95 % CL: 0–4.1 %]). Our sequence was identical to the *D. repens* isolate obtained from the blood of a sled dog in our previous study (accession number KF494237; [8]). *Wolbachia* DNA was detected in 2 out of 147 cats (1.4 % [95 % CL: 0–5.5 %]). Both sequences were identical, displaying the highest homology (>99 %) to the sequence of *Wolbachia*, endosymbiont of *D. repens* (GenBank accession number AJ010273).

The occurrence of *Dirofilaria repens* in dogs from different regions of Poland
Dirofilaria repens
DNA was detected only in dogs from central Poland. None of the samples from the other regions (southern, western or northern Poland) tested positive. The specific diagnostic 320 bp band of the *12S rRNA* gene fragment of *D. repens* was observed in 36 dogs out of 94 healthy dogs that were tested (prevalence 38.3 % [95 % CL: 25.9–51.8 %]). To confirm the specific amplification, 16 (44 % of all positive) randomly selected samples were sequenced, aligned and compared with sequences from the GenBank database. All sequences were identical, displaying the highest homology (295/ 296 identical nucleotides, 99.7 %) to the sequence of *D. repens* isolated from a subcutaneous human case in Russia (accession number KM205374). Our sequences displayed similar high homology (263/265 identical nucleotides, 99.2 %) with the *D. repens* isolate obtained from a sled dog in our previous study (accession number KF494237; [8]).

To test for the occurrence of possible unidentified, asymptomatic co-infections with *B. canis* and *D. repens*, we also analyzed samples from these 94 healthy dogs from central Poland for *Babesia* DNA. Only 1 asymptomatic dog (prevalence 1.06 % [95 % CL: 0–5.2 %]) proved positive for *B. canis* but it was not infected with *D. repens*.

The occurrence of *Dirofilaria repens* in dogs with babesiosis in central Poland
First, to confirm the laboratory diagnosis of *B. canis* infection based on microscopical observation of blood smears, the 560 bp *18S rRNA* gene fragment of *Babesia* was amplified in blood samples from all symptomatic dogs (58/58 = 100 %). Then, the 320 bp *12S rRNA* gene fragment of *D. repens* was amplified with species-specific primers. *Dirofilaria repens* DNA was detected in 52 of 58 dogs with babesiosis (prevalence 89.7 % [95 % CL: 81.6–94.5 %]). The difference in prevalence of *D. repens* between healthy dogs and dogs with babesiosis (38.3 % versus 89.7 %) was highly significant (Fisher's exact test, $P < 0.0001$).

To confirm the occurrence of co-infections of *B. canis* and *D. repens*, respective PCR products were sequenced from 30 double-positive dogs (57.7 % of all double-positive samples). Sequences were aligned and compared with the GenBank database. Sequencing revealed that 30 *Babesia* sequences displayed the highest homology (514/519 identical nucleotides; 99.0 %) to the *B. canis* genotype 2 (EU622793), originally isolated from a dog with babesiosis in Poland [38] and to a *B. canis* isolate from a *D. reticulatus* tick (KT272401; 516/520 = 99 %; [31]).

The sequencing of 30 *D. repens* positive amplicons revealed the presence of a *D. repens* variant identical with isolates obtained in this study from the healthy dogs from the same region of central Poland, displaying the highest homology (97–99 %) to the sequence of *D. repens* isolated from a human case in Russia (KM205374) and to a sequence from one of our dogs deposited earlier (KF494237). Lower homology for several sequences arose through some non-specific background amplification of canine DNA.

The influence of *D. repens* infections on the severity of babesiosis
Various blood parameters were compared between two groups of dogs: 36 or 32 dogs co-infected with *B. canis* and *D. repens* and 5 dogs infected only with *B. canis* (Table 1).

Generally, mean numbers of erythrocytes, leucocytes, thrombocytes and mean values for hematocrit or hemoglobin concentration obtained for all 41 dogs with babesiosis were below reference values, but the majority of these values were lower in dogs with co-infection in comparison to dogs infected only with *B. canis*. However, these differences were significant only for the mean number of thrombocytes and leucocytes (Table 1). Thrombocyte numbers were twice as high in dogs with just *B. canis* compare to those with co-infection.

A contrasting pattern was observed for biochemical parameters. Although overall mean parameter values calculated for all dogs with babesiosis were higher relative to normal levels (values of AST, ALT and ALP and serum urea concentration), the means for dogs only infected with *B. canis* were higher than those of dogs with concurrent *D. repens* (Table 1), indicating a more severe babesiosis in the former dogs with involvement of hepatic and renal failure. Statistically significant differences were observed only for ALP activity (Table 1).

In the next step of analysis, we test our research hypothesis, that severity of babesiosis may be affected by concurrent *D. repens* infection through the negative impact of the presence of microfilariae on a range of blood parameters and the function of vital organs (liver, kidney). The symptoms were compiled to create three general classes of symptoms (anemia, symptoms of hepatic or renal failure; Table 2), each with three severity levels and implemented into statistical models (ANOVAs for specific parameter). Statistical analysis confirmed significant differences between the mean blood parameters of dogs arbitrarily assigned to three classes of severity (Table 2) and revealed some interesting effects of the interaction between the presence of *D. repens* and severity of general symptoms on mean values of selected parameters (Table 3). Contrary to our expectations, among the different parameters the values that were profoundly above normal level were observed in dogs assigned to class 2 and infected only with *B. canis*, and the range of means in three severity classes was generally lower in dogs with co-infections (i.e. differences in leucocytes, ALP, serum creatinine or urea concentrations between two groups of dogs in class 2; Table 3).

In the final step of our analysis, we examined associations between the prevalence of *D. repens* and the severity scores for babesiosis, anemia, symptoms of hepatic or renal dysfunction (between 3 respective classes). No statistically significant associations were obtained in these analyses. The only observed trend was for the association between the presence of *D. repens* and hepatic dysfunction classes ($\chi^2 = 3.69$, df = 2, $P = 0.158$). Prevalence of *D. repens* was highest in class 0 (normal) with all dogs co-infected with filariae (100 %); was 91 % in class 1 (abnormal) and the lowest (70 %) in dogs assigned to severity class 2 (hepatic failure), indicating an opposite association to that predicted in our research hypothesis.

Discussion

The main aims of this study were to estimate the prevalence of *D. repens* in cats and dogs from different regions of Poland and to evaluate the influence of this nematode infection on concurrent canine babesiosis. We confirmed the high prevalence of *D. repens* infection in the recently established endemic region in central Poland and found no infected dogs outside this area. Interestingly, although the prevalence of *D. repens* was more than twice as high in dogs with babesiosis in comparison to healthy animals, statistical analyses of a range of blood parameters revealed a diverse influence of concurrent *D. repens* infection on measures of pathology in babesiosis.

In our study *D. repens* DNA was found only in dogs and in one cat from the area of Warsaw, spanning a radius of about 60 km from the city center in the region of Mazovia (Masovian voivodeship). To our knowledge, this is the first finding of *D. repens* in a cat in central Europe. Interestingly, detection of the filarial endosymbiotic bacterium, *Wolbachia*, proved to be a more sensitive detection technique than the direct detection of *D. repens* DNA, detecting 2 and 1 positive cat, respectively, but this conclusion needs further confirmation due to the very limited number of positive samples in our study.

Mazovia was first recognized as a new endemic region for canine dirofilariosis in Poland [14, 25] and recent studies, including the present one, confirm the stable continuous transmission of parasites in this region [8, 9]. The prevalence of *D. repens* recorded in this study in dogs (38 %) is within the range of previously reported rates in this area (20–60 %) and is typical for endemic regions in much warmer climates [2]. Such a high prevalence in dogs indicates a high risk of emergence of human dirofilariosis in the region, as seroprevalence of *D. repens* in humans may reach the same values as prevalence in dogs in some locations [1, 2]. Interestingly, all the dogs included in this study were 'healthy', as were the dogs in previous studies [9, 19], so no directed treatment to control microfilaraemia in these dogs had been implemented, creating a continuous source of infection for the vectors.

We were unable to discover *D. repens* DNA in more than 100 dogs from three other macroregions of Poland. This is generally in agreement with the results of a previous study on 1588 dogs from Poland, reporting a much lower prevalence of *D. repens* in dogs from northern, western and southern Poland, spanning a range of just 0–10 % [10, 21]. Demiaszkiewicz et al. [10] reported higher prevalence in dogs from eastern Poland, ranging between 13–16 % for Podlaskie and Lubelskie voivodeships, in regions not included in the present study. However, the well-established endemic area in central Poland may serve as the source of the spread of the parasite to new regions in Poland, due to translocation of asymptomatic but nevertheless infected dogs.

Central and eastern Poland are also endemic regions for canine babesiosis and we discovered a positive association between infection with these two vector-borne parasites. Prevalence of *D. repens* was 2.5 times higher in dogs with babesiosis than in representatives of a healthy population from the same region and this association was highly significant. Although *D. repens* infections are more prevalent, but generally asymptomatic, in dogs in central Poland, infection with *B. canis* rarely remains asymptomatic [29, 39] although the course of babesiosis may differ from moderate to severe and sometimes even fatal. All the dogs involved in this phase of our study were infected with *B. canis*, presenting a range of symptoms and typically characteristic changes in blood parameters [40–44]. Additionally, to check if there were any asymptomatic co-infections of *B. canis* and *D. repens*, we tested 94 healthy dogs from Mazovia by the same molecular techniques. Despite the high prevalence of *D. repens* (38 %) in these dogs, we detected only one dog from this group as positive for *B.canis* DNA and this individual was free of *D. repens*, so no asymptomatic co-infections were found. However, in 366 microfilaraemic but clinically healthy working dogs in Slovakia, 14 cases of co-infection of *B. canis* and *D. repens* were confirmed [19]. The other explanation can be that the high rate of co-infection between mosquito-borne dirofilariosis and tick-borne babesiosis is the result of generally higher exposure of the dogs to these vectors, i.e. through their spatio-temporal activity patterns or the lack of treatment for ectoparasites in this group of dogs.

The possible mechanisms underlying the impact of *D. repens* on the course of babesiosis are currently unknown. In a recent review on common features in malaria and babesiosis, two principal factors linked to pathogenecity were identified, one associated with immunological stimulation and the second with adhesion and sequestration of infected RBC [45]. Heavy burdens of microfilariae in capillary vessels may interfere with RBC adhesion, disturbing blood flow through vital organs. In our study, analyses of various blood parameters revealed a quite different pattern for parameters associated with blood morphology and anemia and for biochemical parameters. In the first instance, as we might have expected, the most pronounced changes were observed in dogs with co-infection compared with dogs infected only by *B. canis* (lower numbers of thrombocytes, hematocrit, hemoglobin concentration), but of these only the number of thrombocytes was significantly lower. Contrary to our expectation, the biochemical parameters displayed more pronounced changes in dogs infected solely by *B. canis*, implying that these animals were experiencing more severe episodes of babesiosis with hepatic and renal failure. This finding has similarities to the conclusions of a long-term study on malaria and intestinal helminths in humans from Thailand [46, 47]. Observational studies in Thailand have shown that although the incidence of *Plasmodium falciparum* malaria was twice as high in helminth-infected patients, there was a 64 % reduction of cerebral malaria and an 84 % reduction of acute renal failure in patients co-infected with malaria and helminths in comparison to those without helminths [46]. Although fever was lower in patients with co-infections, they suffered from more severe anemia, but generally it was concluded that helminth invasions had a protective effect against severe and fatal course of *P. falciparum* malaria.

The possible mechanisms underlying these phenomena (higher susceptibility to *B. canis* infection but less severe babesiosis) require further investigation. The higher probability of developing babesiosis after *B. canis* infection in *D. repens*-infected dogs, may be the result of a depression of the immune response against pre-erythrocytic stages (sporozoites), as proposed for *P. falciparum* [46, 47]. As helminths, including *D. repens*, are long-lived parasites stimulating a Th-2 type response profile with low production of pro-inflammatory cytokines, they have a marked depressive effect on other immune pathways including the Th-1 type responses that are considered to be host protective in the case of intracellular parasites such as *Babesia* spp. [45]. Suppression of the Th-1 arm of the immune system would inevitably reduce pathology associated with effector mechanisms unleashed during Th-1 driven immune responses [45].

The much lower counts of thrombocytes in dogs with co-infection, may be associated with the recently discovered significant role of these cells in both innate and adaptive immunity against a range of pathogens [48]. Recruitment of platelets in a response targeting *B. canis*-infected RBCs and microfilariae may be the cause of the considerable reduction in their numbers in the circulation of dogs with co-infections. However, although in our study the differences in several blood parameters (i.e. ALP) were significant or showed borderline significance (i.e. for AST, ALT), the group of dogs with the single infection was quite small ($n = 5$) and the output of these analyses should be treated with some degree of caution at this stage.

Our study has several limitations. The sensitivity of PCRs was not determined so prevalence of *D. repens* could be underestimated. The number of sampled dogs outside the Warsaw area is limited. The data on blood parameters was available only for dogs suspected of babesiosis and similar data is missing for dogs infected only with *D. repens*. The main reason for this lack is that dirofilariosis is a relatively new health problem and is very rarely diagnosed and treated in routine vet care of pet dogs. Thus, it was impossible to include a group of samples from dogs with clinical symptoms suspected of suffering only from dirofilariosis. We have data on blood parameters only for two dogs infected solely with *D. repens* (within normal ranges for the majority of parameters as follows: mean RBC = 7.12 T/l; mean leucocytes = 6.15 G/l; mean hemoglobin = 10.8 mmol/l; mean hematocrit = 0.495 l/l; mean thrombocytes = 295.5 G/l; mean AST = 27 U/l; mean ALT = 43 U/l; mean ALP = 37 U/l, mean creatinine = 1.15 mg/dl; mean serum urea = 50.5 mg/dl). Not much conclusions can be drawn from these values and further study is needed to fill this gap.

Conclusions

In summary, a very high rate of co-infection with *B. canis* and *D. repens* in dogs treated for babesiosis and the lack of asymptomatic co-infections in healthy dogs suggest that microfilaremic dogs are more prone to developing symptomatic babesiosis. However, contrary to our predictions, the values of biochemical parameters in dogs with co-infection were closer to those of healthy dogs than those solely infected with *B. canis* suggesting milder babesiosis in these animals. These findings are important due to the current spread of dirofilariosis and babesiosis in central Europe, which being mostly undiagnosed has resulted in large numbers of untreated microfilaraemic dogs in the region, which may be more prone to babesiosis. The possible protective effect of the nematode infection on hepatic or renal dysfunction in canine babesiosis is intriguing and its mechanisms require further investigations.

Acknowledgements
The authors would like to acknowledge the owners of dogs and cats for their kind cooperation. We are grateful to the director and veterinary services of local shelter, Malgorzata and Iza Szmurlo, for providing the blood samples from the dogs under their care.

Funding
The study was partially supported by the National Science Center (NCN) grant Sonata Bis no. 2014/14/E/NZ7/00153 (AB) and by the Ministry of Science and Higher Education through the Faculty of Biology, University of Warsaw intramural grant DSM 501/86-104924 (RWF).

Authors' contributions
AB and RWF conceived, designed, and conducted the study, analyzed the data, and wrote the paper. EJM conducted the study and wrote the paper. AR and KT contributed to acquisition of data, analyzed the data and revised the paper. All authors read and approved the final manuscript.

Competing interests
The authors declare that they have no competing interests.

Consent for publication
Not applicable.

Author details
[1]Department of Parasitology, Institute of Zoology, Faculty of Biology, University of Warsaw, 1 Miecznikowa Street, 02-096 Warsaw, Poland. [2]Department of Pathology and Veterinary Diagnostics, Warsaw University of Life Sciences- SGGW, 159c Nowoursynowska Street, 02-766 Warsaw, Poland. [3]Lab-Wet, Veterinary Diagnostic Laboratory, ul. Wita Stwosza 30, 02-661 Warsaw, Poland.

References
1. Genchi C, Kramer LH, Rivasi F. Dirofilarial infections in Europe. Vector Borne Zoonotic Dis. 2011;11(10):1307–17.
2. Simon F, Morchon R, Gonzalez-Miguel J, Marcos-Atxutegi C, Siles-Lucas M. What is new about animal and human dirofilariosis? Trends Parasitol. 2009;25(9):404–9.
3. Simon F, Siles-Lucas M, Morchon R, Gonzalez-Miguel J, Mellado I, Carreton E, Montoya-Alonso JA. Human and animal dirofilariasis: the emergence of a zoonotic mosaic. Clin Microbiol Rev. 2012;25(3):507–44.
4. Tasic-Otasevic SA, Trenkic Bozinovic MS, Gabrielli SV, Genchi C. Canine and human Dirofilaria infections in the Balkan Peninsula. Vet Parasitol. 2015;209(3-4):151–6.
5. Masny A, Golab E, Cielecka D, Salamatin R. Vector-borne helminths of dogs and humans - focus on central and eastern parts of Europe. Parasit Vectors. 2013;6:38.
6. Sałamatin RV, Pavlikovska TM, Sagach OS, Nikolayenko SM, Kornyushin VV, Kharchenko VO, Masny A, Cielecka D, Konieczna-Sałamatin J, Conn DB, et al. Human dirofilariasis due to Dirofilaria repens in Ukraine, an emergent zoonosis: epidemiological report of 1465 cases. Acta Parasitol. 2013;58(4):592–8.
7. Ermakova LA, Nagorny SA, Krivorotova EY, Pshenichnaya NY, Matina ON. Dirofilaria repens in the Russian Federation: current epidemiology, diagnosis, and treatment from a federal reference center perspective. Int J Infect Dis. 2014;23:47–52.
8. Bajer A, Mierzejewska EJ, Rodo A, Bednarska M, Kowalec M, Welc-Faleciak R. The risk of vector-borne infections in sled dogs associated with existing and new endemic areas in Poland: Part 1: A population study on sled dogs during the racing season. Vet Parasitol. 2014;202(3-4):276–86.
9. Demiaszkiewicz AW, Polanczyk G, Osinska B, Pyziel AM, Kuligowska I, Lachowicz J, Sikorski A. Prevalence and distribution of Dirofilaria repens Railliet et Henry, 1911 in dogs in Poland. Pol J Vet Sci. 2014;17(3):515–7.
10. Demiaszkiewicz AW, Polanczyk G, Osinska B, Pyziel AM, Kuligowska I, Lachowicz J, Sikorski A. The prevalence and distribution of Dirofilaria repens in dogs in the Mazovian Province of central-eastern Poland. Ann Agric Environ Med. 2014;21(4):701–4.
11. Miterpáková M, Antolová D, Hurníková Z, Dubinský P. Dirofilariosis in Slovakia - a new endemic area in Central Europe. Helminthologia. 2008;45(1):20–3.
12. Miterpakova M, Antolova D, Hurnikova Z, Dubinsky P, Pavlacka A, Nemeth J. Dirofilaria infections in working dogs in Slovakia. J Helminthol. 2010;84(2):173–6.
13. Tappe D, Plauth M, Bauer T, Muntau B, Diessel L, Tannich E, Herrmann-Trost P. A case of autochthonous human Dirofilaria infection, Germany, March 2014. Euro Surveill. 2014;19(17):2–4.
14. Masny A, Lewin T, Salamatin R, Golab E. Autochthonous canine Dirofilaria repens in the vicinity of Warsaw. Pol J Vet Sci. 2011;14(4):659–61.
15. Czajka C, Becker N, Jost H, Poppert S, Schmidt-Chanasit J, Kruger A, Tannich E. Stable transmission of Dirofilaria repens nematodes, northern Germany. Emerg Infect Dis. 2014;20(2):328–31.
16. Sassnau R, Daugschies A, Lendner M, Genchi C. Climate suitability for the transmission of Dirofilaria immitis and D. repens in Germany. Vet Parasitol. 2014;205(1–2):239–45.
17. Rossi A, Peix A, Pavlikovskaya T, Sagach O, Nikolaenko S, Chizh N, Kartashev V, Simon F, Siles-Lucas M. Genetic diversity of Dirofilaria spp. isolated from subcutaneous and ocular lesions of human patients in Ukraine. Acta Trop. 2015;142:1–4.
18. Petry G, Genchi M, Schmidt H, Schaper R, Lawrenz B, Genchi C. Evaluation of the Adulticidal Efficacy of Imidacloprid 10 %/Moxidectin 2.5 % (w/v) Spot-on (Advocate(R), Advantage(R) Multi) against Dirofilaria repens in Experimentally Infected Dogs. Parasitol Res. 2015;114 Suppl 1:S131–44.
19. Vichova B, Miterpakova M, Iglodyova A. Molecular detection of co-infections with Anaplasma phagocytophilum and/or Babesia canis canis in Dirofilaria-positive dogs from Slovakia. Vet Parasitol. 2014;203(1-2):167–72.
20. Tarello W. Clinical aspects of dermatitis associated with Dirofilaria repens in pets: a review of 100 canine and 31 feline cases (1990-2010) and a report of a new clinic case imported from Italy to Dubai. J Parasitol Res. 2011;2011:7.
21. Osińska B, Demiaszkiewicz AW, Pyziel AM, Dolka I. Prevalence of Dirofilaria repens in dogs in central-eastern Poland and histopathological changes caused by this infection. Bull Vet Inst Pulawy. 2014;58(1):35–9.
22. Kronefeld M, Kampen H, Sassnau R, Werner D. Molecular detection of Dirofilaria immitis, Dirofilaria repens and Setaria tundra in mosquitoes from Germany. Parasit Vectors. 2014;7:30.
23. Sassnau R, Dyachenko V, Pantchev N, Stöckel F, Dittmar K, Daugschies A. Dirofilaria-repens-Befall in einem Schlittenhunde-Rudel im Land Brandenburg - Diagnose und Therapie der kaninen kutanen Dirofilariose. Tierärztliche Praxis Kleintiere. 2009;37(2):95–101.
24. Bockova E, Rudolf I, Kocisova A, Betasova L, Venclikova K, Mendel J, Hubalek Z. Dirofilaria repens microfilariae in Aedes vexans mosquitoes in Slovakia. Parasitol Res. 2013;112(10):3465–70.
25. Demiaszkiewicz AW, Polanczyk G, Pyziel AM, Kuligowska I, Lachowicz J. The first foci of dirofilariosis of dogs evoked by Dirofilaria repens Railliet et Henry, 1911 in central Poland. Wiad Parazytol. 2009;55(4):367–70.
26. Cielecka D, Zarnowska-Prymek H, Masny A, Salamatin R, Wesolowska M, Golab E. Human dirofilariosis in Poland: the first cases of autochthonous infections with Dirofilaria repens. Ann Agric Environ Med. 2012;19(3):445–50.
27. Bourdoiseau G. Canine babesiosis in France. Vet Parasitol. 2006;138(1-2):118–25.

28. Mierzejewska EJ, Pawelczyk A, Radkowski M, Welc-Faleciak R, Bajer A. Pathogens vectored by the tick, Dermacentor reticulatus, in endemic regions and zones of expansion in Poland. Parasit Vectors. 2015;8:490.
29. Bajer A, Mierzejewska EJ, Rodo A, Welc-Faleciak R. The risk of vector-borne infections in sled dogs associated with existing and new endemic areas in Poland. Part 2: Occurrence and control of babesiosis in a sled dog kennel during a 13-year-long period. Vet Parasitol. 2014;202(3-4):234–40.
30. Trzeszczkowski AK, Kiziewicz B. The tick-borne diseases occuring among dogs and cats of Wysokie Mazowieckie county and Siemiatycze county. In: Buczek A, Blaszak C, editors. Arthropods in the contemporary word. Lublin: Koliber; 2015.
31. Mierzejewska EJ, Welc-Faleciak R, Karbowiak G, Kowalec M, Behnke JM, Bajer A. Dominance of Dermacentor reticulatus over Ixodes ricinus (Ixodidae) on livestock, companion animals and wild ruminants in eastern and central Poland. Exp Appl Acarol. 2015;66(1):83–101.
32. Bonnet S, Jouglin M, L'Hostis M, Chauvin A. Babesia sp. EU1 from roe deer and transmission within Ixodes ricinus. Emerg Infect Dis. 2007;13(8):1208–10.
33. Bonnet S, Jouglin M, Malandrin L, Becker C, Agoulon A, L'Hostis M, Chauvin A. Transstadial and transovarial persistence of Babesia divergens DNA in Ixodes ricinus ticks fed on infected blood in a new skin-feeding technique. Parasitology. 2007;134(Pt 2):197–207.
34. Gioia G, Lecova L, Genchi M, Ferri E, Genchi C, Mortarino M. Highly sensitive multiplex PCR for simultaneous detection and discrimination of Dirofilaria immitis and Dirofilaria repens in canine peripheral blood. Vet Parasitol. 2010; 172(1-2):160–3.
35. Turba ME, Zambon E, Zannoni A, Russo S, Gentilini F. Detection of Wolbachia DNA in blood for diagnosing filaria-associated syndromes in cats. J Clin Microbiol. 2012;50(8):2624–30.
36. Welc-Faleciak R, Bajer A, Bednarska M, Paziewska A, Sinski E. Long term monitoring of Babesia microti infection in BALB/c mice using nested PCR. Ann Agric Environ Med. 2007;14(2):287–90.
37. Tamura K, Stecher G, Peterson D, Filipski A, Kumar S. MEGA6: Molecular Evolutionary Genetics Analysis version 6.0. Mol Biol Evol. 2013;30(12):2725–9.
38. Adaszek L, Winiarczyk S. Molecular characterization of Babesia canis canis isolates from naturally infected dogs in Poland. Vet Parasitol. 2008;152(3-4):235–41.
39. Leschnik M, Feiler A, Duscher GG, Joachim A. Effect of owner-controlled acaricidal treatment on tick infestation and immune response to tick-borne pathogens in naturally infested dogs from Eastern Austria. Parasit Vectors. 2013;6:62.
40. Adaszek L, Winiarczyk S, Skrzypczak M. The clinical course of babesiosis in 76 dogs infected with protozoan parasites Babesia canis canis. Pol J Vet Sci. 2009;12(1):81–7.
41. Zygner W, Gojska O, Rapacka G, Jaros D, Wedrychowicz H. Hematological changes during the course of canine babesiosis caused by large Babesia in domestic dogs in Warsaw (Poland). Vet Parasitol. 2007;145(1-2):146–51.
42. Zygner W, Gójska-Zygner O, Bąska P, Długosz E. Increased concentration of serum TNF alpha and its correlations with arterial blood pressure and indices of renal damage in dogs infected with Babesia canis. Parasitol Res. 2014;113(4):1499–503.
43. Zygner W, Gojska-Zygner O, Wedrychowicz H. Strong monovalent electrolyte imbalances in serum of dogs infected with Babesia canis. Ticks Tick Borne Dis. 2012;3(2):107–13.
44. Gojska-Zygner O, Zygner W. Hyperaldosteronism and its association with hypotension and azotaemia in canine babesiosis. Vet Q. 2015;35(1):37–42.
45. Krause PJ, Daily J, Telford SR, Vannier E, Lantos P, Spielman A. Shared features in the pathobiology of babesiosis and malaria. Trends Parasitol. 2007;23(12):605–10.
46. Nacher M. Worms and malaria: blind men feeling the elephant? Parasitology. 2008;135(7):861–8.
47. Nacher M. Interactions between worms and malaria: good worms or bad worms? Malar J. 2011;10:259.
48. Semple JW, Freedman J. Platelets and innate immunity. Cell Mol Life Sci. 2010;67(4):499–511.

17

The recovery of added nematode eggs from horse and sheep faeces by three methods

Antonio Bosco[1], Maria Paola Maurelli[1*] , Davide Ianniello[1], Maria Elena Morgoglione[1], Alessandra Amadesi[1], Gerald C. Coles[2], Giuseppe Cringoli[1] and Laura Rinaldi[1]

Abstract

Background: Nematode infections in horses are widespread across the world. Increasing levels of anthelmintic resistance, reported worldwide in equine parasites, have led to the creation of programs for the control of nematodes based on faecal egg counts (FEC). To improve nematode egg counting in equine faecal samples and establish whether the matrix of equine faeces or the eggs affect the counts, the analytical sensitivity, accuracy and precision of Mini-FLOTAC (combined with Fill-FLOTAC), McMaster and Cornell-Wisconsin techniques were compared. Known numbers of eggs extracted from equine or ovine faeces were added to egg free ovine and equine faeces to give counts of 10, 50, 200 and 500 eggs per gram (EPG) of faeces.

Results: The Cornell-Wisconsin significantly underestimated egg counts and McMaster showed a low analytical sensitivity, revealing 100% of sensitivity only for concentrations greater than 200 EPG. EPG values detected by Mini-FLOTAC did not differ significantly from expected counts at any level of egg density.

Conclusions: Mini-FLOTAC combined to Fill-FLOTAC which provides an accurate method of weighing without need for a balance and filtering out debris, could be used for FEC on the farm as well as in the laboratory.

Keywords: Mini-FLOTAC, Fill-FLOTAC, Nematodes, Horses, Sheep

Background

Nematodes which infect horses are clinically important across the world and anthelmintic resistance (AR) is becoming increasingly prevalent [1]. The problem of AR has led to the creation of programs for the control of nematodes based on faecal egg counts (FEC). More accurate and precise FEC methods need to be included in studies evaluating any parasite control program, emphasizing the requirement for simple, reliable and sensitive diagnostic tools and preferably suitable to assess both the intensity of infections and the efficacy of drugs on horse farms [1]. Sources of potential error include the method of sampling, flotation solution used, sample dilution, counting procedures [2–4], faecal moisture [5], and the storage or preservation of faeces [3, 6].

In order to evaluate which FEC technique is characterized by higher analytical sensitivity (the smallest number of parasitic elements in a sample that can be detected accurately by a given technique), accuracy (how well the observed value agrees with the 'true' value) and precision (how well repeated observations agree with one another), eggs extracted from equine and ovine faecal samples and added to egg free samples were counted by three FEC techniques: Mini-FLOTAC, modified McMaster and Cornell-Wisconsin.

Methods

Faecal samples with positive and negative FEC were collected from adult sheep and horses stabled in paddock of farms located in southern Italy. Each sample was analyzed 5 times by the FLOTAC basic technique [7] with an analytical sensitivity of 1 egg per gram (EPG) of faeces to determine the presence/absence of nematode eggs, i.e. cyathostomes for horses and gastrointestinal nematodes

* Correspondence: mariapaola.maurelli@unina.it
[1]Department of Veterinary Medicine and Animal Production, University of Naples Federico II, CREMOPAR Campania Region, Naples, Italy
Full list of author information is available at the end of the article

(*Trichostrongylus*, *Haemonchus* and *Teladorsagia*) for sheep. Nematode eggs were extracted from the positive samples using the mass recovery method, i.e., a method that employs 4 sieves of different dimension (1 mm, 250 μm, 212 μm and 38 μm) in order to separate the eggs from the faeces. Then ten aliquots of 0.1 ml each were taken and the number of eggs counted [8]. A series of cross-contaminations were performed: nematode extracted from horses' faeces were used to contaminate negative horse and sheep faeces and *vice versa*. The egg suspensions were added to the negative faeces (250 g) and thoroughly homogenized to give four faecal samples (250 g each) for each EPG level (10, 50, 200 and 500).

Each sample was analyzed using satured sodium chloride solution (specific gravity = 1.200) by three FEC techniques: Mini-FLOTAC combined with Fill-FLOTAC [9–11], modified McMaster technique [12] and Cornell-Wisconsin technique [13]. After a thorough homogenization from each faecal sample for each EPG level, 60 g were weighted for Mini-FLOTAC, 36 g for McMaster chamber, 36 g for McMaster grid and 60 g for Cornell-Wisconsin. In total twelve replicates were used for each method and for each EPG level (10, 50, 200 and 500) using single faecal samples. The weight of faeces used, dilution ratio, reading volume and analytical sensitivity of each technique are shown in Table 1. Fill-FLOTAC enables the first four step of the Mini-FLOTAC technique i.e. sample collection and weighing, homogenization, filtration and filling of Mini-FLOTAC chamber [9, 11]. The repeatability of the 5 g size of Fill-FLOTAC to measure 5 g of faeces using horse and sheep samples was measured 10 times.

Statistical analysis

A coefficient of variation [(standard deviation divided by mean count times) *100] was calculated for each set of replicate counts for each method and level of EPG. The coefficient of variation showed the precision of the method [14] that refers to the closeness of two or more measurements to each other. Mean of eggs (X) showed the accuracy of the method that describe the closeness of a measurement to the true value.

The raw counts from each sample were multiplied by the appropriate multiplication factor (5 for Mini-FLOTAC, 50 for McMaster grid, 15 for McMaster chamber and 1 for Cornell-Wisconsin), and then, the mean of the replicate counts for each sample was calculated.

The analytical sensitivity of tests across the different levels of egg excretion for each technique was evaluated using line graphs.

Boxplots (indicating median, percentiles and outliers) were used to estimate the precision and accuracy of each technique for each of the four levels of egg cross-contamination. A no parametric test, i.e. Spearman rank correlation (*rho*), was used to examine any association between true and observed egg counts. For each FEC technique at each level of egg count, the percentage recovery was calculated to assess the level of over- or under- estimation of FEC result (measurement error) using the following formula: % egg recovery = 100 - (true FEC - observed FEC) / true FEC * 100. Significance testing was set at $p < 0.05$. Statistical analysis was performed in IBM SPSS Statistics 20.

Results

The study involving 768 counts showed that at all egg concentrations the Mini-FLOTAC and Cornell-Wisconsin had 100% analytical sensitivity (using either sheep or horse faeces contaminated with nematode eggs). Instead, McMaster grid and chamber showed an analytical sensitivity of 100% only for concentrations greater than 200 EPG (the analytical sensitivity ranged from 8.3% to 75.0% at lowest concentration of eggs) (Fig. 1a, b). Spearman's rank correlation showed a significant ($p < 0.05$) positive relationship between observed EPG values and true EPG values for all methods and for all types of cross-contamination, but the Rho values ranged from 0.91 for McMaster grid to 0.97 for Mini-FLOTAC. Additional files show mean of eggs (X), standard deviation (SD) and coefficient of variation (CV%) recovered by Mini-FLOTAC, McMaster and Cornell-Wisconsin for each EPG level and for each contamination [see Additional files 1, 2]. The mean of precision (CV%) and accuracy (X) for each method is presented in Tables 2 and 3.

Fig. 2a-d show the boxplot of the observed EPG at each level of egg excretion for Mini-FLOTAC, McMaster grid, McMaster chamber and Cornell-Wisconsin, respectively. The length of boxplots of Mini-FLOTAC

Table 1 Schematic features of Mini-FLOTAC, McMaster (grid and chamber) and Cornell-Wisconsin techniques

FEC Techniques	Amount of faeces used (grams)	Dilution Ratio	Reading Volume (ml)	Reading Area (mm^2)	Analytical sensitivity (EPG)
Mini-FLOTAC	5	1:10	2.0	648	5
McMaster *grid*	3	1:15	0.30	200	50
McMaster *chamber*	3	1:15	1.0	648	15
Cornell-Wisconsin	5	1:10	10	324	1

The weight of faeces used for each replicate, dilution ratio, reading volume, reading area and analytical sensitivity of Mini-FLOTAC, two versions of McMaster (grid and chamber) and Cornell-Wisconsin egg counting

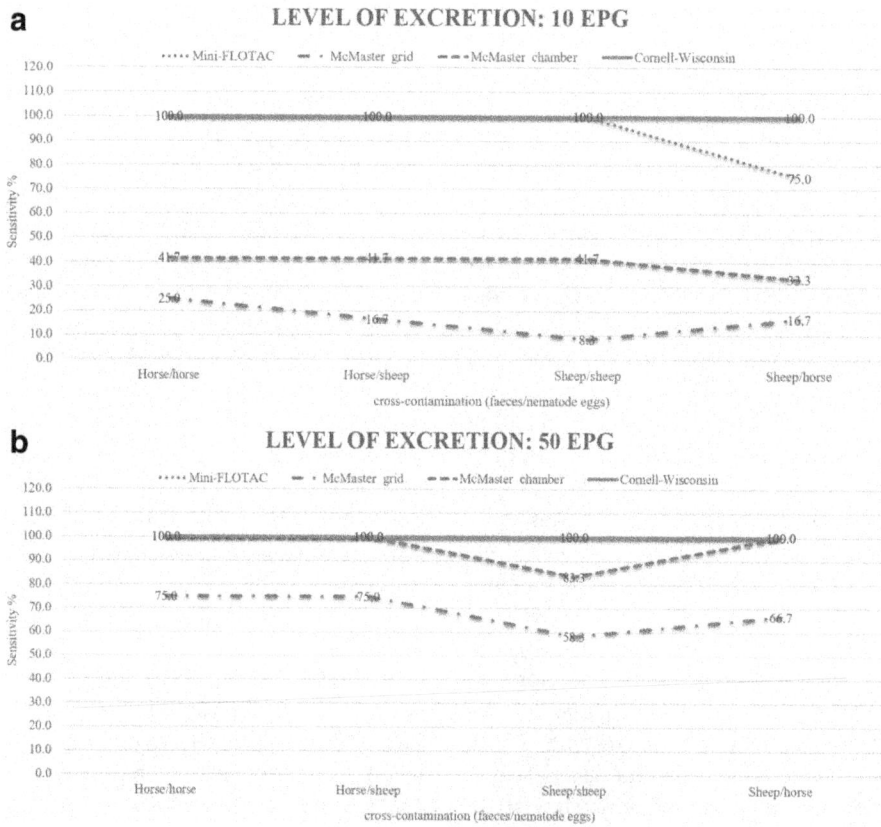

Fig. 1 Analytical sensitivity (% of positive test results across the replicates) of each FEC technique using nematode egg suspensions of 10 EPG for the four cross-contaminations (**a**) and of 50 EPG for the four cross-contaminations (**b**)

technique was very narrow for each contamination level and for all cross-contaminations showing a high precision and accuracy compared to the other techniques.

Sheep faeces had a mean (± standard deviation, SD) of 5.1 ± 0.14 g (maximum 5.1 g, minimum 4.8 g), while horse faeces had an average (± SD) of 5.0 ± 0.11 (maximum 5.2 g, minimum 4.9 g), thus demonstrating a good repeatability of the Fill-FLOTAC for weighing faecal samples..

At the lower level of eggs (10 EPG), CV% was high and exceeded 100% in McMaster grid and chamber methods. Furthermore, using McMaster grid and chamber methods were found negative results from the analysis of replicates, whereas the other methods never detected negative results.

Discussion

Regarding the recovery of eggs, 100% of nematode eggs from sheep were recovered when added to egg-free sheep faeces, but only 91.0% were recovered from horse faeces. There was a significant difference between recovery of nematode eggs of sheep from sheep faeces and from horse faeces. When nematode eggs from horses were added to sheep faeces the recovery was 95.9%, but reduced egg counts (90.5%) were found when added to horse faeces. Noel et al. [15] performed a study on the percentage of recovery of eggs using Mini-FLOTAC technique for the diagnosis of equine strongyles and recovered 42.6% of the eggs. As discussed by Cringoli et al. [11], various factors might explain the difference between results presented in

Table 2 Mean CV% for Mini-FLOTAC, McMaster and Cornell-Wisconsin at the different egg count levels and for each method evaluated in this study

Method	10 EPG	50 EPG	200 EPG	500 EPG
Mini-FLOTAC	49.6%	10.9%	8.1%	3.1%
McMaster grid	248.6%	90.5%	39.9%	17.3%
McMaster chamber	135.6%	51.4%	23.1%	10.9%
Cornell-Wisconsin	33.4%	16.6%	51.8%	5.2%

Table 3 Mean number of detected eggs for Mini-FLOTAC, McMaster and Cornell-Wisconsin at the different egg count levels and for each method evaluated in this study

Method	10 EPG	50 EPG	200 EPG	500 EPG
Mini-FLOTAC	9	45	192	409
McMaster grid	8	49	179	492
McMaster chamber	7	39	167	461
Cornell-Wisconsin	4	19	104	248

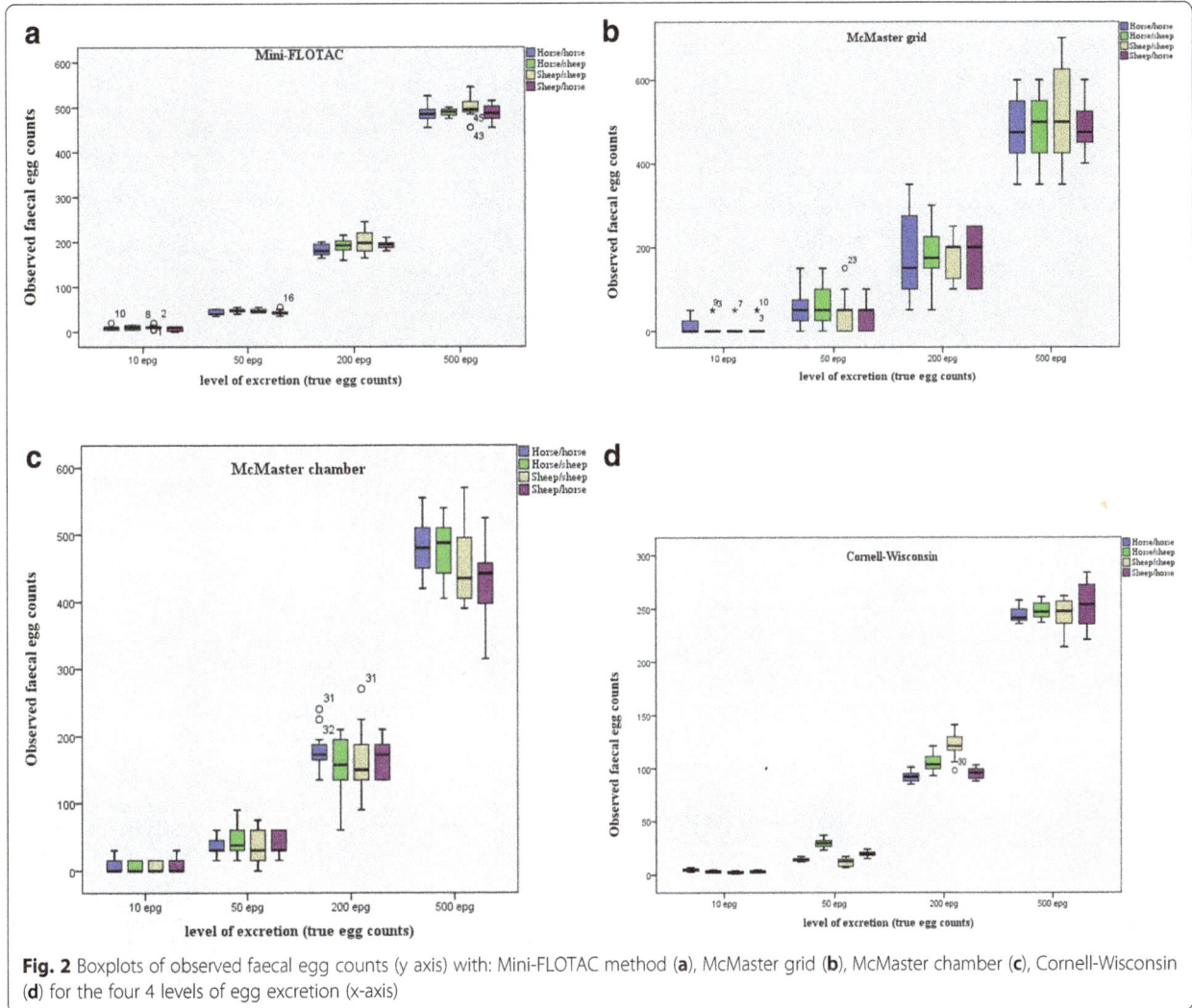

Fig. 2 Boxplots of observed faecal egg counts (y axis) with: Mini-FLOTAC method (**a**), McMaster grid (**b**), McMaster chamber (**c**), Cornell-Wisconsin (**d**) for the four 4 levels of egg excretion (x-axis)

this study and results presented by Noel et al. [15]; in fact, one of the main limitations of Mini-FLOTAC technique, as with any copromicroscopic technique based on flotation (e.g. simple flotation, Wisconsin, and McMaster), is that the selection of fixative and duration of faecal preservation before Mini-FLOTAC analysis, the procedure of egg isolation and the choice of the flotation solution might influence the performance of the Mini-FLOTAC technique, specifically affecting the percentage of parasitic elements recovered [11]. The very poor performance of the Cornell-Wisconsin method indicates that this should not be used in future for counting equine nematode eggs, a conclusion also reached for bovine nematodes [4]. The McMaster technique is adequate if egg counts are greater than 50 EPG, but it is not satisfactory for lower counts which could be important if looking for the beginning AR. These results are similar to Vadlejch et al. [16] who compared the accuracy and precision of different McMaster methods for diagnosis of *Teladorsagia circumcincta* in sheep and confirmed that this method detected negative

samples at lower concentrations. Under-estimation of FEC occurred when the entire McMaster chamber was examined rather than limited to the gridded area (Fig. 2b, c) whereas over-estimation of FEC occurred when the gridded area was examined, due to high multiplication factor. This is in agreement with Cringoli et al. [2] who observed aggregation of eggs to the center of McMaster slides, Morgan et al. [17] who described the Poisson distribution of nematode eggs in faecal suspensions and Kochanowsky et al. [14] that showed that the best limit of detection and analytical sensitivity and the lowest coefficients of variation were obtained with the use of the whole McMaster chamber variant. Only counting eggs in the gridded area appears to account for this aggregation at higher levels of egg densities; the number of eggs present at lower densities, however, was still underestimated. Finally CVs for McMaster grid and chambers were higher than other techniques for ovine and equine faeces, especially for lower counts, as yet reported by Noel et al. [15]. Also Dias de Castro et al. [18] and Scare et al. [19] showed that SD and CV values for significantly lower for Mini-FLOTAC than McMaster for detection of gastrointestinal nematode eggs in cattle and horses.

Conclusions

In conclusion, Mini-FLOTAC combined with Fill-FLOTAC which provides an accurate method of weighing without need for a balance and filtering out debris, could be used for FEC on the farm as well as in the laboratory.

Additional files

Additional file 1: Mean of eggs (X), Standard Deviation (SD), Coefficient of variation (CV%) recovered by Mini-FLOTAC, McMaster and Cornell-Wisconsin from horse faeces containing a predetermined number of nematode eggs extracted from horse and sheep faeces. (DOCX 14 kb)

Additional file 2: Mean of eggs (X), Standard Deviation (SD), Coefficient of variation (CV%) recovered by Mini-FLOTAC, McMaster and Cornell-Wisconsin from sheep faeces containing a predetermined number of nematode eggs extracted from horse and sheep faeces. (DOCX 14 kb)

Abbreviations
EPG: Eggs per gram; FEC: Faecal egg counts; SD: Standard deviation

Acknowledgements
The Authors would like to express sincere appreciation to Paola Pepe, Mario Parrilla and Mirella Santaniello for their technical collaboration.

Funding
No funding was obtained for this study.

Authors' contributions
Conceived, designed and coordinated the study: GC and LR. Performed sampling and laboratory analyses: AB, MPM, DI, MEM, AA and GCC. All the authors contributed to the data analysis and interpretation, to preparation and final approval of the manuscript.

Consent for publication
Not applicable

Competing interests
The FLOTAC and Mini-FLOTAC apparatus have been developed and are patented by G. Cringoli, but the patent will be handed over to the University of Naples Federico II. The fact that one of the authors is the current patent holder of the FLOTAC and Mini-FLOTAC apparatus played no role in the preparation and submission of the manuscript.
Laura Rinaldi is a member of the editorial board (Section Editor) for BMC Veterinary Research, it didn't influence the reviewers.
The remaining authors have no competing financial interests.

Author details
[1]Department of Veterinary Medicine and Animal Production, University of Naples Federico II, CREMOPAR Campania Region, Naples, Italy. [2]University of Bristol, School of Veterinary Sciences, Langford House, Bristol BS40 5DU, UK.

References
1. Andersen UV, Howe DK, Olsen SN, Nielsen MK. Recent advances in diagnosing pathogenic equine gastrointestinal helminths: the challenge of prepatent detection. Vet Parasitol. 2013;192:1–9.
2. Cringoli G, Rinaldi L, Veneziano V, Capelli G, Scala A. The influence of flotation solution, sample dilution and the choice of McMaster slide area (volume) on the reliability of the McMaster technique in estimating the faecal egg counts of gastrointestinal strongyles and *Dicrocoelium dendriticum* in sheep. Vet Parasitol. 2004; 131:121.
3. Rinaldi L, Coles GC, Maurelli MP, Musella V, Cringoli G. Calibration and diagnostic accuracy of simple flotation, McMaster and FLOTAC for parasite egg counts in sheep. Vet Parasitol. 2011;177:345–52.
4. Levecke B, Rinaldi L, Charlier J, Maurelli MP, Bosco A, Vercruysse J, Cringoli G. The bias, accuracy and precision on faecal egg count reduction test results in cattle using McMaster, Cornell-Wisconsin and FLOTAC egg counting methods. Vet Parasitol. 2012;188:194–9.
5. Roeber F, Jex AR, Gasser RB. Advances in the diagnosis of key gastrointestinal nematode infections of livestock, with an emphasis on small ruminants. Biotechnol Adv. 2013;31:1135–52.
6. Crawley JA, Chapman SN, Lummaa V, Lynsdale CL. Testing storage methods of faecal samples for subsequent measurement of helminth egg numbers in the domestic horse. Vet Parasitol 2016;221: 130-133.
7. Cringoli G, Rinaldi L, Maurelli MP, Utzinger J. FLOTAC: new multivalent techniques for qualitative and quantitative copromicroscopic diagnosis of parasites in animals and humans. Nat Protoc. 2010;5:503–15.
8. Godber OF, Phythian CJ, Bosco A, Ianniello D, Coles G, Rinaldi L, Cringoli G. A comparison of the FECPAK and mini-FLOTAC faecal egg counting techniques. Vet Parasitol. 2015;30:342–5.
9. Cringoli G, Rinaldi L, Albonico M, Bergquist R, Utzinger J. Geospatial (s)tools: integration of advanced epidemiological sampling and novel diagnostics. Geospat Health. 2013;7:399–404.
10. Rinaldi L, Levecke B, Bosco A, Ianniello D, Pepe P, Charlier J, Cringoli G, Vercruysse J. Comparison of individual and pooled faecal samples in sheep for the assessment of gastrointestinal strongyle infection intensity and anthelmintic drug efficacy using McMaster and mini-FLOTAC. Vet Parasitol. 2014;205:216–23.
11. Cringoli G, Maurelli MP, Levecke B, Bosco A, Vercruysse J, Utzinger J, Rinaldi L. The mini-FLOTAC technique for the diagnosis of helminth and protozoan infections in humans and animals. Nat Protoc. 2017;12:1723–32.
12. Whitlock HV. Some modifications of the McMaster helminth egg-counting technique and apparatus. J Counc Sci Ind Res. 1948;21:177–80.
13. Egwang TG, Slocombe JO. Evaluation of the Cornell-Wisconsin centrifugal flotation technique for recovering trichostrongylid eggs from bovine feces. Can J Vet Res. 1982;46:133–7.
14. Kochanowsky M, Dabrowska J, Karamon J, Cencek T, Osinski Z. Analysis of the accuracy and precision of the McMaster method in detection of the eggs of *Toxocara* and *Trichuris* species (Nematoda) in dog faeces. Folia Parasitologica (Praha). 2013;60:264–72.
15. Noel ML, Scare JA, Bellaw JL, Nielsen MK. Accuracy and precision of mini-FLOTAC and McMaster techniques for determining equine strongyle egg count. J Equin Vet Sci. 2017;48:182–187e.
16. Vadlejch J, Petrtyl M, Zaichenko I, Cadkova Z, Jankovska I, Langrova I, Moravec M. Which McMaster egg counting technique is the most reliable? Parasitol Res. 2011;109:1387–94.
17. Morgan ER, Cavill L, Curry GE, Wood RM, Mitchell ESE. Effects of aggregation and sample size on composite faecal egg counts in sheep. Vet Parasitol. 2005;131:79–87.
18. Dias de Castro L, Abrahao CLH, Buzatti A, Molento MB, Bastianetto E, Rodrigues DS, Lopes L, Xavier Silva M, Green de Freitas M, Conde MH, Borges F. Comparison of McMaster and mini-FLOTAC fecal egg counting techniques in cattle and horses. Vet Parasitol Reg Studies and Re. 2017;10: 132–5.

18

Protective immunity induced by *Eimeria* common antigen 14–3-3 against *Eimeria tenella*, *Eimeria acervulina* and *Eimeria maxima*

Jianhua Liu[1], Lianrui Liu[1], Lingjuan Li[2], Di Tian[1], Wenyu Li[1], Lixin Xu[1], Ruofeng Yan[1], Xiangrui Li[1] and Xiaokai Song[1*] ⓘ

Abstract

Background: Avian coccidiosis is often caused by co-infection with several species of *Eimeria* worldwide. Developing a multivalent vaccine with an antigen common to multiple *Eimeria* species is a promising strategy for controlling clinical common co-infection of *Eimeria*. In the previous study, 14–3-3 was identified as one of the immunogenic common antigen in *E. tenella*, *E. acervulina* and *E. maxima*. The aim of the present study was to evaluate the immunogenicity and protective efficacy of Ea14–3-3 in the form of DNA vaccine against infection with three species of *Eimeria* both individually and simultaneously.

Results: After vaccination with pVAX-Ea14–3-3, the Ea14–3-3 gene was transcribed and expressed in the injected muscles. Vaccination with pVAX-Ea14–3-3 significantly increased the proportion of CD4[+] and CD8[+] T lymphocytes and produced a strong IgY response in immunized chickens. Similarly, pVAX-Ea14–3-3 stimulated the chicken's splenocytes to produce high levels of Th1-type (IFN-γ, IL-2) and Th2-type (IL-4) cytokines. The vaccine-induced immune response was responsible to increase weight gain, decreased the oocyst output, and alleviated enteric lesions significantly in immunized chickens as compared to control group, in addition to induce moderate anti-coccidial index (ACI).

Conclusion: These results indicate that Ea14–3-3 is highly immunogenic and capable to induce significant immune responses. Furthermore, Ea14–3-3 antigen can provide effective protection against infection with *Eimeria tenella*, *Eimeria acervulina*, *Eimeria maxima* both individually and in combination with three *Eimeria* species. Significant outcomes of our study provide an effective candidate antigen for developing a multivalent *Eimeria* vaccine against mixed infection with various *Eimeria* species under natural conditions.

Keywords: Chicken coccidian, Common antigen 14–3-3, Mixed infection, Immunogenicity, DNA vaccine

Background

Avian coccidiosis is one of the most widespread and economically detrimental diseases in the poultry industry. It causes severe damage to the host intestine, resulting in impaired feed intake, increased mortality and increased susceptibility to other disease agents [1, 2]. It has been estimated that the annual loss due to coccidiosis exceeds $3 billion USD globally [3]. Primarily, control of avian coccidiosis is based on the use of anti-coccidial drugs and live vaccines [1]. Although these two approaches have been generally effective for controlling the disease, the drawbacks of these two approaches, such as drug resistance and residue, high cost and lack of uniformity in vaccination have prompted the search for new generation vaccines including subunit vaccines and DNA vaccines [3–6]. The causes of clinical coccidiosis in the intensive farming are infection by various *Eimeria* species [3, 7]. The species of *Eimeria tenella*, *E. acervulina* and *E. maxima* are commonly found in all commercial birds [1, 8, 9]. Thus, applied vaccines should contain protective antigens

* Correspondence: songxiaokai@njau.edu.cn
[1]MOE Joint International Research Laboratory of Animal Health and Food Safety, College of Veterinary Medicine, Nanjing Agricultural University, Nanjing 210095, People's Republic of China
Full list of author information is available at the end of the article

common to relevant species and confer effective protection against mixed infection with *Eimeria* species [10].

Several antigens common to *Eimeria* have been reported previously. Talebi et al. [11] found an immunogenic protein (45 kDa) among five *Eimeria* species. While, Sasai et al. [12] observed a common antigen present on conoid of six chicken's *Eimeria* sporozoites. Additionally, Constantinoiu et al. [13] reported highly conserved apical antigens among subjected *Eimeria* species. However, the reported common antigens were not well identified by sequencing and their protective efficacies have not been evaluated. In the earlier study of our lab, Ea14–3-3 antigen was identified as one of the common immunodominant antigens from *E. tenella*, *E. acervulina* and *E. maxima* [14]. It has been documented that 14–3-3 proteins are involved in many patho-physiological and cellular immune processes by triggering or interfering with the activity of specific protein associates [15]. In apicomplexan parasites, the 14–3-3 protein plays a vital role in parasite invasion, molecular and biological processes with immuno-protective responses [16–20]. Moreover, in *E. tenella*, 14–3-3 antigen was proven to interact with telomerase activity and involved in the process of coccidia development [17].

The 14-3-3 proteins have been showed an immunogenic response, and able to stimulate the host immune activity in some parasites. Schechtman et al. [21] reported that the 14–3-3 antigen of *Schistosoma mansoni* influenced the significant humoral and cellular responses and induced moderate protection against challenged infection. In *Toxoplasma gondii*, the 14–3-3 protein induced effective immune responses in BALB/c mice and was suggested as a novel DNA vaccine candidate against toxoplasmosis [20]. Besides that, 14–3-3 antigens in *Trichinella spiralis* and *Echinococcus* were documented to be highly immunogenic and described as promising vaccine targets against infections [22, 23]. Therefore, 14–3-3 protein may be potential vaccine candidates against these parasites.

In the current study, the immunogenicity and protective efficacy of Ea14–3-3 against *E. tenella*, *E. acervulina* and *E. maxima* was further investigated. Results of this study may provide an effective candidate antigen for developing a multivalent *Eimeria* vaccine against mixed infection with multiple species of *Eimeria* under natural conditions.

Results

Sequence analysis and eukaryotic expression plasmid construction of Ea14-3-3 gene

The ORF of Ea14–3-3 gene was cloned into pMD18-T and confirmed by sequencing. The ORF of Ea14–3-3 gene is composed of 837 nucleotides with predicted molecular weights of 31.77 kDa (Additional file 1: Figure S1). Sequence analysis showed that Ea14–3-3 has similarity of 100% in nucleotides and amino acid sequences with the genes in NCBI (XM_013394831). Ea14–3-3 has a high

amino acid similarity of more than 94% among the four chicken coccidia species (Additional file 2: Table S1). The constructed pVAX-Ea14–3-3 plasmid was confirmed by endonuclease cleavage and sequence analysis. Endonuclease cleavage with *Bam*H I /*Xho* I produced a band of about 837 bp, which is equal to the size of the inserted gene *Ea14–3-3* (Additional file 3: Figure S2 lane 2). The fragment was extracted from the gel and sequenced. The sequence analysis revealed that the inserted gene has 100% similarity of nucleotides and amino acid sequences with the Ea14–3-3 gene.

Ea14–3-3 was transcribed and expressed in the injected site of chickens

RT-PCR assay was employed with the specific primers for Ea14–3-3 to detect transcriptions of the Ea14–3-3 gene in the injected muscles. Agarose electrophoresis showed a band of approximately 837 bp from the muscle injected with pVAX-Ea14–3-3 (Fig. 1a, lane 1). No specific DNA bands were detected in pVAX1 injected and non-injected control sample (Fig. 1a, lane 2 and 3). These results indicate that Ea14–3-3 was transcribed in the injected site muscles of chickens.

Western blot assay was employed with primary antibody of anti-*E. acervulina* chicken sera to detect the expressed proteins. As shown in Fig. 1b, in pVAX-Ea14–3-3 injected muscle anti-*E. acervulina* chicken sera reacted with a protein band of approximately 32 kDa (Fig. 1b, lane 1). No specific band was detected in non-injected control and

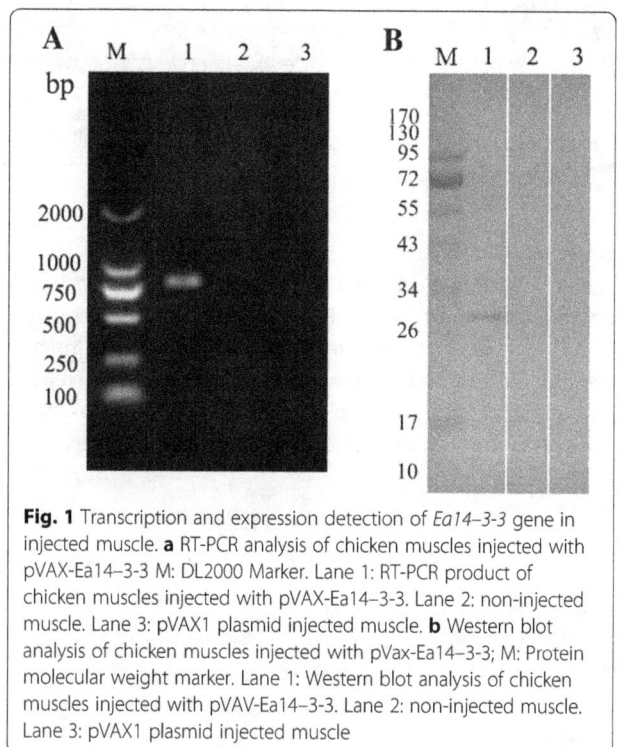

Fig. 1 Transcription and expression detection of *Ea14–3-3* gene in injected muscle. **a** RT-PCR analysis of chicken muscles injected with pVAX-Ea14–3-3 M: DL2000 Marker. Lane 1: RT-PCR product of chicken muscles injected with pVAX-Ea14–3-3. Lane 2: non-injected muscle. Lane 3: pVAX1 plasmid injected muscle. **b** Western blot analysis of chicken muscles injected with pVax-Ea14–3-3; M: Protein molecular weight marker. Lane 1: Western blot analysis of chicken muscles injected with pVAV-Ea14–3-3. Lane 2: non-injected muscle. Lane 3: pVAX1 plasmid injected muscle

vector control samples (Fig. 1b, lane 2 and 3). These results indicate that Ea14–3-3 was expressed in the injected site muscles of chickens.

Ea14–3-3 induced significant cellular immune responses in chickens

The proportions of CD4$^+$/CD3$^+$ and CD8$^+$/CD3$^+$ splenic T lymphocytes from vaccinated chickens were determined by flow cytometry assay. As per depicted in Fig. 2, 1 week after the primary and booster dose of vaccination, the proportions of CD4$^+$/CD3$^+$ and CD8$^+$/CD3$^+$ splenic T lymphocytes from vaccinated chickens were significantly higher than those from PBS and pVAX1 empty plasmid control chickens ($p < 0.05$). No significant difference was observed between the pVAX1 and PBS control chickens ($p > 0.05$). The results demonstrated that Ea14–3-3 effectively promoted the T lymphocyte responses in chickens. The mRNA levels of IFN-γ, IL-2, IL-4, TNFSF15, IL-17D

and TGF-β4 cytokines from vaccinated chickens were determined by qPCR. As shown in Fig. 3, 1 week after the primary and booster dose of immunization, the production of IFN-γ, IL-2, IL-4 TNFSF15, IL-17D and TGF-β4 was significantly increased in pVAX-Ea14–3-3-vaccinated chickens as compared to pVAX1-vaccinated and PBS control chickens ($p < 0.05$). No significant difference was observed between pVAX1 and PBS control chickens ($p > 0.05$). These results indicated that Ea14–3-3 effectively promoted the production of cytokines in chickens.

In a word, the *Eimeria* common antigen 14–3-3 effectively induced the secretion of cytokines in chickens.

Ea14–3-3 induced a significant serum antibody response in chickens

The indirect ELISA method was employed to determine the antibody response induced by Ea14–3-3. As shown in Fig. 4, from 1 week to 6 weeks post-booster vaccination,

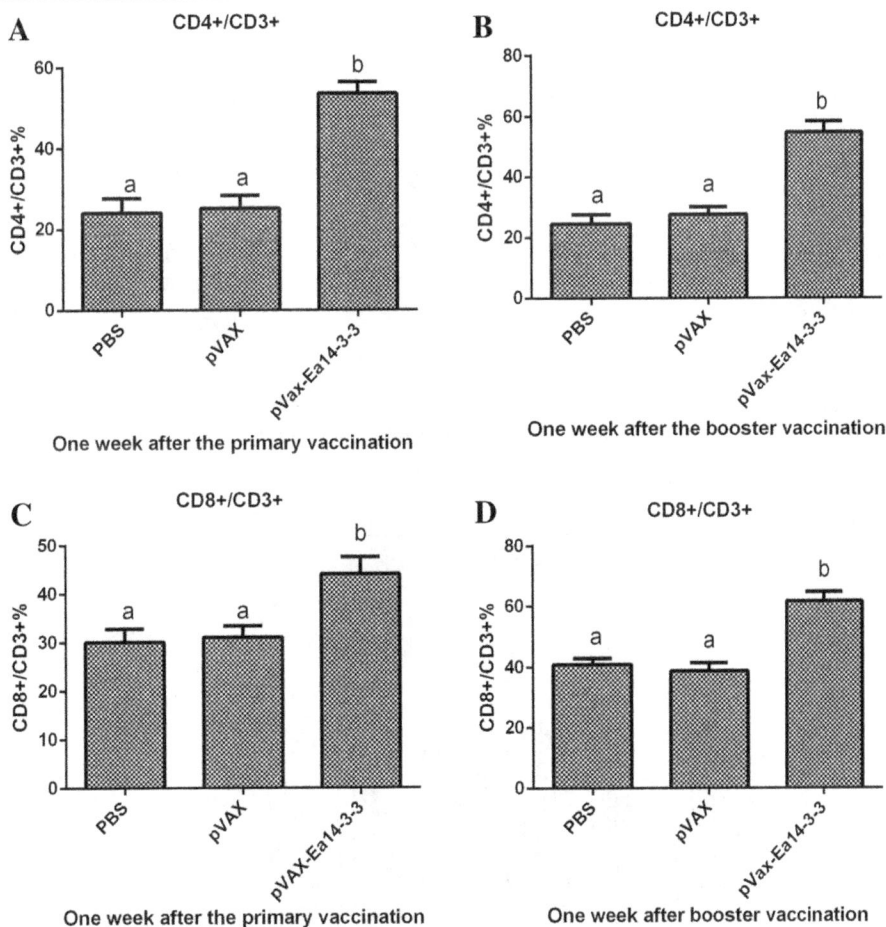

Fig. 2 Changes of proportion of CD4$^+$/CD3$^+$ and CD8$^+$/CD3$^+$ T cells in spleens of the chickens vaccinated with pVAX-Ea14–3-3. (**a**) Proportion of CD4$^+$/CD3$^+$ T cells in spleens of the chickens 1 week after the primary vaccination; (**b**) proportion of CD4$^+$/CD3$^+$ T cells in spleens of the chickens 1 week after the booster vaccination; (**c**) proportion of CD8$^+$/CD3$^+$ T cells in spleens of the chickens 1 week after the primary vaccination; (**d**) proportion of CD8$^+$/CD3$^+$ T cells in spleens of the chickens 1 week after the booster vaccination; significant difference ($p < 0.05$) between numbers with different letters; non-significant difference ($p > 0.05$) between numbers with the same letter

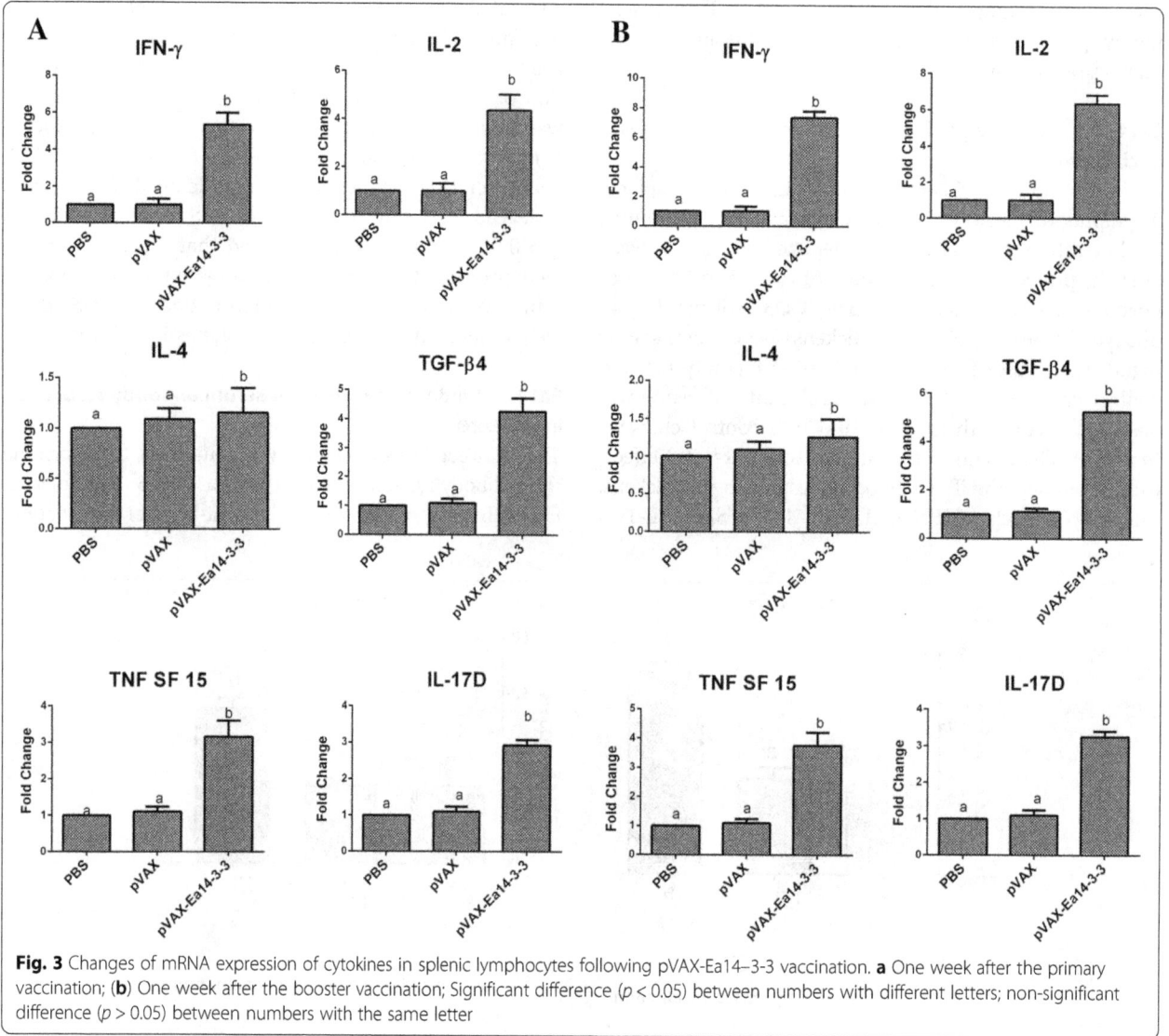

Fig. 3 Changes of mRNA expression of cytokines in splenic lymphocytes following pVAX-Ea14–3-3 vaccination. **a** One week after the primary vaccination; (**b**) One week after the booster vaccination; Significant difference (p < 0.05) between numbers with different letters; non-significant difference (p > 0.05) between numbers with the same letter

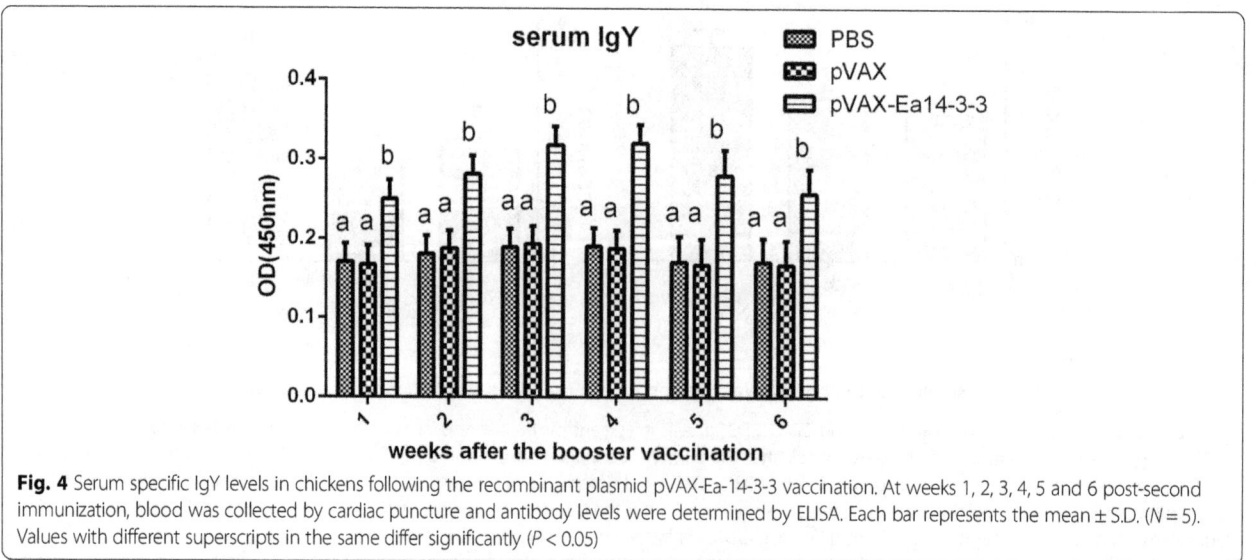

Fig. 4 Serum specific IgY levels in chickens following the recombinant plasmid pVAX-Ea-14-3-3 vaccination. At weeks 1, 2, 3, 4, 5 and 6 post-second immunization, blood was collected by cardiac puncture and antibody levels were determined by ELISA. Each bar represents the mean ± S.D. (N = 5). Values with different superscripts in the same differ significantly (P < 0.05)

the induced antibody titers of all pVAX-Ea14–3-3 vaccinated groups were significantly higher as compared to the PBS and pVAX1 empty plasmid control groups. No significant difference was observed between the pVAX1 and PBS control group ($p > 0.05$). The antibody titers of vaccinated groups increased slowly from the first week to the third week post-booster immunization, peaked at the fourth week, and then decreased gradually PBS and pVAX1 empty plasmid groups were not detected any specific antibodies. The results showed that Ea14–3-3 significantly induced significant serum antibody response in chickens.

Ea14–3-3 induced effective protection against *E. tenella*, *E. acervulina* and *E. maxima*

To evaluate the protective efficacy of pVAX-Ea14–3-3, groups of chickens were challenged with *E. tenella*, *E. acervulina*, *E. maxima* or mixed oocysts of the three *Eimeria* species. As shown in Table 1, vaccination with pVAX-Ea14–3-3 significantly increased the body weight gains, decreased the oocyst output, and alleviated the enteric lesions of vaccinated groups as compared to PBS control and pVAX1 control groups ($p < 0.05$). No significant difference was observed between the pVAX1 and PBS control group ($p > 0.05$). The vaccination resulted in ACIs of 171.31(*E. acervulina*), 161.03(*E. maxima*), 178.29 (*E. tenella*) and 170.92 (mixed *Eimeria*). This result indicates that Ea14–3-3 provided effective protections against

challenge with *E. tenella*, *F. acervulina*, *E. maxima* and mixed infection of the three *Eimeria* species.

Discussion

Avian coccidiosis, one of the most potential destructive diseases in birds, is caused by several *Eimeria* species under natural conditions. Thus an ideal field *Eimeria* vaccine should provide effective protection against co-infection with mixed *Eimeria* species [2, 9, 24–26]. Common antigens shared among *Eimeria* species are extremely promising for the development of multivalent *Eimeria* vaccines against multiple *Eimeria* species. Previous studies have revealed such a few common antigens among *Eimeria* which had serological cross reactions among certain species [13]. For example, Talebi [11] found a few shared proteins between species and at least one protein band (45 kDa) was conserved among the five species. The conserved protein band of all these species could be recognized by chicken anti-*E. maxima* sera. Sasai et al. [12] identified a common conoid sporozoites antigen among 6 different *Eimeria* species (*E. brunetti*, *E. maxima*, *E. mitis*, *E. necatrix*, *E. praecox* and *E. tenella*) by confocal laser scanning microscopy using a chicken monoclonal antibody (mAb) 6D12-G10 against *E. acervulina* sporozoite. Constantinoiu et al. [13] analyzed cross-reactivity of five chicken mAb against *E. acervulina* sporozoites using confocal laser immunofluorescence assay and found mAb 8E-1 recognized an

Table 1 Protective efficacy of common antigen *Ea14–3-3* against challenge with *E. tenella*, *E. acervulina*, *E. maxima* and mixed oocysts of the three *Eimeria* species

Group	Challenge with *Eimeria* spp.	Average body weight gain (g)	Relative body weight gain (%)	Mean lesion scores	Oocyst decrease ratio (%)	ACI
pVAX-Ea14–3-3	E. tenella	53.26 ± 11.52[b]	87.49	0.42 ± 0.52[b]	58.79	178.29
pVAX1 control	E. tenella	35.26 ± 9.89[a]	58.00	3.59 ± 0.51[c]	−0.61	112.1
Challenged control	E. tenella	32.58 ± 10.29[a]	53.11	3.78 ± 0.67[c]	0.00	105.41
Unchallenged control*	PBS	61.30 ± 9.29[c]	100	0 ± 0[a]	100	200
pVAX-Ea14–3-3	E. acervulina	53.96 ± 12.0[b]	88.51	1.62 ± 0.54[b]	77.05	171.31
pVAX1 control	E. acervulina	38.41 ± 10.93[a]	63.20	3.01 ± 0.81[c]	12.67	93.1
Challenged control	E. acervulina	37.38 ± 10.27[a]	62.37	3.26 ± 0.67[c]	0.00	89.77
Unchallenged control*	PBS	61.30 ± 8.89[c]	100	0 ± 0[a]	100	200
pVAX-Ea14–3-3	E. maxima	52.96 ± 11.91[b]	88.23	1.72 ± 0.64[bc]	72.04	161.03
pVAX1 control	E. maxima	35.39 ± 11.52[a]	58.62	2.56 ± 0.71[c]	12.19	93.02
Challenged control	E. maxima	35.18 ± 12.21[a]	57.18	2.90 ± 0.67[c]	0.00	88.18
Unchallenged control*	PBS	61.30 ± 9.29[c]	100	0 ± 0[a]	100	200
pVAX-Ea14–3-3	Mixed oocysts	52.98 ± 11.54[b]	86.82	0.59 ± 0.51[b]	39.33	170.92
pVAX1 control	Mixed oocysts	35.10 ± 10.81[a]	57.57	3.58 ± 0.61[c]	−1.69	111.77
Challenged control	Mixed oocysts	33.08 ± 11.09[a]	53.77	3.70 ± 0.57[c]	0.00	106.77
Unchallenged control*	PBS	61.30 ± 9.29[c]	100	0 ± 0[a]	100	200

Significant difference ($p < 0.05$) between numbers with different letters. No significant difference ($p > 0.05$) between numbers with the same letter
*unchallenged control was shared among the groups challenged with different *Eimeria* species
Mixed oocysts: mixed oocysts of *E. tenella*, *E. acervulina* and *E. maxima*

apical tip molecule present on all chicken *Eimeria* sporozoites. However, these above studies merely revealed molecular weight or fluorescence localization of the common antigens. They did not further identify the specific common antigen by individual sequencing. In our previous study, at least 5 specific *Eimeria* common immunodominant antigens among three *Eimeria* species have been identified by immuno-proteomic analysis and LC-MS/MS technique [13]. The 14–3-3, one of the five identified *Eimeria* common immunogenic antigens is highly conserved among three *Eimeria* species (Additional file 2: Table S1). In the present observation, we further evaluated immunogenicity and protective efficacy of common antigen of 14–3-3 against challenge with *E. tenella*, *E. acervulina* and *E. maxima*. We found that vaccination with the common antigen Ea14–3-3 contributed effective protection not only against individual infection with *E. tenella*, *E. acervulina*, or *E. maxima*, but also against the co-infections with corresponding species. Hence, these findings provide a promising common antigen for developing a vaccine against clinical co-infection by multiple *Eimeria* species.

Cellular immune responses play a dominant role in the immunity against coccidiosis [27]. In this study, the cellular immune responses induced by *Ea*-14-3-3 were assessed. The results showed that the proportions of spleen T lymphocyte subpopulations of CD4$^+$ and CD8$^+$ were significantly increased. High levels of Th1-type (IFN-γ, IL-2) and Th2-type (IL-4) cytokines were produced. These vaccine-induced immune responses resulted in effective protections against *Eimeria*. These results are consistent with other reported findings. Bessay et al. [28] found that *E. acervulina* infection induced a significant increase in the proportion of CD4$^+$ and CD8$^+$ in the duodenal intraepithelial leucocytes (IEL) from day 4 to day 8 post infection (pi). Min et al. [29] found that the ratios of CD4$^+$/CD3$^+$ and CD8$^+$/CD3$^+$ were remarkably increased after immunizing chickens with a pcDNA3-1E vaccine.

Several cytokines have been shown to be involved in immune responses to *Eimeria* infection [27, 30]. Th1-type cytokines such as IFN-γ and IL-2 are responsible for cellular immunity and dominant during *Eimeria* infection [27, 30]. The cytokine IFN-γ has been demonstrated to be important in immuno-regulation in coccidial infections [26, 31]. Recombinant chicken IFN-γ could inhibit the intracellular development of *E. tenella* in vitro and reduce oocyst production and body weight loss following *E. acervulina* challenge infection [30, 32]. IL-2 is considered as a potent growth factor for T-cell differentiation, B-cell development and NK-cell activation [30, 33]. IL-2 mRNA transcripts level in the spleen and intestine was significantly enhanced after infections with *E. acervulina*. IL-2 has been demonstrated to be able to significantly improve the protective

effect of recombinant coccidia genes by DNA vaccination [29, 34]. In this study, the mRNA transcripts level of IFN-γ and IL-2 were significantly increased by vaccination with pVAX-Ea14–3-3 (Fig. 3). Furthermore, proportions of CD4$^+$/CD3$^+$ and CD8$^+$/CD3$^+$ T lymphocytes were significantly increased (Fig. 2). The increasing trend of CD4$^+$/CD3$^+$ and CD8$^+$/CD3$^+$ T lymphocytes in accordance with IFN-γ and IL-2, indicating that T-cell immune response might be prompted by Th1-type cytokines. IL-4, a typical Th2-type cytokine, is responsible for regulating humoral immunity [35]. In this study, the mRNA transcripts level of IL-4 was significantly increased by vaccination with pVAX-Ea14–3-3 (Fig. 3), which in accordance with high level of antibody response in the vaccinated chickens. IL-17D produced by Th17 cells, participates in the induction of inflammation during protozoan infection. After infection with *E. maxima* and *E. tenella*, the expression of IL-17 increased significantly in lymphocytes of the spleen [36, 37]. In this study, the mRNA transcripts level of IL-17D was significantly increased by vaccination with pVAX-Ea14–3-3 (Fig. 3). TGF-β is an anti-inflammatory cytokine that downregulate inflammatory responses and promote repair of damaged mucosal epithelial integrity following injury [30, 38]. After infected with *E. acervulina*, the mRNA level of TGF-β4 in spleen and intestinal epithelial endothelial cells was significantly higher than that in uninfected chickens [39]. In this study, the mRNA level of TGF-β4 was significantly increased by vaccination with pVAX-Ea14–3-3. The high level of TGF-β4 might help repair the mucous membrane damaged by *Eimeria* parasites. TNF is able to promote the proliferation and differentiation of IL-2 and IFN-γ, enhancing the stimulation of antigen on B cells [40]. In vivo experiments revealed that TNFSF15 gene was highly increased following primary infections with *Eimeria* [41]. In this study, the mRNA level of TNFSF15 was significantly increased following vaccination with pVAX-Ea14–3-3. In short, vaccination with pVAX-Ea14–3-3 induced high level of IFN-γ, IL-2, IL-4, TNFSF15, IL17D and TGF-β, playing important roles in immune responses against *Eimeria* infection.

Although the Ea14–3-3 DNA vaccine provided effective protection against *Eimeria*, some measures could be taken to improve protection and to make it more practical for use in fields [42]. The protective efficacy of the DNA vaccine could be enhanced by co-injection with plasmids encoding immune stimulating cytokines (IFN-γ, IL-2) [29, 34, 43]. The sugarcane (*Saccharum officinarum* L.) bagasse-derived polysaccharides could be used as native immunomodulatory candidate to improve the protective efficacy of the DNA vaccine [44].

In the current study, an optimal vaccination procedure including two injections was used to obtain best efficacy for the DNA vaccine. However, on commercial broiler poultry farms, farmers prefer to administer single vaccinations via non-injection delivery routes at day 1 of age. Hence, the vaccination procedure must be further optimized to make vaccination with pVAX-Ea14–3-3 more practical, for example, identify the minimal vaccination age and evaluate the efficacy of a single vaccination and non-injection delivery routes [45].

Conclusion

The coccidal common antigen of Ea14–3-3 induced significant humoral and cellular immune response against *Eimeria* infection. Vaccinations with DNA vaccine of Ea14–3-3 had significant ability to induce effective protection against infection of individual *Eimeria* species (*E. tenella*, *E. acervulina* and *E. maxima*), while, also in the mixed infection of these species. Our study indicates that effective common antigen of 14–3-3 could be used in the development of multivalent vaccine against co-infections of multiple *Eimeria* species in commercial poultry industry.

Methods

Chicken, parasite and vector

One-day-old Hy-Line layer chickens were conventionally reared in standardized and sterilized wire cages to prevent intensive contact with any contamination. The birds were given with coccidiostat-free feed and water ad-libitum. Animal experiment was approved by the Institutional Animal Care and Use Committee of Nanjing Agricultural University (approval number: 2012CB120762). Oocysts of *E. tenella*, *E. acervulina* and *E. maxima* used in challenged infection were propagated, harvested and sporulated 7 days prior to the challenged infection, using a previously described protocol [46]. The eukaryotic expression vector pVAX1 was purchased from Invitrogen (Carlsbad, California, USA).

Antisera preparation

Two-week-old chickens were orally inoculated with 1×10^4 sporulated oocysts of *E. acervulina* 3–5 times per bird by the interval of 3-days. Negative control birds were inoculated with distilled water. One week post the third inoculation, wing vein blood was collected and determined by ELISA. Forth to fifth dose was given to chickens unless titers of the sera antibody were beyond 1: 64. Serum was stored at – 20 °C for Western blot analysis, while negative control serum was collected from negative control chickens.

Cloning of the *14–3-3* gene

Micro glass beads were used to break the *E. acervulina* sporulated oocysts via whirl mix [46]. Briefly, equal volume of 0.5-mm-diameter glass beads and oocysts were mixed in a tube and agitated on a whirl mix with the maximum speed for about 8–10 bursts of 1 s each. At the interval of every 4 bursts, supernatant sample was

scrutinized by microscopic examination to ensure that most of the oocysts were broken and sporocysts were intact. Subsequently, the sporocysts were recovered from the glass beads by repeated additions of medium. The sporozoites were released from the sporocysts by in vitro excystation with trypsin 0.25% (*w/v*) and taurocholic acid 1% (w/v) at 41 °C. Finally, the sporozoites were purified over nylon wool and DE-52 cellulose columns according to the manufacturer's instructions [46]. Total RNA was extracted from *E. acervulina* sporozoites using E.Z.N.A. TM Total RNA Kit I (OMEGA, Norcross, Georgia, USA) according to the manufacturer's instructions. Reverse transcription reaction (RT) was performed to produce cDNA with Oligo (dT) as primers [47]. With the complementary DNA (cDNA) as a template, the complete open reading frame (ORF) of the Ea14–3-3 gene (GenBank Accession No. XM_013394831) was amplified by polymerase chain reaction (PCR) using specific primers designed for Ea14–3-3 ORF (*BamH* I anchored forward primer 5'-CGCGGATCCATGATTGAGGACATCAAGACTCTT -3', *Xho* I anchored reverse primer 5'-CCGCTCGAG CTACTGCTGCTCAGTAGTAGCTT-3'). The PCR products were cloned into pMD18-T vector (TaKaRa Biotech, Dalian, China) to produce pMD18-T-Ea14–3-3. The resultant plasmid was identified by endonuclease digestion and sequencing. Basic local alignment search tool (BLAST) (http://www.ncbi.nlm.nih.gov/BLAST/) was used to analyze the nucleotide sequence.

Construction of eukaryotic expression plasmid pVAX-Ea14–3-3

The ORF of *Ea14–3-3* was cloned into eukaryotic expression vector pVAX1 to construct pVAX-Ea14–3-3. Briefly, fragments of Ea14–3-3 were excised from the pMD18-T-Ea14–3-3 by *BamH* I and *Xho* I digestion and ligated into pVAX1 at the same enzyme sites to construct pVAX-Ea14–3-3. The resulting plasmid was confirmed by endonuclease cleavage and sequence analysis.

Transcription detection of the Ea14–3-3 gene by RT-PCR in chickens

Two-week-old chickens were vaccinated with 100 μg dose of the recombinant plasmid pVAX-Ea14–3-3 through intramuscular injection in the thigh region. While, control group chickens were injected with the pVAX1 vector as described above. A small circle was marked on the injection site and kept clear until the cutting of muscle sample. One week later, injected site muscle sample (~ 0.5 g) was excised from each chicken for mRNA extraction. Potential residual plasmids were removed by DNase I (TaKaRa) digestion. RT-PCR was employed with the RNA product as template using the specific primers for Ea14–3-3 ORF. Electrophoresis in 1% agarose gel was subsequently performed to detect the Ea14–3-3 fragment. Muscles from the corresponding site of non-injected chickens were also lacerated as control samples.

Expression detection of Ea14–3-3 gene by Western blot in chickens

Two-week-old chickens were immunized with 100 μg dose of the recombinant plasmid pVAX-Ea14–3-3 or pVAX1 vector as mentioned previously. One week later, a sample of each injected muscles (about 0.5 g) was obtained as before, and treated with RIPA lysis buffer (0.1 mol/L phenyl-methylsulfonyl fluoride (PMSF), 50 mmol/L Tris–HCl, 150 mmol/L NaCl, 1% Nonnidet P-40, 0.1% SDS) for 3 h. The muscle sample from the corresponding site of each non-injected chicken was used as the control. The samples were centrifuged at 13,000 rpm for 10 min, and the supernatant was collected for Western blot analysis. For detection of expressed proteins, Western blot assay was performed using anti-*E. acervulina* chicken sera as primary antibody as previously reported method [48, 49].

Immunogenicity evaluation of Ea14–3-3 in chickens
Experimental design

Two-week-old chickens were randomly divided into 3 groups of 40 chickens in each group. As described previously, experimental groups of chickens were vaccinated with 100 μg of recombinant plasmid pVAX-Ea14–3-3. Vector control group chickens were injected with 100 μg of empty pVAX1, and the PBS control group chickens were injected with same volume of sterile PBS (pH 7.4). One week later, all chickens were received booster injection. One week after the primary and booster immunizations, 5 chickens from each group were euthanized by cervical dislocation for evaluation of T lymphocyte sub-populations and cytokines production separately. Blood sera were collected from the rest of 30 chickens in each group for specific antibody determination.

Flow Cytometry analysis of T lymphocyte subpopulations

Ea14–3-3 antigen induced changes in T lymphocyte subpopulations were determined using flow cytometry. Spleens from 5 euthanized chickens of each group were collected to evaluate spleen's T lymphocyte subpopulation proportions of CD4[+] and CD8[+]. The spleens were cut into pieces and gently pushed through a mesh (250 μm pore size). Spleen lymphocyte suspensions were prepared as described previously [50]. The cells (1×10^6 cells/ml) were dually stained with mouse anti-chicken CD3-PE/Cy5, mouse anti-chicken CD8α-FITC, and mouse anti-chicken CD3-PE/Cy5 + mouse anti-chicken CD4-FITC at room temperature in the dark for 30 min. After 3 washes twice PBS by centrifugation (2000 rpm for 5 min at 4 °C), splenocytes population were determined by FACScan flow cytometer and analyzed with Cell Quest software (BD Biosciences, Franklin Lakes, NJ, USA).

Determination of cytokine transcription by quantitative real-time PCR

Spleen lymphocytes from the vaccinated chickens (five per group) were prepared as previously described [50]. Total RNA was extracted from spleen lymphocytes using an E.Z.N.A.® Total RNA Kit Maxi Kit (OMEGA). The cDNA was then generated using RT-PCR. Quantitative real-time PCR (qPCR) was employed to determine IFN-γ, IL-2, IL-4 TNFSF15, IL-17D and TGF-β4 mRNA levels in immunized chickens. The qPCR was carried out with an initial denaturation at 95 °C for 30 s, followed by 40 cycles at 95°C for 10 s, at 60 °C for 30 s and followed by a melting curve program at 95°Cfor 15 s, at 60°Cfor 15 s, at 95 °Cfor 15 s, using an ABI PRISM 7500 Fast Real-Time PCR System (Applied Biosystems, Carlsbad, CA,United States). The chicken GAPDH gene was used as an internal control. The primers for qPCR are shown in Table 2 [51]. The same cDNA sample (without dilution) was used for all cytokines and GAPDH to normalize and standardize the data. The relative quantification of cytokine gene mRNA was determined via comparison the internal control gene of GAPDH using the $2^{-\Delta\Delta CT}$ method as previously described [52]. A validation experiment was performed by running a dilution series of the cDNA to evaluate the amplification efficiencies of the cytokine genes and internal control gene [51]. The qPCR efficiencies (E) were calculated using the following formula: $E = 10^{-1/slope} - 1$ [53]. Pfaffl correction was conducted for these qPCR analyses.

Determination of serum antibody level

Blood samples were collected from the wing vein of each chicken at 1-week intervals for 6-weeks post-booster vaccination. Sera were collected for determining Ea14–3-3-specific antibody levels through indirect ELISA as previously described [49]. In brief, 96-well microtiter plates (Corning-Costar NY, USA) were coated overnight at 4 °C with 10 μg/ml *E. acervulina* sporozoites (100 μl protein solution per well) in 0.05 M carbonate buffer (pH 9.6). The plates were washed 3 times with PBST, blocked with 5% Bovine Serum Albumin (BSA) for 2 h at 37 °C and then incubated with chicken serum diluted 1:50 in PBS for 1 h at 37 °C. A 1: 3000 dilution of horseradish peroxidase-conjugated donkey anti-chicken IgY anti-body (Sigma) in 5% SMP was added as the secondary antibody (100 ml/well) to detect bound antibodies, and the plates were again incubated for 1 h at 37 °C. Finally, the complexes were developed by incubation with 3, 3, 5, 5-tetramethylbenzidine (TMB) for 15 min. The reaction was stopped by adding 50 μL of 2 M H_2SO_4 to each well, and the absorbance was measured at 450 nm (OD_{450}) using an automated ELISA reader.

Table 2 Primers used for the quantitative RT-PCR

RNA target	Primer sequence	Accession NO.	Amplification efficiency (%)[a]	Correlation coefficients (r^2)
IFN-γ	Forward: 5′-AGCTGACGGTGGACCTATTATT-3′	Y07922	99.16	0.9976
	Reverse: 5′-GGCTTTGCGCTGGATTC-3′			
IL-2	Forward: 5′-TCTGGGACCACTGTATGCTCT-3′	AF000631	98.53	0.9932
	Reverse: 5′-ACACCAGTGGGAAACAGTATCA-3′			
TNFSF15	Forward:5′-CCTGAGTTATTCCAGCAACGCA-3′	NM_001024578	98.51	0.9992
	Reverse: 5′-ATCCACCAGCTTGATGTCACTAAC-3′			
IL-17D	Forward:5′-GCTGCCTCATGGGGATCTTTGGTG-3′	EF570583	98.18	0.9954
	Reverse: 5′-CGATGACGGCTTGTTCTGGTTGAC-3′			
TGF-β4	Forward: 5′-CGGGACGGATGAGAAGAAC-3′	M31160	97.39	0.9981
	Reverse: 5′-CGGCCCACGTAGTAAATGAT-3′			
IL-4	Forward: 5′-ACCCAGGGCATCCAGAAG-3′	AJ621735	99.41	0.9996
	Reverse: 5′-CAGTGCCGGCAAGAAGTT-3′			
GAPDH	Forward: 5′-GGTGGTGCTAAGCGTGTTAT-3′	K01458	95.48	0.9994
	Reverse: 5′-ACCTCTGTCATCTCTCCACA-3′			

[a]Amplification efficiency (%) = $(10^{-1/slope} - 1) \times 100$

Evaluation of immune protection

At 14 days of age, chickens were weighed and randomly divided into 13 groups with 30 chickens per group. Experimental group chickens were immunized with 100 μg of pVAX-Ea14–3-3 via intramuscular injection in thigh region. The challenged control group and unchallenged control chickens were injected with sterile PBS. The empty vector control group was immunized with 100 μg pVAX1 as mentioned above. A booster immunization was given at 7 day after the first immunization. At 28 days of age, the chickens were challenged with freshly sporulated oocyst of *E. tenella* (5×10^4/chicken), *E. acervulina* (1×10^5/chicken) and *E. maxima* (1×10^5/chicken) and mixed sporulated oocysts (5×10^4 *E. tenella* /chicken, 1×10^5 *E. acervulina* /chicken, 1×10^5 *E. maxima* /chicken) separately except the non-immunized and non-challenged group [54]. Six days post-challenged infection, all the chickens were slaughtered. Average body weight gain, oocyst decrease ratio, lesion score, and anti-coccidial index (ACI) were calculated.

The protective efficacy was evaluated based on body weight gain, lesion score, oocyst output, oocyst decrease ratio and ACI [55, 56]. Body weight gain was determined by weighing the chickens at the end of the experiment and deducing the weight of the same chickens at the time of challenge. Lesion scores were observed and recorded consistent with the method described by Reid and Johnson [57]. The intestinal contents from the whole guts of chickens in all groups were collected and oocysts per gram of content (OPG) were determined via McMaster's counting technique. ACI is a comprehensive index for assessing the protective effect of immune protection and is calculated as follow: (survival rate + relative rate of weight gain) - (lesion value + oocyst value). According to McManus [58], an ACI ≥180 is considered as high performance, an ACI between 160 and 179 is considered effective, while value of ACI < 160 is considered ineffective. All the chickens in this study were euthanized by CO_2 inhalation. Briefly, CO_2 was delivered from compressed gas canister with flowmeter and pressure regulator. After opening the switch, CO_2 would be steadily flowing into the euthanasia chamber. The number of animals put in the euthanasia chamber depended on the size of the box to avoid crowding. The entire body of the animal must go into the euthanasia chamber. The gas was delivered with a displacement rate of 20% of the euthanasia chamber volume per minute. After the animal loses consciousness, a secondary physical method of euthanasia of cervical dislocation was performed.

Statistical analysis

Non-normally distributed ANOVA with Tamhane's T2 multiple range tests were applied for the determination of statistical significance through SPSS statistical package (SPSS Inc., Chicago, IL, USA). The differences between all groups were tested and $p < 0.05$ value was considered as to indicate a significant difference.

Additional files

Additional file 1: Figure S1. Open reading frames (ORFs) and deduced amino acid sequence of common antigen 14–3-3. (TIF 12897 kb)

Additional file 2: Table S1. Amino acid similarities of 14–3-3 between *E. acervulina*, *E. maxima*, *E. tenella*, *E. necatrix* (%). 1.Ea14–3-3 = 14–3-3 of *E. acervulina*; Em14–3-3 = 14–3-3 of *E. maxima*; Et14–3-3 = 14–3-3 of *E. tenella*; En14–3-3 = 14–3-3 of *E. necatrix*. (DOCX 16 kb)

Additional file 3: Figure S2. Identification of recombinant plasmid pVAX-Ea14–3-3 digested by *BamH I/Xho I*. M: DNA molecular weight marker DL 2000. Lane 1: pVAX-Ea14–3-3. Lane 2: pVAX-Ea14–3-3 digested by *BamH I/Xho I*. (TIF 62 kb)

Abbreviations

ACI: Anti-coccidial index; *E. acervulina*: *Eimeria acervulina*; *E. maxima*: *Eimeria maxima*; *E. tenella*: *Eimeria tenella*; Ea14-3-3: *Eimeria acervulina* 14-3-3 protein; FITC: Fluorescein isothiocyanate; ORF: Open reading frame; PE: P-phycoerythrin; qPCR: quantitative real-time PCR; RT-PCR: transcription-polymerase chain reaction

Acknowledgments

We gratefully thank Jianmei Huang, Zhouyang Zhou for sample collection and valuable suggestions. We also gratefully thank Mr. Muhammad Haseeb and Muhammad Waqqas Hasan for their carful polish in the language of the manuscript.

Fundings

This work was supported by the National Key R&D Program of China (Grant No. 2017YFD0500401), the National Natural Science Foundation of China (Grant No. 31672545), the Fundamental Research Funds for the Central Universities (Grant No. KYZ201631), the Natural Science Foundation of Jiangsu Province of China (Grant No. BK20161442) and the Priority Academic Program Development of Jiangsu Higher Education Institutions (PAPD).

Authors' contributions

SXK designed the study and critically revised the manuscript. LXR, YRF and XLX helped in the study design and analyzed the data. LJH contributed to the main experiment and wrote the draft. LLR performed the laboratory tests. LLJ, TD and LWY contributed to the effective protection experiment. All authors read and approved the final manuscript.

Consent for publication

Not applicable.

Competing interests

The authors declare that they have no competing interests.

Author details

[1]MOE Joint International Research Laboratory of Animal Health and Food Safety, College of Veterinary Medicine, Nanjing Agricultural University, Nanjing 210095, People's Republic of China. [2]Henan Muxiang Veterinary Pharmaceutical Co., ltd, Zhengzhou 450000, People's Republic of China.

References

1. Williams R. Anticoccidial vaccines for broiler chickens: pathways to success. Avian pathol. 2002;31(4):317–53.
2. Morris G, Gasser R. Biotechnological advances in the diagnosis of avian coccidiosis and the analysis of genetic variation in *Eimeria*. Biotechnol Adv. 2006;24(6):590–603.
3. Blake DP, Tomley FM. Securing poultry production from the ever-present *Eimeria* challenge. Trends Parasitol. 2014;30(1):12–9.
4. Vermeulen A. Progress in recombinant vaccine development against coccidiosis a review and prospects into the next millennium. Int J Parasitol. 1998;28(7):1121–30.
5. Clarke L, Fodey TL, Crooks SR, Moloney M, O'Mahony J, Delahaut P, O'Kennedy R, Danaher M. A review of coccidiostats and the analysis of their residues in meat and other food. Meat Sci. 2014;97(3):358–74.
6. Meunier M, Chemaly M, Dory D. DNA vaccination of poultry: the current status in 2015. Vaccine. 2016;34(2):202–11.
7. Reid AJ, Blake DP, Ansari HR, Billington K, Browne HP, Bryant J, Dunn M, Hung SS, Kawahara F, Miranda-Saavedra D. Genomic analysis of the causative agents of coccidiosis in domestic chickens. Genome Res. 2014; 24(10):1676–85.
8. You M-J. The comparative analysis of infection pattern and oocyst output in *Eimeria tenella*, *E. maxima* and *E. acervulina* in young broiler chicken.[J]. Vet World. 2014;7(7):542–47.
9. Awais MM, Akhtar M, Iqbal Z, Muhammad F, Anwar MI. Seasonal prevalence of coccidiosis in industrial broiler chickens in Faisalabad, Punjab, Pakistan. Trop Anim Health Prod. 2012;44(2):323–8.
10. Del Cacho E, Gallego M, Lee SH, Lillehoj HS, Quilez J, Lillehoj EP, Sánchez-Acedo C. Induction of protective immunity against *Eimeria tenella*, *Eimeria maxima*, and *Eimeria acervulina* infections using dendritic cell-derived exosomes. Infect Immun. 2012;80(5):1909–16.
11. Talebi A. Protein profiles of five avian *Eimeria* species. Avian Pathol. 1995; 24(4):731–5.
12. Sasai K, Lillehoj HS, Hemphill A, Matsuda H, Hanioka Y, Fukata T, Baba E, Arakawa A. A chicken anti-conoid monoclonal antibody identifies a common epitope which is present on motile stages of *Eimeria*, *Neospora*, and *Toxoplasma*. J Parasitol. 1998;84(3):654–6.
13. Constantinoiu C, Lillehoj H, Matsubayashi M, Hosoda Y, Tani H, Matsuda H, Sasai K, Baba E. Analysis of cross-reactivity of five new chicken monoclonal antibodies which recognize the apical complex of *Eimeria* using confocal laser immunofluorescence assay. Vet Parasitol. 2003;118(1):29–35.
14. Liu L, Huang X, Liu J, Li W, Ji Y, Tian D, Tian L, Yang X, Xu L, Yan R. Identification of common immunodominant antigens of *Eimeria tenella*, *Eimeria acervulina* and *Eimeria maxima* by immunoproteomic analysis. Oncotarget. 2017;8(21):34935.
15. Cau Y, Valensin D, Mori M, Draghi S, Botta M. Structure, function, involvement in diseases and targeting of 14-3-3 proteins: an update. Curr Med Chem. 2017;24(999):1.
16. Lalle M, Curra C, Ciccarone F, Pace T, Cecchetti S, Fantozzi L, Ay B, Breton CB, Ponzi M. Dematin, a component of the erythrocyte membrane skeleton, is internalized by the *malaria* parasite and associates with *Plasmodium* 14-3-3. J Biol Chem. 2011;286(2):1227–36.
17. Zhao N, Gong P, Cheng B, Li J, Yang Z, Li H, Yang J, Zhang G, Zhang X. *Eimeria tenella*: 14-3-3 protein interacts with telomerase. Parasitol Res. 2014; 113(10):3885–9.
18. Inoue M, Nakamura Y, Yasuda K, Yasaka N, Hara T, Schnaufer A, Stuart K, Fukuma T. The 14-3-3 proteins of *Trypanosoma brucei* function in motility, cytokinesis, and cell cycle. J Biol Chem. 2005;280(14):14085–96.
19. Assossou O, Besson F, Rouault JP, Persat F, Ferrandiz J, Mayencon M, Peyron F, Picot S. Characterization of an excreted/secreted antigen form of 14-3-3 protein in *Toxoplasma gondii* tachyzoites. FEMS Microbiol Lett. 2004;234(1):19–25.
20. Meng M, He S, Zhao G, Bai Y, Zhou H, Cong H, Lu G, Zhao Q, Zhu X-Q. Evaluation of protective immune responses induced by DNA vaccines encoding *Toxoplasma gondii* surface antigen 1 (SAG1) and 14-3-3 protein in BALB/c mice. Parasit Vectors. 2012;5(1):273.
21. Schechtman D, Tarrab-Hazdai R, Arnon R. The 14-3-3 protein as a vaccine candidate against schistosomiasis. Parasite Immunol. 2001;23(4):213–7.
22. Yang J, Zhu W, Huang J, Wang X, Sun X, Zhan B, Zhu X. Partially protective immunity induced by the 14-3-3 protein from *Trichinella spiralis*. Vet Parasitol. 2016;231:63–8.
23. Siles-Lucas M, Merli M, Gottstein B. 14-3-3 proteins in *Echinococcus*: their role and potential as protective antigens. Exp Parasitol. 2008;119(4):516–23.
24. Shirley MW, Smith AL, Tomley FM. The biology of avian *Eimeria* with an emphasis on their control by vaccination. Adv Parasitol. 2005;60:285–330.
25. Carvalho FS, Wenceslau AA, Teixeira M, Matos Carneiro JA, Melo ADB, Albuquerque GR. Diagnosis of *Eimeria* species using traditional and molecular methods in field studies. Vet Parasitol. 2011;176(2):95–100.
26. Ogedengbe JD, Hunter DB, Barta JR. Molecular identification of *Eimeria* species infecting market-age meat chickens in commercial flocks in Ontario. Vet Parasitol. 2011;178(3):350–4.
27. Chapman HD. Milestones in avian coccidiosis research: a review. Poult Sci. 2014;93(3):501–11.
28. Bessay M, Le Vern Y, Kerboeuf D, Yvore P, Quéré P. Changes in intestinal intra-epithelial and systemic T-cell subpopulations after an *Eimeria* infection in chickens: comparative study between *E. acervulina* and *E. tenella*. Vet Res. 1996;27(4-5):503–14.
29. Min W, Lillehoj HS, Burnside J, Weining KC, Staeheli P, Zhu JJ. Adjuvant effects of IL-1beta, IL-2, IL-8, IL-15, IFN-alpha, IFN-gamma TGF-beta4 and lymphotactin on DNA vaccination against *Eimeria acervulina*. Vaccine. 2001; 20(1–2):267–74.

30. Diloul RA, Lillehoj HS. Poultry coccidiosis: recent advancements in control measures and vaccine development. Expert Rev Vaccines. 2006;5(1):143–63.

31. Rose ME, Wakelin D, Hesketh P. Interferon-gamma-mediated effects upon immunity to coccidial infections in the mouse. Parasite Immunol. 1991;13(1):63–74.

32. Lillehoj HS, Choi KD. Recombinant chicken interferon-γ-mediated inhibition of Eimeria tenella development in vitro and reduction of oocyst production and body weight loss following Eimeria acervulina challenge infection. Avian Dis. 1998;42(2):307–14.

33. Jang SI, Lillehoj HS, Lee SH, et al. Eimeria maxima recombinant Gam82 gametocyte antigen vaccine protects against coccidiosis and augments humoral and cell-mediated immunity. Vaccine. 2010;28(17):2980–5.

34. Song X, Huang X, Yan R, Xu L, Li X. Efficacy of chimeric DNA vaccines encoding Eimeria tenella 5401 and chicken IFN-gamma or IL-2 against coccidiosis in chickens. Exp Parasitol. 2015;156:19–25.

35. Inagaki-Ohara K, Dewi FN, Hisaeda H, Smith AL, Jimi F, Miyahira M, Abdel-Aleem AS, Horii Y, Nawa Y. Intestinal intraepithelial lymphocytes sustain the epithelial barrier function against Eimeria vermiformis infection. Infect Immun. 2006;74(9):5292–301.

36. Kim W H, Jeong J, Park A R, et al. Chicken IL-17F: Identification and comparative expression analysis in Eimeria- infected chickens[J]. Dev Comp Immunol. 2012;38(3):401–9.

37. Zhao GH, Cheng WY, Wang W, et al. The expression dynamics of IL-17 and Th17 response relative cytokines in the trachea and spleen of chickens after infection with Cryptosporidium baileyi. Parasit Vectors. 2014;7(1):1–7.

38. Strober W, Kelsall B, Fuss I, Marth T, Ludviksson B, Ehrhardt R, Neurath M. Reciprocal IFN-gamma and TGF-beta responses regulate the occurrence of mucosal inflammation. Immunol Today. 1997;18(2):61–4.

39. Jakowlew SB, Mathias A, Lillehoj HS. Transforming growth factor-beta isoforms in the developing chicken intestine and spleen: increase in transforming growth factor-beta 4 with coccidia infection. Vet Immunol Immunopathol. 1997;55(4):321–39.

40. Shalaby MR, Aggarwal BB, Rinderknecht E, et al. Activation of human polymorphonuclear neutrophil functions by interferon-gamma and tumor necrosis factors. J Immunol. 1985;135(3):2069.

41. Park SS, Lillehoj HS, Hong YH, Lee SH. Functional characterization of tumor necrosis factor superfamily 15 (TNFSF15) induced by lipopolysaccharides and Eimeria infection. Dev Comp Immunol. 2007;31(9):934–44.

42. Ivory C, Chadee K. DNA vaccines: designing strategies against parasitic infections. Genet Vaccines Ther. 2004;2(1):17.

43. Lillehoj H, Min W, Dalloul R. Recent progress on the cytokine regulation of intestinal immune responses to Eimeria. Poultry Sci. 2004;83(4):611–23.

44. Awais MM, Akhtar M, Anwar MI, Khaliq K. Evaluation of Saccharum officinarum L. bagasse-derived polysaccharides as native immunomodulatory and anticoccidial agents in broilers. Vet Parasitol. 2018;249:74–81.

45. Song X, Xu L, Yan R, Huang X, Shah MAA, Li X. The optimal immunization procedure of DNA vaccine pcDNA–TA4–IL-2 of Eimeria tenella and its cross-immunity to Eimeria necatrix and Eimeria acervulina. Vet Parasitol. 2009; 159(1):30–6.

46. Tomley F. Techniques for isolation and characterization of apical organelles from Eimeria tenella Sporozoites. Methods. 1997;13(2):171–6.

47. Sambrook J, Russell DW. Molecular cloning: a laboratory manual[M]. Cold Spring Harbor Laboratory. 2001;675.

48. Song H, Qiu B, Yan R, et al. The protective efficacy of chimeric SO7/IL-2 DNA vaccine against coccidiosis in chickens. Res Vet Sci. 2013;94(3):562–7.

49. Song X, Zhao X, Xu L, Yan R, Li X. Immune protection duration and efficacy stability of DNA vaccine encoding Eimeria tenella TA4 and chicken IL-2 against coccidiosis. Res Vet Sci. 2017;111:31–5.

50. Sasai K, Aita M, Lillehoj H, Miyamoto T, Fukata T, Baba E. Dynamics of lymphocyte subpopulation changes in the cecal tonsils of chickens infected with Salmonella enteritidis. Vet Microbiol. 2000;74(4):345–51.

51. Song H, Song X, Xu L, Yan R, Shah MAA, Li X. Changes of cytokines and IgG antibody in chickens vaccinated with DNA vaccines encoding Eimeria acervulina lactate dehydrogenase. Vet Parasitol. 2010;173(3):219–27.

52. Livak KJ, Schmittgen TD. Analysis of relative gene expression data using real-time quantitative PCR and the $2^{-\Delta\Delta CT}$ method. Methods. 2001;25(4): 402–8.

53. Sanchez H, Chapot R, Banzet S, Koulmann N, Birot O, Bigard AX, Peinnequin A. Quantification by real-time PCR of developmental and adult myosin mRNA in rat muscles. Biochem Biophys Res Commun. 2006;340(1):165–74.

54. Holdsworth PA, Conway DP, Mckenzie ME, Dayton AD, Chapman HD, Mathis GF, Skinner JT, Mundt HC, Williams RB. World Association for the Advancement of veterinary parasitology (WAAVP) guidelines for evaluating the efficacy of anticoccidial drugs in chickens and turkeys. Vet Parasitol. 2004;121(3–4):189.

55. Morehouse NF, Baron RR. Coccidiosis: evaluation of coccidiostats by mortality, weight gains, and fecal scores. Exp Parasitol. 1970;28(1):25–9.

56. Chapman H, Shirley M. Sensitivity of field isolates of Eimeria species to monensin and lasalocid in the chicken. Res Vet Sci. 1989;46(1):114–7.

57. Johnson J, Reid WM. Anticoccidial drugs: lesion scoring techniques in battery and floor-pen experiments with chickens. Exp Parasitol. 1970;28(1):30–6.

58. McManus EC, Campbell WC, Cuckler AC. Development of resistance to quinoline coccidiostats under field and laboratory conditions. Int J Parasitol. 1968;54(6):1190–3.

19

White-nose syndrome detected in bats over an extensive area of Russia

Veronika Kovacova[1]* iD, Jan Zukal[2,3], Hana Bandouchova[1], Alexander D. Botvinkin[4], Markéta Harazim[2,3], Natália Martínková[2,5], Oleg L. Orlov[6,7], Vladimir Piacek[1], Alexandra P. Shumkina[8], Mikhail P. Tiunov[9] and Jiri Pikula[1]

Abstract

Background: Spatiotemporal distribution patterns are important infectious disease epidemiological characteristics that improve our understanding of wild animal population health. The skin infection caused by the fungus *Pseudogymnoascus destructans* emerged as a panzootic disease in bats of the northern hemisphere. However, the infection status of bats over an extensive geographic area of the Russian Federation has remained understudied.

Results: We examined bats at the geographic limits of bat hibernation in the Palearctic temperate zone and found bats with white-nose syndrome (WNS) on the European slopes of the Ural Mountains through the Western Siberian Plain, Central Siberia and on to the Far East. We identified the diagnostic symptoms of WNS based on histopathology in the Northern Ural region at 11° (about 1200 km) higher latitude than the current northern limit in the Nearctic. While body surface temperature differed between regions, bats at all study sites hibernated in very cold conditions averaging 3.6 °C. Each region also differed in *P. destructans* fungal load and the number of UV fluorescent skin lesions indicating skin damage intensity. *Myotis bombinus, M. gracilis* and *Murina hilgendorfi* were newly confirmed with histopathological symptoms of WNS. Prevalence of UV-documented WNS ranged between 16 and 76% in species of relevant sample size.

Conclusions: To conclude, the bat pathogen *P. destructans* is widely present in Russian hibernacula but infection remains at low intensity, despite the high exposure rate.

Keywords: Chiroptera, Hibernation, *Pseudogymnoascus destructans*, Prevalence, Distribution

Background

Any infectious disease determinants associated with the host(s), the agent and the environment will vary geographically [1]. Geographic distribution of infectious diseases is modulated by climate-associated factors inducing changes in the host-pathogen system [2–4]. Variation in the host-pathogen system attributable to climate includes changes in virulence, adaptation of the pathogen to hosts and vectors, the pathogen's ability to survive in the environment after being shed from the host, along with host population ecology, susceptibility and immune function [5]. Generally speaking, anthropogenic, environmental and ecological factors are drivers of infectious disease emergence [6]. Spatial and temporal distribution data related to infectious diseases are

necessary to increase our understanding of population health in wild animals, to identify populations and species at risk, to trace disease origin, to predict and model disease spread and dynamics and to propose effective control measures.

While bats have been recognised as important reservoir hosts for a great variety of emerging infectious agents [7], the fungus *Pseudogymnoascus destructans* [8, 9], causative agent of white-nose syndrome (WNS), is the first pathogen to threaten chiropteran biodiversity [10, 11] in the temperate zone. Constrained by temperature [12] and humidity [13], WNS emerged in a specific niche, i.e. underground bat hibernacula [14]. Breaking out as a point epidemic in eastern North America in 2006 [10], *P. destructans* infection has gradually been recognized as a panzootic in bats of the northern hemisphere [10, 15–21].

Success in WNS surveillance depends on the use of accurate tools and timing of sampling, along with knowledge on the seasonality and natural history of the disease. In addition to qualitative fungus identification

* Correspondence: kovacovav@vfu.cz
[1]Department of Ecology and Diseases of Game, Fish and Bees, University of Veterinary and Pharmaceutical Sciences Brno, Palackého tř. 1946/1, 612 42 Brno, Czech Republic
Full list of author information is available at the end of the article

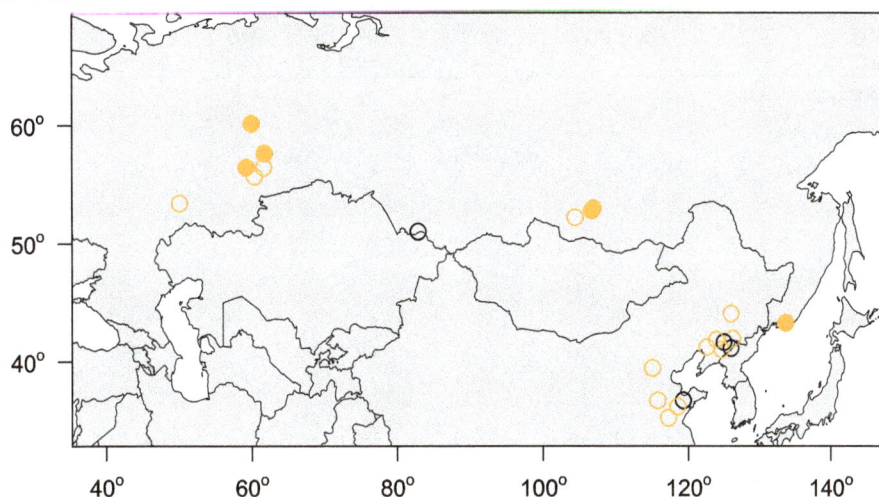

Fig. 1 Distribution of study sites in the central and eastern parts of the Russian Federation. Closed circles = this study, open circles = previously published sites [21, 28], orange = *Pseudogymnoascus destructans* infection confirmed with quantitative PCR, black = *P. destructans* not detected

using culture and polymerase chain reaction (PCR) [8], quantitative methods such as qPCR [22] and image analysis of photographs taken via trans-illumination of wing membranes with UV light [23] can also be used to evaluate infection intensity [21]. In fact, modification of the Wood's lamp for UV light diagnostics of WNS is one of the most useful tools allowing immediate recognition of infected bats, the method being highly sensitive and specific in targeting skin lesions for biopsy collection under field conditions. As UV lamp is a non-lethal diagnostic tool allowing rapid examination, it is applicable for the examination of protected bat species. UV transillumination also allows the researcher to distinguish between invasive infection and skin surface colonisation in *P. destructans*-exposed bats [24, 25] as it functions by fluorescing skin lesions laden with vitamin B_2, that are characteristic of *P. destructans* infection [26].

WNS skin infection has recently been recognised in the West Siberian Plain of Russian Asia [21] and north-eastern China [19]. Widespread endemicity of the WNS fungus in the Palearctic suggests that bat tolerance to this infection probably became established due to long-term co-evolution [21, 27]. Interestingly, presence of the pathogen has also been identified in historic bat populations and the regions of Samara and Irkutsk (European and Asian parts of Russia, respectively) using ethanol-stored samples of bat ectoparasites [28]. Here we further address the infection status of bats over an extensive geographic area of Russia, extending the known northern and eastern geographic limits of the disease and detailing site- and species-dependent differences in epidemiological characteristics.

Methods

Bat sampling sites and procedures

Between 2014 and 2017 we sampled 188 bats (11 species) at 11 hibernation sites from the European slopes of the Ural Mountains through the Western Siberian Plain, Siberia and the Russian Far East (Fig. 1; Table 1). Bats were sampled during the late hibernation season (April and May) and all bats were later released at the capture site. Bat body temperature was measured individually with a Raynger MX2 non-contact IR thermometer (Raytek Corporation, USA) by focusing the laser beam at the central part of bat's body. Following hand capture, the

Table 1 Number of bats sampled in Russia

Species	Gender			Total
	Females	Males	NA	
Eptesicus nilssonii	9	22		31
Myotis bombinus	1	2		3
Myotis brandtii	7	11	1	19
Myotis dasycneme	30	19		49
Myotis daubentonii	1	2		3
Myotis gracilis	2	32		34
Myotis macrodactylus	1			1
Myotis petax	2			2
Murina hilgendorfi	19	17		36
Plecotus auritus		1		1
Plecotus ognevi		8	1	9
Total	80	106	2	188

Gender and species data were obtained for bats included in the study. While each bat was sexed by inspection of external genitalia, species identification was based on morphological traits and/or sequencing the mitochondrial gene for cytochrome b (mtcyb)

Table 2 Differences in bat communities, hibernation temperature and infection status between sites

Region	Locality	Number of bats	Number of species	WNS UV lesions	WNS qPCR assay	WNS histo-positivity	Median temperature (°C)
Southern Ural	Slyudorudnik mine	12	4	+	+	+	3.95
Middle Ural	Arakaevskaja cave	10	2	+	+	+	1.25
	Smolinskaja cave	21	3	+	+	+	4.70
	Šajtanskaja cave	25	4	+	+	–	1.40
Northern Ural	Dačnaja cave	1	1	–	–	–	3.50
	Komsomolskaja cave	18	3	+	+	+	2.70
	Partizanskaja cave	16	2	+	+	+	3.45
Baikal	Aja cave	2	1	N.A.	+	N.A.	N.A.
	Mečta cave	31	3	+	+	+	1.00
	Cave Vologodskovo	10	1	+	+	+	4.70
Far East	Primorskij Velikan cave	42	5	+	+	+	4.40
Total number of positive bats				78	135	48	

Apart from hibernation conditions (body surface temperature of bats), the table includes data concerning bat biodiversity and qualitative measures of *Pseudogymnoascus destructans* infection status

dorsal side of the left wing was swabbed with a nylon swab (FLOQ Swabs, Copan Flock Technologies srl, Brescia, Italy) for qPCR diagnosis. Presence and quantity of *P. destructans* was assessed using a TaqMan® Universal Master Mix II with UNG (Life Technologies, Foster City, CA, USA) using the dual-probe assay [22]. Optimisation of the PCR reaction and calculation of fungal load was in accordance with Zukal et al. [21] for samples taken between 2014 and 2016 and Zahradníková et al. [28] for samples from 2017. The diagnostic symptoms of WNS were confirmed by current standards. For histopathology analysis, we selected orange-yellow fluorescing spots observed over a 368 nm UV lamp [23]. Suspect wing tissues were biopsied and stored in 10% formalin. The

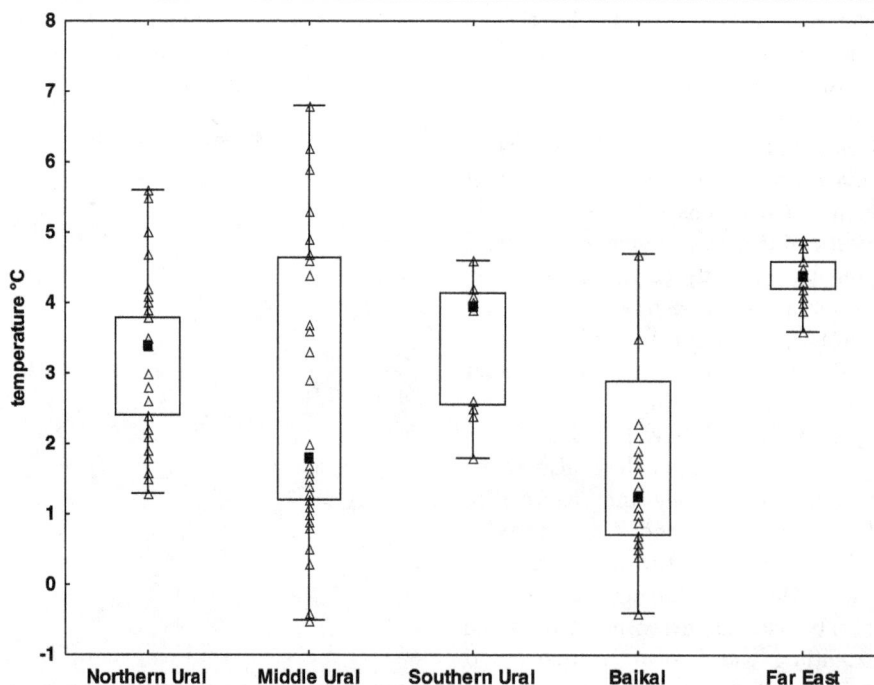

Fig. 2 Body temperature of hibernating bats in the study regions. *Explanation*: black square mid-point = median; box = inter-quartile range; whiskers = minimum/maximum range, empty triangles = particular samples

formalin-fixed skin samples were then embedded in paraffin and stained for fungi with periodic acid-Schiff stain. Histological observation took place under an Olympus BX51 light microscope (Olympus Corporation, Tokyo, Japan). Yellow-orange fluorescing WNS lesions on the right wing were manually enumerated on trans-illuminated photographs using the ImageJ counting tool [29].

Phylogenetic reconstruction

We sequenced the mitochondrial gene for cytochrome b (mtcyb) in 77 bats in order to validate species identification in newly sampled regions. DNA was isolated from the wing punch biopsies using the DNeasy Blood & Tissue Kit (Qiagen, Halden, Germany), according to the manufacturer's protocol. We amplified the mtcyb gene with the

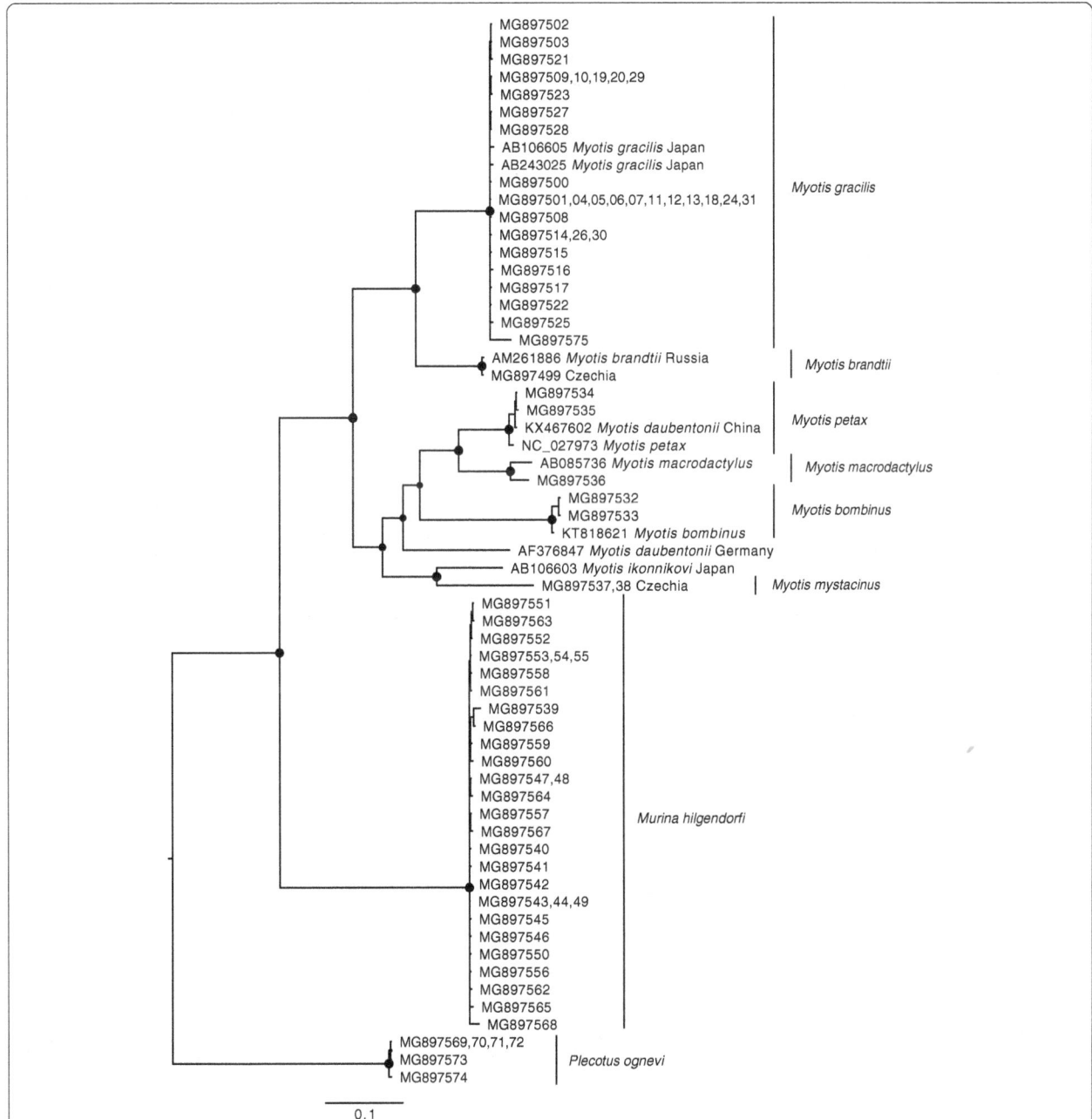

Fig. 3 Bayesian inference phylogeny of bats from the Eastern Palearctic based on partial mtcyb gene sequences. Circles at nodes indicate Bayesian posterior probability >0.95; species reported in this study are indicated with vertical bars. Specimen vouchers are listed for newly sequenced individuals, where numbers in curly brackets represent multiple vouchers. Previously published sequences are reported with their accession numbers, species designation in GenBank and country of sample origin

mammalian primers L7 (ACCAATGACATGAAAAATC ATCGTT) and H6 (TCTCCATTTCTGGTTTACA AGAC) [30], supplied at 0.2 μM concentration in a reaction mix containing 1× buffer, 0.2 mM of dNTPs, 2 mM MgCl$_2$ and 0.1 U Platinum Taq polymerase (Invitrogen, Life Technologies, Carlsbad, CA, USA). The cycling conditions included a 3 min denaturation step at 95 °C, followed by 36 cycles of 40 s at 95 °C, 50 s at 53 °C and 80s at 72 °C. The reaction was finalised with a 3 min extension at 72 °C. We purified the PCR products through EXO-CIP enzymatic purification and sequenced them commercially with amplification primers from both directions. The chromatograms were assembled in CodonCode Aligner 7.1 (CodonCode, Centerville, MA, USA). Together with mtcyb sequences from GenBank, we aligned the sequences in MAFFT 7.3 [31] and reconstructed the phylogenetic relationships in MrBayes 3.2 [32] using Markov chain Monte Carlo (MCMC) sampling over two independent runs. The MCMC used the HKY + Γ substitution model run for 1 million generations with 30% of initial sampled states discarded as burn in. The settings enabled MCMC convergence and trees in the posterior were summarised with 50% majority-rule consensus.

Statistical analysis

The common logarithm of *P. destructans* load and the number of UV-documented skin lesions were used for statistical analysis as these variables did not meet normality (Shapiro-Wilk test, $p < 0.05$). Differences between regions and bat species were tested using ANOVA. Body surface temperature could not be transformed to normality; hence, non-parametric Kruskal-Wallis ANOVA was used for the comparison of body surface temperature between regions and bat species. Pearson's correlation

coefficient was used to evaluate the relationship between *P. destructans* load and the number of UV-identified skin lesions. All analyses were performed using Statistica for Windows 12.0 (StatSoft, USA).

Results
Locality-dependent differences

WNS positive bats (both *P. destructans*-positive on qPCR and WNS-positive on UV and histopathology) were confirmed in all study regions (Fig. 1) and at all hibernation sites (Table 2) except the Dachnaya cave, where a single bat was checked with no signs of WNS and negative qPCR results. The sample sites covered the whole of the Asian part of Russia, with additional new sites in the European part. Sites situated in the Northern Ural region were approximately 1200 km further north than any previous site with confirmed WNS in the world. Bats at all study sites hibernated in very cold climatic conditions (median 3.6 °C, min − 0.5 °C, max 6.8 °C), with warmest conditions recorded near the coast at the Primorskiy Velikan cave in the Primorskiy region (Fig. 2). Body surface temperatures differed significantly between regions, with a significant correlation observed between body surface temperature and ambient temperature (Kruskal-Wallis test: $H_{4, 185} = 39.35$, $p < 0.001$). Regions also differed significantly in *P. destructans* fungal load (ANOVA: $F_{4,130} = 17.11$, $p < 0.001$) and number of UV fluorescent skin lesions (ANOVA: $F_{4,66} = 17.54$, $p = 0.001$), with bats hibernating in the Baikal having lowest values of both disease parameters (Table 2).

Differences between species of hibernating bats

Samples were analysed from 11 bat species covering most of the hibernating bat diversity in the Eastern Palearctic region. Of the 77 bats sequenced (European

Table 3 Prevalence (percentage) with confidence interval of *Pseudogymnoascus destructans* infection in Russian bats

Species	WNS UV-documented skin lesions				WNS qPCR assay				Histo-positivity
	Negative	Positive	Analyzed	Prevalence	Negative	Positive	Analyzed	Prevalence	
Eptesicus nilssonii	26	5	31	16.1 ± 12.9	26	5	31	16.1 ± 12.9	+
Myotis bombinus	1	1	2	50.0 ± 69.3		3	3	100.0 ± 0.0	+
Myotis brandtii	10	9	19	47.4 ± 22.5	7	12	19	63.2 ± 21.7	−
Myotis dasycneme	12	37	49	75.5 ± 12.0	7	41	48	85.4 ± 10.0	+
Myotis daubentonii	2	1	3	33.3 ± 53.3	2	1	3	33.3 ± 53.3	N.A.
Myotis gracilis	26	7	33	21.2 ± 13.9	5	29	34	85.3 ± 11.9	+
Myotis macrodactylus	1		1	0.0 ± 0.0		1	1	100.0 ± 0.0	N.A.
Myotis petax		2	2	100.0 ± 0.0		1	1	100.0 ± 0.0	+
Murina hilgendorfi	21	15	36	41.7 ± 16.1		36	36	100.0 ± 0.0	+
Plecotus auritus		1	1	100.0 ± 0.0		1	1	100.0 ± 0.0	+
Plecotus ognevi	7		7	0.0 ± 0.0	3	5	8	62.5 ± 33.5	N.A.
Total	106	78	184		50	135	185		8 species

Numbers of positive bats were determined using qualitative characteristics of *P. destructans* infection status examination

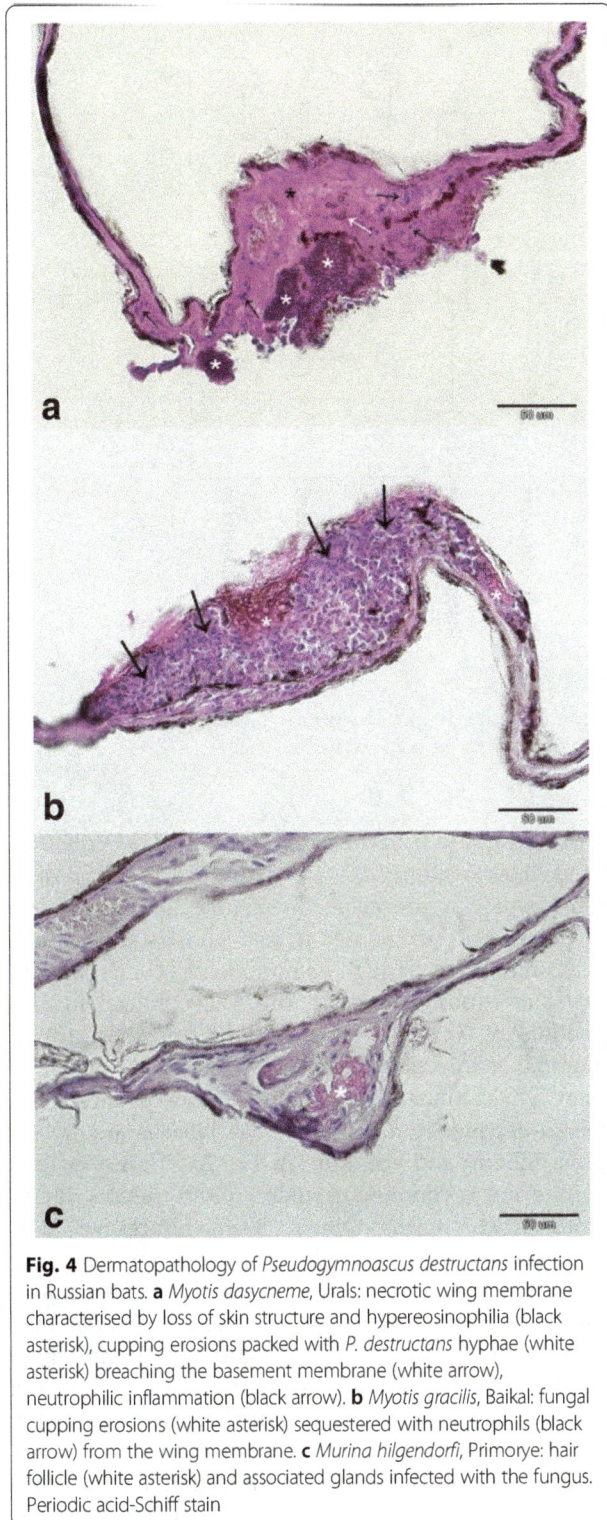

Fig. 4 Dermatopathology of *Pseudogymnoascus destructans* infection in Russian bats. **a** *Myotis dasycneme*, Urals: necrotic wing membrane characterised by loss of skin structure and hypereosinophilia (black asterisk), cupping erosions packed with *P. destructans* hyphae (white asterisk) breaching the basement membrane (white arrow), neutrophilic inflammation (black arrow). **b** *Myotis gracilis*, Baikal: fungal cupping erosions (white asterisk) sequestered with neutrophils (black arrow) from the wing membrane. **c** *Murina hilgendorfi*, Primorye: hair follicle (white asterisk) and associated glands infected with the fungus. Periodic acid-Schiff stain

phylogenetic reconstruction (Fig. 3), we confirmed that bat genetic diversity based on the mtcyb gene is consistent with known bat diversity in the Eastern Palearctic.

With the exception of *Myotis macrodactylus* and *Plecotus ognevi*, where only *P. destructans* DNA material was found on the wings, all the bat species monitored were confirmed as both *P. destructans* and WNS positive (Table 3). Three bat species (*M. bombinus*, *M. gracilis* and *Murina hilgendorfi*) are newly confirmed with WNS histopathological symptoms identical with those shown by European and North American bats (Fig. 4). Prevalence of *P. destructans* infection (qPCR) and WNS (expressed as UV fluorescent skin lesions) varied between species (Table 3), with WNS prevalence ranging between 16 and 76% in samples with more than five specimens. Similarly, both WNS impact parameters, i.e. *P. destructans* load (ANOVA: $F_{8,126} = 9.41$, $p < 0.001$; Additional file 1: Figure S1 and Fig. 5) and number of UV fluorescent skin lesions (ANOVA: $F_{7,63} = 3.32$, $p = 0.005$) differed significantly between bat species. There was also a significant correlation between fungal load and number of UV fluorescent skin lesions ($r = 0.40$, $p < 0.05$).

Discussion

Russia's enormous size and the geographic remoteness of many hibernacula makes active surveillance for bat diseases a difficult task in the Eastern Palearctic. The resulting poor knowledge of bat community infection status over such an extensive understudied territory means that impacts of wildlife conservation concern often go undetected. Further, while single visits to hibernation sites provide static data, they cannot evaluate disease dynamics or changes in bat abundance. However, long-term monitoring of hibernating bats in caves in the study regions have yet to report any mass mortalities or dramatic declines in bat abundance [33–36].

Since 2008, presence of *P. destructans* and/or WNS has been confirmed over an area stretching from Portugal to Turkey [17, 18, 37, 38]. By extending our knowledge on the distribution range of *P. destructans* to the Northern Ural region (forming the boundary between the European and Asian continents) and on to the southern part of the Russian Far East, we come close to covering the geographic limits of bat hibernation in the Palearctic temperate zone [21, 39–41]. In light of current data, the last remaining biogeographic questions regarding WNS distribution in the Palearctic are its presence or absence in Japan, Sakhalin, the Kuril Islands or the Kamchatka Peninsula. Based on its presence in both Continental Europe and the British Isles [42], it is quite likely that *P. destructans* will be found in islands off the mainland of Far Eastern Asia. Furthermore, we were able to confirm histopathological symptoms of WNS (Fig. 4a; [24, 43]) in bats at an 11° (ca. 1200 km) higher latitude than the previous highest finding in the Canadian provinces [44].

Nucleotide Archive: MG897500 – MG897575), 25 were identical to others in the dataset. We added nine previously published sequences in order to obtain an alignment containing 60 unique haplotypes of partial mtcyb sequences 1061 bp long. Using Bayesian inference

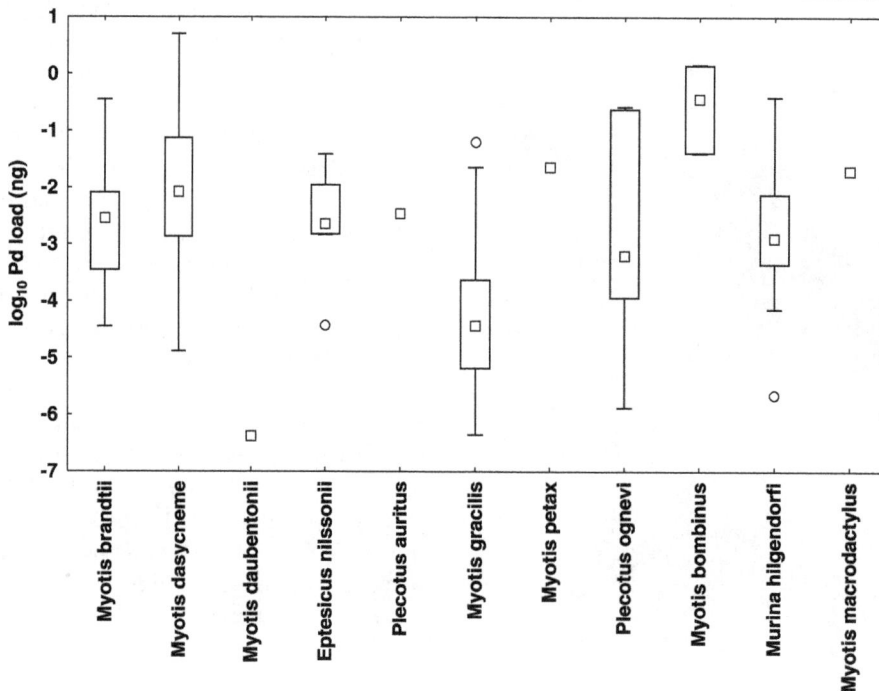

Fig. 5 Infection intensity, measured as fungal load in nanograms on a $\log_{10}$ scale, for *Pseudogymnoascus destructans* positive bats. *Explanation:* mid-point = median; box = inter-quartile range; whiskers = non-outlier minimum/maximum range; dots = outliers

In contrast with sites in North America, *P. destructans* in the Palearctic region does not appear to be associated with dramatic bat mortalities [15, 19, 21], despite the number of *P. destructans* or WNS positive bat species being higher in the Palearctic than Nearctic (Additional file 2: Table S1). As previously predicted by Zukal et al. [40], three Asian vespertilionid bat species were newly confirmed with pathognomonic skin lesions induced by *P. destructans* infection in the present study (e.g. Fig. 4b, c). Paired data on identification of *P. destructans* with qPCR and WNS diagnostics on histopathology, supported with host molecular genetic phylogeny from the Eastern Palearctic [45], indicates that WNS affects *M. bombinus, M. brandtii, M. dasycneme, M. gracilis, M. petax, Eptesicus nilssonii, Murina hilgendorfi* and *Plecotus auritus* in Russia. Both *M. daubentonii* and *M. macrodactylus* were found to be infected with *P. destructans*, though WNS has not yet been confirmed on histopathology. Russian Siberian bats invaded by the fungus show clearly visible orange–yellow fluorescence of wing membrane skin lesions under UV light, documenting that this diagnostic tool [23] is applicable throughout the known distribution range of the pathogen and, moreover, that Russian *P. destructans* strains hyperproduce vitamin B_2, a WNS virulence factor [26].

The WNS fungus is a generalist pathogen of hibernating vespertilionid and rhinolophid bats [40]. Assuming that all bats (with species-specific behavioural and roosting variation) that enter a *P. destructans*-contaminated hibernaculum have an equal chance of exposure to the pathogen, prevalence (percentage of bats positive for the agent) documented in Russian bats should then be an indicator of a high environmental contamination level and exposure rate. In this study, fungal load, a function of variables such as the infectious dose, duration of infection and growth rate of the agent in given environmental conditions, showed site- and species-dependent differences. Bat hibernation in the Urals, Siberia and the Russian Far East lasts up to 7 months and is confined to underground shelters due to strong frosts during winter. Temperatures in such hibernacula do not exceed 5 °C throughout the year [33–36]; hence, Russian bats should show lower fungal loads than European and North American bats as they hibernate under colder microclimatic conditions, which lead to slow temperature-dependent growth of the pathogen [12]. The prevalence of UV-documented skin lesions and histopathological positivity in this study signifies species susceptibility to infection. As the probability of serious wing membranes damage increases with increasing fungal load [25], and a lowered fungal load is linked with lower WNS impact (expressed as reduced UV fluorescent lesions, similar to [21]), we suggest that bats hibernating in such cold climatic conditions have a higher probability of surviving infection than elsewhere [46].

Conclusion

While it is not known how long the *P. destructans* fungal pathogen has been present in the Palearctic region, or whether there were periods of mass mortality associated with infection in the past (cf. [15]), our data suggest that its geographic expansion apparently covers the whole Palearctic niche of bat hibernation. The circumstances that influence its potential to cause morbidity and/or mortality in bats in Palearctic Russia are poorly understood; however, *P. destructans* is a significant disease-causing pathogen of hibernating bats, discovery of which warrants development of active surveillance programmes to better understand its epizootiology and to protect wildlife in general. This programme could be combined with testing for other agents of zoonotic importance, such as rabies.

Additional files

Additional file 1: Figure S1. Infection intensity, measured as fungal load in nanograms on a $\log_{10}$ scale, for particular regions. *Explanation*: mid-point = median; box = inter-quartile range; whiskers = non-outlier minimum/maximum range; dots = outliers; stars = extremes. (DOCX 21 kb)

Additional file 2: Table S1. Bat species from Palearctic and Nearctic regions with confirmed WNS or *Pseudogymnoascus destructans* infection. Summarized from [10, 16, 19, 21, 40, 47]. (XLSX 13 kb)

Additional file 3: Table S2. Datasets used and analyzed during the current study and not included in Tables 1, 2 and 3. (XLSX 31 kb)

Abbreviations

MCMC: Markov chain Monte Carlo; UV: Ultraviolet; WNS: White-nose syndrome

Acknowledgements

We would like to thank Masha Orlova Jr., Alexander Osintsev, Alexander Stashkin and Julia Kosheleva for their help with field research. We are grateful to Dr. Kevin Roche for his correction and improvement of the English text.

Funding

This research was supported by the Grant Agency of the Czech Republic (Grant No. 17-20286S) and through institutional support from the Institute of Vertebrate Biology of the Czech Academy of Sciences, v.v.i. (RVO: 68081766). The funders had no role in the study design, data analysis, and decision to publish, or preparation of the manuscript.

Authors' contributions

JP and JZ designed the study and participated in field research, with help from HB, AB, VK, NM, OO, VP, AS, MT. JP, VK and MH performed the laboratory analyses. JZ and NM analysed the data. JZ, JP and VK wrote the manuscript, with contributions from all authors. All authors read and approved the final manuscript.

Consent for publication

Not applicable.

Competing interests

The authors declare that they have no competing interests.

Author details

[1]Department of Ecology and Diseases of Game, Fish and Bees, University of Veterinary and Pharmaceutical Sciences Brno, Palackého tř. 1946/1, 612 42 Brno, Czech Republic. [2]Institute of Vertebrate Biology of the Czech Academy of Sciences, v.v.i., Květná 8, 603 65 Brno, Czech Republic. [3]Institute of Botany and Zoology, Masaryk University, Kotlářská 267/2, 611 37 Brno, Czech Republic. [4]Irkutsk State Medical University, Krasnogo Vosstania street 1, Irkutsk, Russian Federation664003. [5]Institute of Biostatistics and Analyses, Masaryk University, Kamenice 126/3, 625 00 Brno, Czech Republic. [6]International Complex Research Laboratory for Study of Climate Change, Land Use and Biodiversity, Tyumen State University, Volodarckogo 6, 625003 Tyumen, Russia. [7]Department of Biochemistry, Ural State Medical University, Repina 3, 620014 Ekaterinburg, Russia. [8]Western Baikal protected areas, Federal State Budgetary Institution "Zapovednoe Pribaikalye", Baikalskaya st. 291B, 664050 Irkutsk, Russia. [9]Institute of Biology and Soil Science, Far East Branch of the Russian Academy of Sciences, Pr-t 100-letiya Vladivostoka 159, 690022 Vladivostok, Russia.

References

1. Pikula J, Treml F, Beklová M, Holešovská Z, Pikulová J. Ecological conditions of natural foci of tularaemia in the Czech Republic. Eur J Epidemiol. 2003;18:1091–5.
2. Rosenthal J. Climate change and the geographic distribution of infectious diseases. Eco Health. 2009;6:489–95.
3. Bandouchova H, Bartonička T, Berkova H, Brichta J, Kokurewicz T, Kovacova V, Linhart P, Piacek V, Pikula J, Zahradníková A Jr, Zukal J. Alterations in the health of hibernating bats under pathogen pressure. Sci Rep. 2018;8:6067.
4. Swaminathan A, Viennet E, McMichael AJ, Harley D. Climate change and the geographical distribution of infectious diseases. In: Petersen E, Chen LH, Schlagenhauf-Lawlor P, editors. Infectious diseases: a geographic guide: John Wiley & Sons Ltd; 2017. p. 470–80.
5. Tack AJ, Thrall PH, Barrett LG, Burdon JJ, Laine A-L. Variation in infectivity and aggressiveness in space and time in wild host-pathogen systems - causes and consequences. J Evol Biol. 2012;25:1918–36.
6. Jones KE, Patel NG, Levy MA, Storeygard A, Balk D, Gittleman JL, Daszak P. Global trends in emerging infectious diseases. Nature. 2008;451:990–3.
7. Calisher CH, Childs JE, Field HE, Holmes KV, Schountz T. Bats: important reservoir hosts of emerging viruses. Clin Microbiol Rev. 2006;19:531–45.
8. Gargas A, Trest MT, Christensen M, Volk TJ, Blehert DS. *Geomyces destructans* sp. nov associated with bat white-nose syndrome. Mycotaxon. 2009;108:147–54.
9. Minnis AM, Linder DL. Phylogenetic evaluation of *Geomyces* and allies reveals no close relatives of *Pseudogymnoascus destructans*, comb nov, in bat hibernacula of eastern North America. Fungal Biol. 2013;117:638–49.
10. Blehert DS, Hicks AC, Behr M, Meteyer CU, Berlowski-Zier BM, Buckles EL, Coleman JT, Darling SR, Gargas A, Niver R, Okoniewski JC, Rudd RJ, Stone WB. Bat white-nose syndrome: an emerging fungal pathogen? Science. 2009;323:227.
11. Frick WF, Pollock JF, Hicks AC, Langwig KE, Reynolds DS, Turner GG, Butchkoski CM, Kunz TH. An emerging disease causes regional population collapse of a common north American bat species. Science. 2010;329:679–82.
12. Verant ML, Boyles JG, Waldrep W Jr, Wibbelt G, Blehert DS. Temperature-dependent growth of *Geomyces destructans*, the fungus that causes bat white-nose syndrome. PLoS One. 2012;7:e46280.
13. Marroquin CM, Lavine JO, Windstam ST. Effect of humidity on development of *Pseudogymnoascus destructans*, the causal agent of bat white-nose syndrome. Northeast Nat. 2017;24:54–64.
14. Perry RW. A review of factors affecting cave climates for hibernating bats in temperate North America. Environ Rev. 2012;21:28–39.
15. Martínková N, Bačkor P, Bartonička T, Blažková P, Červený J, Falteisek L, Gaisler J, Hanzal V, Horáček D, Hubálek Z, Jahelková H, Kolařík M, Korytár L, Kubátová A, Lehotská B, Lehotský R, Lučan RK, Májek O, Matějů J, Řehák Z, Šafář J, Tájek P, Tkadlec E, Uhrin M, Wagner J, Weinfurtová D, Zima J, Zukal J, Horáček I. Increasing incidence of *Geomyces destructans* fungus in bats from the Czech Republic and Slovakia. PLoS One. 2010;5:e13853.

16. Wibbelt G, Kurth A, Hellmann D, Weishaar M, Barlow A, Veith M, Pruger J, Gorfol T, Grosche L, Bontadina F, Zophel U, Seidl H-P, Cryan PM, Blehert DS. White-nose syndrome fungus (*Geomyces destructans*) in bats, Europe. Emerg Infect Dis. 2010;16:1237–43.

17. Puechmaille SJ, Wibbelt G, Korn V, Fuller H, Forget F, Mühldorfer K, Kurth A, Bogdanowicz W, Borel C, Bosch T, Cherezy T, Drebet M, Görföl T, Haarsma AJ, Herhaus F, Hallart G, Hammer M, Jungmann C, Le Bris Y, Lutsar L, Masing M, Mulkens B, Passior K, Starrach M, Wojtaszewski A, Zöphel U, Teeling EC. Pan-European distribution of white-nose syndrome fungus (*Geomyces destructans*) not associated with mass mortality. PLoS One. 2011;6:e19167.

18. Pikula J, Bandouchova H, Novotny L, Meteyer CU, Zukal J, Irwin NR, Zima J, Martínková N. Histopathology confirms white-nose syndrome in bats in Europe. J Wildl Dis. 2012;48:207–11.

19. Hoyt JR, Sun K, Parise KL, Lu G, Langwig KE, Jiang T, Yang S, Frick WF, Kilpatrick AM, Foster JT, Feng J. Widespread bat white-nose syndrome fungus, northeastern China. Emerg Infect Dis. 2016;22:140–2.

20. Lorch JM, Palmer JM, Lindner DL, Ballmann AE, George KG, Griffin K, Knowles S, Huckabee JR, Haman KH, Anderson CD, Becker PA, Buchanan JB, Foster JT, Blehert DS. First detection of bat white-nose syndrome in western North America. mSphere. 2016;1:e00148–16.

21. Zukal J, Banďouchová H, Brichta J, Cmokova A, Jaroň KS, Kolařík M, Kovacova V, Kubatova A, Novakova A, Orlov O, Pikula J, Presenik P, Suba J, Zahradnikova A, Martínková N. White-nose syndrome without borders: *Pseudogymnoascus destructans* infection tolerated in Europe and Palearctic Asia but not in North America. Sci Rep. 2016;6:19829.

22. Shuey MM, Drees KP, Lindner DL, Keim P, Foster JT. Highly sensitive quantitative PCR for the detection and differentiation of *Pseudogymnoascus destructans* and other Pseudogymnoascus species. App Environ Microbiol. 2014;80:1726–31.

23. Turner GG, Meteyer CU, Barton H, Gumbs JF, Reeder DA, Overton B, Bandouchova H, Bartonička T, Martínková N, Pikula J, Zukal J, Blehert DS. Nonlethal screening of bat-wing skin with the use of ultraviolet fluorescence to detect lesions indicative of white-nose syndrome. J Wildl Dis. 2014;50:566–73.

24. Bandouchova H, Bartonicka T, Berkova H, Brichta J, Cerny J, Kovacova V, Kolarik M, Kollner B, Kulich P, Martínková N, Rehak Z, Turner GG, Zukal J, Pikula J. *Pseudogymnoascus destructans*: evidence of virulent skin invasion for bats under natural conditions, Europe. Transbound Emerg Dis. 2015;62:1–5.

25. Pikula J, Amelon SK, Bandouchova H, Bartonicka T, Berkova H, Brichta J, Hooper S, Kokurewicz T, Kolarik M, Kollner B, Kovacova V, Linhart P, Piacek V, Turner GG, Zukal J, Martínková N. White-nose syndrome pathology grading in Nearctic and Palearctic bats. PLoS One. 2017;12:e018043.

26. Flieger M, Bandouchova H, Cerny J, Chudickova M, Kolarik M, Kovacova V, Martínková N, Novak P, Sebesta O, Stodulkova E, Pikula J. Vitamin B2 as a virulence factor in *Pseudogymnoascus destructans* skin infection. Sci Rep. 2016;6:33200.

27. Campana MG, Kurata NP, Foster JT, Helgen LE, Reeder DAM, Fleischer RC, Helgen KM. White-nose syndrome fungus in a 1918 bat specimen from France. Emerg Infect Dis. 2017;23:1611–2.

28. Zahradníková A Jr, Kovacova V, Orlova MV, Orlov OL, Martínková N, Piacek V, Zukal J, Pikula J. Historic and geographic surveillance of *Pseudogymnoascus destructans* possible from collections of bat parasites. Transbound Emerg Dis. 2018;65:303–8.

29. Schindelin J, Rueden CT, Hiner MC, Eliceiri KW. The ImageJ ecosystem: an open platform for biomedical image analysis. Mol Reprod Dev. 2015;82:518–29.

30. Tougard C, Delefosse T, Hanni C, Montgelard C. Phylogenetic relationships of the five extant Rhinoceros species (Rhinocerotidae, Perissodactyla) based on mitochondrial cytochrome b and 12S rRNA genes. Mol Phylogenet Evol. 2001;19:34–44.

31. Katoh K, Standley DM. MAFFT multiple sequence alignment software version 7: improvements in performance and usability. Mol Biol Evol. 2013;30:772–80.

32. Ronquist F, Teslenko M, van der Mark P, Ayres DL, Darling A, Hohna S, Larget B, Liu L, Suchard MA, Huelsenbeck JP. MrBayes 32: efficient Bayesian phylogenetic inference and model choice across a large model space. Syst Biol. 1990;61:539–42.

33. Bolshakov VN, Orlov OL, Snitko VP. Letučije myši Urala. Akadem kniga Jekatěrinburg; 2005. p. 176. (In Russian).

34. Botvinkin AD. Bats in the Lake Baikal region (biology, observation methods, protection). Irkutsk: Veter Stranstviy; 2002. p. 208. (In Russian).

35. Tiunov MP. Distribution of the bats in Russian Far East (problems and questions). In: Proceedings of the Japan-Russia Cooperation Symposium on the Conservation of the Ecosystem in Okhotsk. Published by Office of "Japan-Russia Cooperative Symposium on the Conservation of the Ecosystem in Okhotsk", Sapporo, Japan; 2011. p. 359–369.

36. Tiunov MP. Bats of Russian Far East. Vladivostok: Dalnauka; 1997. p. 134. (in Russian with English summary).

37. Pavia-Cardoso MDN, Morinha F, Barros P, Vale-Goncalves H, Coelho AC, Fernandes L, Travassos P, Faria AS, Bastos E, Santos N, Cabral JA. First isolation of *Pseudogymnoascus destructans* in bats from Portugal. Eur J Wildl Res. 2014;60:645–9.

38. Pavlinić I, Đaković M, Lojkić I. *Pseudogymnoascus destructans* in Croatia confirmed. Eur J Wildl Res. 2015;61:325–8.

39. Ransome RD. The natural history of hibernating bats. London: Christopher Helm; 1990. p. 256.

40. Zukal J, Bandouchova H, Bartonička T, Berkova H, Brack V, Brichta J, Dolinay M, Jaroň KS, Kovacova V, Kovařík M, Martínková N, Ondráček K, Řehák Z, Turner GG, Pikula J. White-nose syndrome fungus: a generalist pathogen of hibernating bats. PLoS One. 2014;9:e97224.

41. Ruf T, Geiser F. Daily torpor and hibernation in birds and mammals. Biol Rev. 2015;90:891–926.

42. Barlow AM, Worledge L, Miller H, Drees KP, Wright P, Foster JT, Sobek C, Borman AM, Fraser M. First confirmation of *Pseudogymnoascus destructans* in British bats and hibernacula. Vet Rec. 2015;177:73.

43. Meteyer CU, Buckles EL, Blehert DS, Hicks AC, Green DE, Shearn-Bochsler V, Thomas NJ, Gargas A, Behr MJ. Histopathologic criteria to confirm white-nose syndrome in bats. J Vet Diag Invest. 2009;21:411–4.

44. Davy CM Donaldson ME, Rico Y, Lausen CL, Dogantzis K, Ritchie K, Willis CKR, Burles DW, Jung TS, McBurney S, Park A, McAlpine DJ, Vanderwolf KF, Kyle CJ. Prelude to a panzootic: gene flow and immunogenetic variation in northern little brown myotis vulnerable to bat white-nose syndrome. FACETS. 2017;2:690–714.

45. Ruedi M, Stadelmann B, Gager Y, Douzery EJP, Francis CM, Lin LK, Guillén-Servent A, Cibois A. Molecular phylogenetic reconstructions identify East Asia asthe cradle for the evolution of the cosmopolitan genus *Myotis* (Mammalia, Chiroptera). Mol Phylogenet Evol. 2013;69:437–49.

46. Grieneisen LE, Brownlee-Bouboulis SA, Johnson JS, Reeder DM. Sex and hibernaculum temperature predict survivorship in white-nose syndrome affected little brown myotis (*Myotis lucifugus*). R Soc Open Sci. 2015;2:140470.

47. US Fish Wildlife Service Online [2017/11/28]. https://www.whitenosesyndrome.org/about/bats-affected-wns.

20

Parasitic pneumonia in roe deer (*Capreolus capreolus*) in Cornwall, Great Britain, caused by *Varestrongylus capreoli* (Protostrongylidae)

Victor R. Simpson[1*] and Damer P. Blake[2]

Abstract

Background: Roe deer (*Capreolus capreolus*) became extinct over large areas of Britain during the post mediaeval period but following re-introductions from Europe during the 1800s and early 1900s the population started to recover and in recent decades there has been a spectacular increase. Many roe deer are shot in Britain each year but despite this there is little published information on the diseases and causes of mortality of roe deer in Great Britain.

Case presentation: The lungs of two hunter-shot roe deer in Cornwall showed multiple, raised, nodular lesions associated with numerous protostrongylid-type nematode eggs and first stage larvae. There was a pronounced inflammatory cell response (mostly macrophages, eosinophils and multinucleate giant cells) and smooth muscle hypertrophy of the smaller bronchioles. The morphology of the larvae was consistent with that of a *Varestrongylus* species and sequencing of an internal transcribed spacer-2 fragment confirmed 100% identity with a published Norwegian *Varestrongylus* cf. *capreoli* sequence. To the best of the authors' knowledge this is the first confirmed record of *V. capreoli* in Great Britain. Co-infection with an adult protostrongylid, identified by DNA sequencing as *Varestrongylus sagittatus*, was also demonstrated in one case.

Conclusions: Parasitic pneumonia is regarded as a common cause of mortality in roe deer and is typically attributed to infection with *Dictyocaulus* sp. This study has shown that *Varestrongylus capreoli* also has the capability to cause significant lung pathology in roe deer and heavy infection could be of clinical significance.

Keywords: Roe deer, *Capreolus*, *Varestrongylus*, Pneumonia, Protostrongylid

Background

Roe deer (*Capreolus capreolus*) and European red deer (*Cervus elaphus elaphus*) are the only species of deer native to the British Isles. Although historically widespread, roe deer became extinct over large areas of Britain during the post mediaeval period, particularly in Wales and the English Midlands [1, 2]. However, following re-introductions from France, Germany, Austria and Siberia during the 1800s and early 1900s [1, 3] roe deer populations in Britain started to recover and it is now believed that all roe deer in southern England are derived from animals introduced from Europe [2]. In recent decades there has been a spectacular increase in the British roe deer population [4] and, with the rate of range expansion recently estimated at 2.3%, per annum, this is expected to expand further for the foreseeable future [5]. The factors that are driving this and other deer population trends in Britain are poorly understood and there is a need for an evidence-based understanding of the mechanisms involved [6]. Increased roe deer density has previously been implicated in the enhanced spread of pathogens such as *Mycobacterium bovis* [7] and might increase the risk of chronic wasting disease (CWD) transmission should it reach the UK [8]. When combined with climate changes which may support larger mollusc populations [9], and a concomitant enhanced

* Correspondence: vic@wildlifevic.org
[1]Wildlife Veterinary Investigation Centre, Chacewater, Truro, Cornwall TR4 8PB, UK
Full list of author information is available at the end of the article

risk of transmission of mollusc-vectored pathogens, there is a greater risk that parasites such as *Varestrongylus capreoli* will become established in the UK. Many roe deer are shot in Britain each year for human consumption and also to limit the damage they do to commercial woodland [10]. Despite this, there is little published information on the diseases and causes of mortality of roe deer in this country.

Case presentation

Samples and sample preparation

The lungs and, in one case the majority of the lung lobes, from two adult male roe deer were submitted to the Wildlife Veterinary Investigation Centre by hunters in April 2015 and April 2017 following the observation of gross abnormalities for the purpose of food safety. Both deer were shot by licenced marksmen as part of estate management strategies at locations denoted by National Grid Reference numbers SX08 64 and SW84 45, respectively. One animal (case #1) had been shot because it was lame, having suffered a recent amputation of the left forelimb distal to the carpus; despite this injury it was in quite good physical condition. The second animal (case #2) was shot for human consumption and was judged to be in good body condition. The lungs in each case were subjected to gross examination and showed multiple swellings in the parenchyma. In order to check for the possible presence of parasite eggs or larvae impression smears from the cut surface of the swellings were made on to microscope slides; a small amount of normal saline was added, a coverslip applied and the specimen examined by direct light microscopy. Duplicate impression smears were mounted in dilute Lactophenol Cotton Blue to clear and stain the characteristic features of any parasitic forms present. In case #1 only an additional smear was air-dried, heat-fixed and stained by Ziehl-Neelson in order to check for the presence of acid-fast organisms such as *Mycobacterium* sp.. Larvae and parasite appendages were measured using an eye-piece micrometer calibrated against a stage micrometer. Representative sections through several parenchymal swellings of both sets of lungs were placed in 10% neutral buffered formalin, dehydrated through graded alcohols, embedded in paraffin wax, sectioned at 5 μm and stained by haematoxylin and eosin (H&E) and periodic acid-Schiff (PAS). Additionally, lungs from case #2 were examined by fine blunt dissection for the presence of adult nematodes. Fragments of dissected lung were pooled, placed in a glass beaker with 2 L of tap water, thoroughly agitated, left to settle and then the sediment examined for parasites or fragments.

Gross pathology

The lungs in case #1 showed multiple tan-coloured, nodular, roughly 2–5 cm diameter swellings located mostly along the margins of the lobes. They were clearly demarcated from the lung parenchyma, had a firm, uniform consistency and frequent small ecchymotic haemorrhages. Also present in the parenchyma were localised areas of atelectasis and haemorrhage (Fig. 1). There was a small number of adult *Dictyocaulus* sp. nematodes present in the bronchi and larger bronchioles. The nodular lung lesions in case #2 were very similar to those in the first case but were often surrounded by a zone of parenchyma that was much paler than elsewhere in the lung.

Bacteriology

No acid-fast organisms were seen in a Ziehl-Neelsen stained, air-dried and heat-fixed impression smear from the cut surface of a lung nodule in case #1.

Histopathology

The nodular lesions in both cases showed dense consolidation with very large numbers of nematode eggs present in various stages of development together with numerous larvae in the bronchioles and the alveolar lumena. Associated with this was a large number of inflammatory cells, mostly macrophages, eosinophils and multinucleate giant cells, and fibrosis of alveolar walls (Fig. 2). The smaller bronchioles showed pronounced smooth muscle hypertrophy and were surrounded by a thick layer of lymphocytes (Fig. 3). No adult nematodes were seen in the nodules or in unaffected lung parenchyma.

Parasitology

There were moderate numbers of adult *Dictyocaulus* sp. in the bronchi and bronchioles of case #1 but none were seen in case #2.

In both cases microscopic examination of wet impression smears from the cut surface of the nodules revealed numerous first stage nematode larvae and embryonated eggs. The larvae had a dorsal spike at the base of the tail

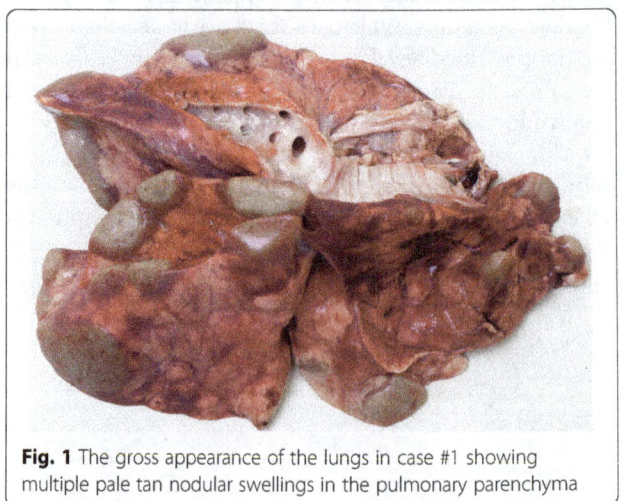

Fig. 1 The gross appearance of the lungs in case #1 showing multiple pale tan nodular swellings in the pulmonary parenchyma

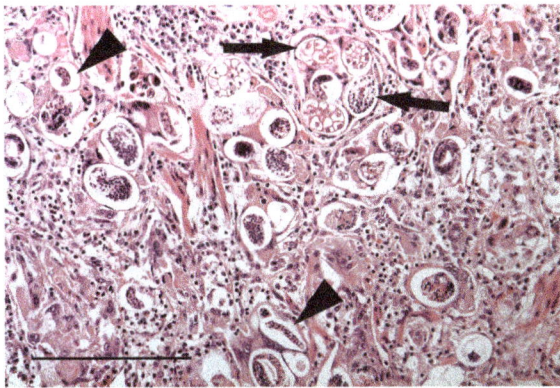

Fig. 2 Histological section through a nodular swelling in the lungs of case #1. Note the eggs in various stages of development (arrows) and first stage larvae (arrow heads) H&E stain. Bar =200 μm

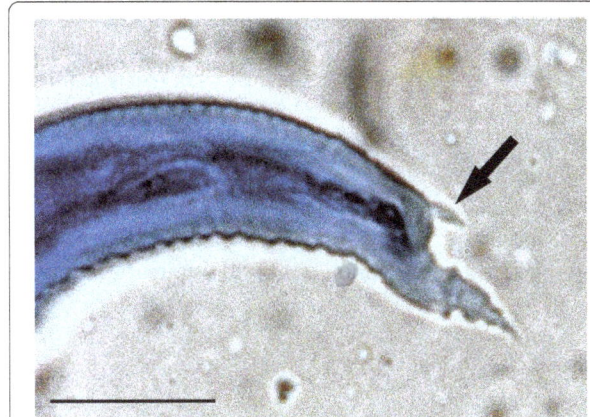

Fig. 4 High power view of the tail appendage with cuticular ridges and the dorsal spine (arrow) of a first stage larva in an impression smear from a lung nodule in case #2. Lactophenol Cotton Blue stain. Bar =25 μm

appendage and the appendage itself had well-developed cuticular folds (Fig. 4). The larvae in case #2 were measured and the mean dimensions ($n = 10$) were length 294.4 μm (standard error 3.3) and width 18.8 μm (0.7).

Blunt dissection of lung parenchyma was carried out in case #2 only. Examination of the sediment after washing the pooled fragments of lung tissue revealed a single male nematode measuring approximately 5 mm in length. It had well developed bursae with radiating rays that did not extend fully to the margins. The spicules were tubular, equal, symmetrical and yellowish brown and measured 258.5 μm (Fig. 5).

Molecular biology

Total genomic DNA was extracted from (i) pooled L1 larvae recovered from an additional unfixed impression smear sample from case #2 only and (ii) a single adult male preserved in 70% (v/v) ethanol, using a Qiagen DNeasy Blood and Tissue kit following the animal tissues spin column protocol as described by the manufacturer

(Qiagen, Hilden, Germany). A fragment of the internal transcribed spacer (ITS)-2 sequence within the nuclear ribosomal DNA was amplified in duplicate and sequenced from each sample using the generic pan-nematode primers NC1 (5′-ACGTCTGGTTCAGGGTTGTT-3′) and NC2 (5′-TTAGTTTCTTTTCCTCCGCT-3′) [11] to confirm parasite identity. Briefly, each PCR reaction contained 3 μl template DNA, 1.5 μl of each of the relevant forward and reverse primers (10 μM stock; Sigma-Aldrich, Poole, UK) and 20.0 μl of MyTaq × 2 mastermix (Bioline, London, UK), made up to a final volume of 40 μl with molecular grade water (Sigma). Molecular grade water was used as a no template negative control. Thermal cycler parameters were: 1 x initial denaturation at 95 °C for 2 min, followed by 35 x (denaturation 30 s at 95 °C, annealing 30 s at 52 °C, extension 30 s at 72 °C), followed by a final extension phase of 72 °C for 7 min. PCR amplicons were resolved by agarose gel electrophoresis using a 1% (w/v)

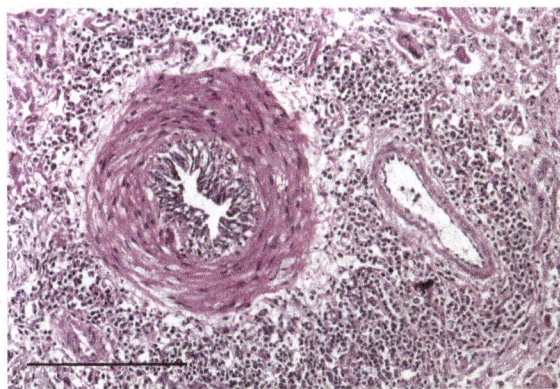

Fig. 3 Histological section through the lung of case #1 showing severe smooth muscle hypertrophy of a small bronchiole and a surrounding rim of lymphocytes. PAS stain. Bar =200 μm

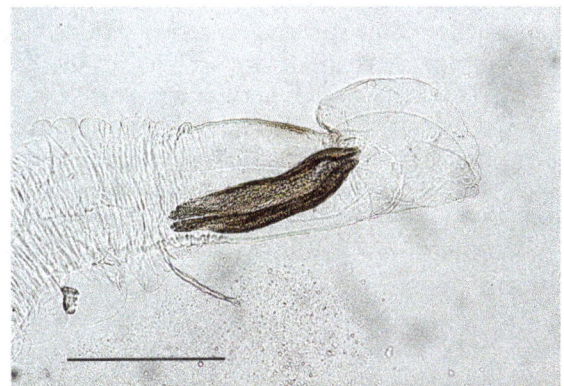

Fig. 5 Caudal end of the male protostrongylid recovered following blunt dissection of lung in case #2. The spicules are tubular, equal size and symmetrical and the bursal rays do not extend fully to the margins. Unstained. Bar =200 μm

UltraPure agarose gel in 1× Tris-borate-EDTA buffer (TBE; all Sigma), including 0.01% (v/v) SafeView nucleic acid stain (NBS Biologicals). The results of electrophoresis were visualised using a U:Genius Gel Documentation System(Syngene). PCR amplicons were purified using a PCR purification kit (Qiagen) and sequenced on both strands using the same primers employed in their original amplification (GATC Biotech, Konstanz, Germany). Sequence assembly, annotation, and interrogation were undertaken with CLC Main Workbench v6.0.2 (CLC Bio, Aarhus, Denmark) using BLASTn against the GenBank non-redundant database to assign identity.

Following these methods partial ITS-2 sequences were derived from L1 larvae and the single adult male worm. In total 449 bp high quality sequence was produced in duplicate from the L1 larvae, with 100% sequence similarity between duplicates (available under accession number LT962658). Comparison with the GenBank non-redundant nucleotide database identified the highest sequence similarity with V. cf. capreoli (accession number KJ452176.1; 100% coverage, 100% identity). Separately, 480 bp sequence was produced in duplicate from the adult male worm (LT962657), with greatest similarity to Varestrongylus sagittatus (KJ439592.1; 100% coverage, 100% identity). Comparison with published V. sagittatus ITS-2 sequences KJ439592–4 and KJ439596–7, revealed 15 copies of the degenerate TCG/CCG triplet repeat, which may provide future value as a genetic marker.

Discussion

The protostrongylid nematode Varestrongylus capreoli is a recognised cause of lung lesions in roe deer in Europe [12–15]. However, prior to the present study it does not appear to have been recorded in roe deer in the British Isles. A histopathological study of roe deer lungs in Scotland described infection with an unidentified protostrongylid nematode but as examination was confined to histopathology no description of the parasite other than the appearance of the eggs and larvae was provided [16]. The paper does not include a description of the gross pathology of the lungs so it is not apparent whether or not there were nodular lesions similar to those seen in the present study. However, the histopathological findings closely resembled those seen in the present Cornish cases with larvae and eggs filling alveolar lumena accompanied by eosinophils, giant cells, alveolar macrophages and some neutrophils, supporting association of the inflammatory response observed with the parasite infection. As in the present study, severe muscular hypertrophy of the smaller bronchiolar walls was a prominent feature [16].

A notable feature in both studies is the absence of adult nematodes in the histological sections. However, adults have been recorded in both alveoli and bronchioles of roe deer elsewhere in Europe [14]. A possible explanation for their absence in some instances is that they may survive for only a short while after egg laying and are phagocytosed. A similar situation exists with Capillaria hepatica infection where eggs often remain in the hepatic parenchyma after the adults have died and been resorbed (Simpson, unpublished data). However, adults of V. sagittatus remain viable for several years [17] and it seems unlikely that V. capreoli would be markedly different from this closely related species. Both deer in the present study were killed in April and showed evidence of active infection with eggs and larvae in varying stages of development. The seasonality of infection for V capreoli does not appear to have been documented but V. sagittatus infection of maral deer (Cervus elaphus maral) peaks during winter and spring [17]; this could possibly be in relation to a period when either the molluscs which act as intermediate hosts become most active or when ingestion of infective larvae is most common. It has been postulated that parasites could infect deer during feeding on dry grass and short shrubs covered by snow in which hibernating snails occur [12, 14]. Also, the presence of immature forms in the lungs could represent a latent phase of infection [12, 14].

The gross appearance of the nodular lung lesions in the present study bore a superficial resemblance to lung lesions due to tuberculosis in roe deer in Spain and Italy [7]. The lesions in those cases included foci in the pulmonary parenchyma that were occasionally calcified and surrounded by a thin layer of epithelioid and multinucleated giant cells. Although no such lesions were seen in the roe deer infected with Varestrongylus sp. it does illustrate the need to examine lung lesions in roe deer for evidence of infection by mycobacteria.

Many conservationists may welcome the re-establishment of a former native species after it had become extinct or extremely rare. However, the recent recolonization of England by roe deer has been dramatic and shows no sign of reducing. This raises concern about an increased risk of disease transmission, such as tuberculosis, due to animals living at a higher population density [7]. In addition there is growing concern that climate change is likely to influence the geographic distribution of diseases such as bluetongue and Lyme disease [6]. There is a need to be aware of these factors from both a conservation viewpoint and also from a zoonotic perspective.

Identification of protostrongylid larvae by morphological features is not generally possible. The first stage larvae of species of the subfamilies Muelleriinae, Elaphostrongylinae and Varestrongylinae all have a dorsal spine and they also have a similar tail appendix [18]. However, the larvae of the various species have a recognised size range and this can assist in identification. In the present study the mean length of the larvae was 294.4 μm and this was within the recorded range of 285–341 μm for Varestrongylus capreoli

[17], although larvae for other *Varestrongylus* spp. fall within the same or similar ranges [15]. Identification was confirmed by sequencing of the ITS-2, which gave a 100% match to a published Norwegian *Varestrongylus* cf. *capreoli* sequence.

The adult male protostrongylid recovered after blunt dissection of the lung was identified by DNA sequencing as *Varestrongylus sagittatus*. This is known to be a common lungworm of European red, maral and fallow (*Dama dama*) deer in Europe and Asia where it produces small nodules in the lungs, similar to those caused by *Muellerius capillaris* in sheep and goats [19]. *Varestrongylus sagittatus*, described using the synonym *Bicaulus sagittatus*, has also been recorded in Britain where it was found in a roe deer buck shot in the New Forest [20]. No morphological or other data was provided to confirm the identification. *Varestrongylus sagittatus* is one of a group of seven *Varestrongylus* species which are characterised by having spicules greater than 200 μm. However, although they measured 258.5 μm in the roe deer specimen in this study, this is significantly shorter than the range normally quoted for *V. sagittatus* (325–433.8 μm) [15]. The total length of the nematode at around 5 mm is also much less than the accepted range for an adult male *V. sagittatus* (14.5–33.8 mm, as well as for a number of other species such as *V. alpenae* (13–15 mm), *V. alces* (11.36–14.7 mm) and *V capricola* (15–18 mm) [15]. A possible explanation for the small size of *V. sagittatus* in this study is that this is typically a parasite of red or fallow deer, not roe deer, and its development may have been restricted in an atypical host.

Conclusions

Verminous pneumonia due to infection with *Dictyocaulus* sp. is considered to be an important cause of mortality in roe deer in Britain [2, 21] and in some areas has been considered to act as the main factor controlling populations [21]. This study has shown that *Varestrongylus capreoli* also has the capability to cause significant lung pathology in roe deer. There is clearly a need to consider the possible involvement of this parasite when investigating lung disease in roe deer, especially as mixed infections with the more obvious *Dictyocaulus* parasite may occur resulting in under diagnosis of *V. capreoli*.

Acknowledgements
The authors wish to thank Adrian Cross and Jeremy Preston for submitting the specimens and Abbey Veterinary Services for histopathological processing and advice. They also express their thanks to Professor Mark Fox from the Royal Veterinary College and Dr. Mark Dagleish from Moredun Research Institute for helpful discussion.

Funding
The study was funded by the Wildlife Veterinary Investigation Centre and the Royal Veterinary College. No external sources of funding were available. This manuscript has been assigned the reference PPS_01724 by the Royal Veterinary College. The funding bodies played no role in the design of the study, the collection, analysis and interpretation of data, or in writing the manuscript.

Authors' contributions
VS performed the gross and histopathological examinations, coordinated the study and drafted the preliminary manuscript. DB carried out the molecular genetic studies. Both authors contributed to writing the draft manuscript and read and approved the final manuscript.

Consent for publication
Not applicable.

Competing interests
The authors declare that they have no competing interests.

Author details
[1]Wildlife Veterinary Investigation Centre, Chacewater, Truro, Cornwall TR4 8PB, UK. [2]Pathobiology and Population Sciences, Royal Veterinary College, Hawkshead Lane, North Mymms, Hertfordshire AL9 7TA, UK.

References
1. Prior R. The roe deer: conservation of a native species. London: Oxford University Press; 1995.
2. Hewison AJM and Staines BW. European roe deer (Capreolus capreolus). In: Harris S, Yalden DW, editors. Mammals of the British isles: handbook, 4th edition. The Mammal Society, Southampton. 2008. p 605–617.
3. Prior R. The roe deer of Cranborne chase. An ecological survey. London: Oxford University Press; 1968.
4. Aebischer NJ, Davey PD & Kingdon NG. National Gamebag Census: Mammal Trends to 2009. Game & Wildlife Conservation Trust, Fordingbridge. 2011. (http://www.gwct.org.uk/ngcmammals). Accessed 22 Dec 2017.
5. Ward AI. Expanding ranges of wild and feral deer in great Britain. Mammal Rev. 2005;35:165–73.
6. Newman C & Macdonald D W. Biodiversity Climate change impacts report card Technical paper 2015 https://nerc.ukri.org/research/partnerships/ride/lwec/report-cards/biodiversity-source02/. Accessed 15 Apr 2018.
7. Balseiro A, Oleaga A, Orusa R, Robetto S, Zoppi S, Dondo A, Goria M, Gortázar C, Marín JF, Domenis L. Tuberculosis in roe deer from Spain and Italy. Vet Rec. 2009;164:468–70.
8. Storm DJ, Samuel MD, Rolley RE, Shelton P, Keuler NS, Richards BJ, Van Deelen TR. Deer density and disease prevalence influence transmission of chronic wasting disease in white-tailed deer. Ecosphere. 2013;4:10.
9. Sternberg M. Terrestrial gastropods and experimental climate change: a field study in a calcareous grassland. Ecol Res. 2000;15:73–81.
10. Fuller RJ, Gill RMA. Ecological impacts of increasing numbers of deer in British woodland. In: Fuller RJ, RMA G, editors. Special Issue, Forestry, vol. 74; 2001. p. 193–9.
11. Gasser RB, Chilton NB, Hoste H, Beveridge I. Rapid sequencing of rDNA from single worms and eggs of parasitic helminths. Nucleic Acids Res. 1993;21: 2525–6.
12. Aguirre AA, Bröjer C, Mörner T. Descriptive epidemiology of roe deer mortality in Sweden. J Wildlife Dis. 1999;35:753–62.
13. Dacal V, Vázquez L, Javier Pato F, Cienfuegos S, Panadero R, López C, Diez-Baños P, Morrondo P. Cambios de la capacidad pulmonar en corzos (Capreolus capreolus) del noroeste de España infectados por nematodos broncopulmonares. Galemys. 2010;22(n° especial):233–42.
14. Švarc R, Pajerský A. Pathomorphological changes of roe deer lungs in the ontogeny of Varestrongylus capreoli (Stroh et Schmid 1938) Docherty, 1945. Folia Parasitol. 1990;32:315–21.
15. Verocai GC, Kutz SJ, Simard M, Hoberg EP. Varestrongylus eleguneniensis sp. n. (Nematoda: Protostrongylidae): a widespread, multi-host lungworm of wild north American ungulates, with an emended diagnosis for the genus and explorations of biogeography. Parasit Vectors. 2014; https://doi.org/10.1186/s13071-014-0556-9.
16. Munro R, Hunter AR. Histopathological findings in the lungs of Scottish red and roe deer. Vet Rec. 1983;112:194–7.
17. Anderson RC. Nematode Parasites of Vertebrates, Their Development and Transmission. 2nd ed. Wallingford: CABI Publishing; 2000.

18. Kafle P, Lejeune M, Verocai GG, Hoberg EP, Kutz SJ. Morphological and morphometric differentiation of dorsal-spined first stage larvae of lungworms (Nematoda: Protostrongylidae) infecting muskoxen (*Ovibos moschatus*) in the Central Canadian Arctic. IJP-PAW. 2015;4:283–90.

19. Mason P. *Elaphostrongylus cervi* and its close relatives; a review of protostrongylids (Nematoda, Metastrongyloidea) with spiny-tailed larvae. Surveillance. 1995;22:19–24.

20. McDiarmid A. Appendix I. Some Parasites and Diseases of Roe Deer with Particular Reference to the Cranborne Chase Population. In: Prior R, editor. The Roe deer of Cranborne Chase. An Ecological Survey. London: Oxford University Press; 1968. p. 183–209.

21. McDiarmid A. Some disorders of wild deer in the United Kingdom. Vet Rec. 1975;97:6–9.

Pathogenic variability among *Pasteurella multocida* type A isolates from Brazilian pig farms

João Xavier de Oliveira Filho[1], Marcos Antônio Zanella Morés[2], Raquel Rebellato[2], Jalusa Deon Kich[2*], Maurício Egidio Cantão[2], Catia Silene Klein[2], Roberto Maurício Carvalho Guedes[3], Arlei Coldebella[2], David Emílio Santos Neves de Barcellos[1] and Nelson Morés[2]

Abstract

Background: *Pasteurella multocida* type A (PmA) is considered a secondary agent of pneumonia in pigs. The role of PmA as a primary pathogen was investigated by challenging pigs with eight field strains isolated from pneumonia and serositis in six Brazilian states. Eight groups of eight pigs each were intranasally inoculated with different strains of PmA (1.5 mL/nostril of 10e7 CFU/mL). The control group ($n = 12$) received sterile PBS. The pigs were euthanized by electrocution and necropsied by 5 dpi. Macroscopic lesions were recorded, and swabs and fragments of thoracic and abdominal organs were analyzed by bacteriological and pathological assays. The PmA strains were analyzed for four virulence genes (*toxA*: toxin; *pfhA*: adhesion; *tbpA* and *hgbB*: iron acquisition) by PCR and sequencing and submitted to multilocus sequence typing (MLST).

Results: The eight PmA strains were classified as follows: five as highly pathogenic (HP) for causing necrotic bronchopneumonia and diffuse fibrinous pleuritis and pericarditis; one as low pathogenic for causing only focal bronchopneumonia; and two as nonpathogenic because they did not cause injury to any pig. PCR for the gene *pfhA* was positive for all five HP isolates. Sequencing demonstrated that the *pfhA* region of the HP strains comprised four genes: *tpsB1*, *pfhA1*, *tpsB2* and *pfhA2*. The low and nonpathogenic strains did not contain the genes *tpsB2* and *pfhA2*. A deletion of four bases was observed in the *pfhA* gene in the low pathogenic strain, and an insertion of 37 kb of phage DNA was observed in the nonpathogenic strains. MLST clustered the HP isolates in one group and the low and nonpathogenic isolates in another. Only the nonpathogenic isolates matched sequence type 10; the other isolates did not match any type available in the MLST database.

Conclusions: The hypothesis that some PmA strains are primary pathogens and cause disease in pigs without any co-factor was confirmed. The *pfhA* region, comprising the genes *tpsB1*, *tpsB2*, *pfhA1* and *pfhA2*, is related to the pathogenicity of PmA. The HP strains can cause necrotic bronchopneumonia, fibrinous pleuritis and pericarditis in pigs and can be identified by PCR amplification of the gene *pfhA2*.

Keywords: Respiratory diseases, Pigs, Bronchopneumonia, Polyserositis, *pfhA*, MLST

* Correspondence: jalusa.kich@embrapa.br
[2]Embrapa Suinos e Aves, P.O. Box 121, Concórdia, Santa Catarina 89700-000, Brazil
Full list of author information is available at the end of the article

Background

Pasteurella multocida capsular type A (*P. multocida* type A) is one of the most common agents associated with bronchopneumonia in pigs [1]. *P. multocida* type A is usually considered a secondary agent of enzootic pneumonia originally caused by *Mycoplasma hyopneumoniae* (*M. hyopneumoniae*) infection [2, 3]. A few studies have reproduced pneumonia, septicemia or pleurisy in pigs by intranasal or intratracheal challenge, commonly with repeated doses of *P. multocida* [3–5]. According to Ross [6], the difficulty of reproducing the disease in the absence of infectious or noninfectious cofactors is a major limitation to demonstrating the primary role of *P. multocida* type A in pneumonic lesions in pigs. However, our group has successfully developed a model to reproduce the disease in pigs inoculated with a field strain of *P. multocida* type A [7]. This model is useful for studying the pathogenicity of other *P. multocida* type A isolates in the specific pig host.

In this context, Pors et al. [8] previously explored the genetic diversity among isolates of *P. multocida* and its association with pathogenicity. Genetic diversity can be assessed using various DNA-based methods. For *P. multocida* studies, Subaaharan et al. [9] proposed multi-locus sequence typing (MLST). The *toxA, tbpA, pfhA* and capsule biosynthesis genes have been suggested as epidemiological markers of virulence-associated genes (VAGs) in *P. multocida* field strains [10], and therefore, multiplex PCR for the *toxA, tbpA, hgbB* and *pfhA* genes was designed for rapid virulence typing [11]. Thus, the objective of the present study was to investigate the capacity of eight *P. multocida* type A field strains to cause disease in healthy pigs.

The *P. multocida* type A strains were screened by PCR for four virulence genes: *toxA*, a protein Gln-deamidating toxin gene; *pfhA*, a filamentous hemagglutinin gene involved in adhesion; and *tbpA* and *hgbB*, transferrin-binding protein and hemoglobin-binding protein genes involved in

iron acquisition. These genes were further analyzed by sequencing, and the strains were compared by MLST of seven housekeeping genes (*adk, aroA, deoD, gdhA, g6pD, mdh,* and *pgi*).

Methods

Animals

Seventy-six 120-day-old pigs each weighing 74 kg were used in this study. The animals were derived from a herd with high health status raised at the facilities of the Embrapa Swine and Poultry Research Center. This herd was populated with caesarean-derived colostrum-deprived animals in 2009. Every six months, the pigs are screened for the pathogens described in Table 1, and this procedure was repeated four days before inoculation. Furthermore, respiratory diseases such as enzootic pneumonia, influenza, polyserositis (Glässer disease), atrophic rhinitis, pleuropneumonia and pasteurellosis have never been diagnosed in the herd. The herd is protected by strict biosecurity guidelines and has health barriers that include closed rooms with positive pressure and visitor restriction.

Animal housing

Four days before inoculation, all animals were transferred from the farm to an isolation unit (biosafety level 2). The animals in each group were housed in different rooms (two pigs per pen) with feed and water provided ad libitum. Access to the animals was restricted to the staff. The internal room temperature was monitored daily.

Strains

Eight strains of *P. multocida* capsular type A from the microorganism collection of the Embrapa Swine and Poultry Research Center were used and are described in Table 2. These strains were isolated from five- to six-month-old pigs with respiratory diseases raised in different herds and were stored in brain-heart infusion

Table 1 Semiannual monitoring of pigs from the high-health-status herd: pathogens and laboratory assays

Microorganisms	Samples	Laboratory tests	References
Mycoplasma hyopneumoniae	Tonsillar swabs	Nested PCR	Yamaguti et al. (2008) [43]
	Serum	ELISA	Herdcheck® *M hyo* ELISA – IDEXX
Actinobacillus pleuropneumoniae	Tonsillar and nostril swabs	Bacterial isolation	Quinn et al. (2011) [12]
	Tonsillar swabs	PCR	Souza et al. (2008) [44]
	Serum	ELISA	APP - ApxIV Ab Test - IDEXX
Haemophilus parasuis	Tonsillar and nostril swabs	Bacterial isolation	Quinn et al. (2011) [12]
	Tonsillar swabs	PCR	Redondo et al. (2003) [45]
Pasteurella multocida	Tonsillar and nostril swabs	Bacterial isolation	Quinn et al. (2011) [12]
	Tonsillar swabs	PCR	Townsend et al. (2001) [15]
PRRS virus	Serum	ELISA	Herdcheck® X3 PRRS ELISA – IDEXX
Influenza virus[a]	Serum	ELISA	AI Multi-Screen Ab test® - IDEXX

[a]Basal levels of circulating antibodies were detected by ELISA. However, genetic material was never detected by RT-PCR

Table 2 *Pasteurella multocida* type A isolates used to challenge the pig groups

Strain BRMSA	Group	Brazil State	Brazil Region	Herd production system	Gross lesion
0496	1	Rio Grande do Sul	South	Farrow to finish	Bronchopneumonia
1196	2	Rio Grande do Sul	South	Farrow to finish	Bronchopneumonia
1113	3	Minas Gerais	Southeast	Finisher	Fibrinous pleuritis
1197	4	Rio Grande do Sul	South	Finisher	Bronchopneumonia
1198	5	Santa Catarina	South	Finisher	Bronchopneumonia
1199	6	Paraná	South	Finisher	Necrosuppurative pleuropneumonia
1200	7	Goiás	Midwest	Finisher	Bronchopneumonia
1201	8	Mato Grosso	Midwest	Finisher	Bronchopneumonia

broth (BHI; OXOID LTD, Basingstoke, Hampshire, England) with sheep blood (1:1) at − 70 °C until use.

The strains were phenotypically and genotypically confirmed as *P. multocida* type A. The phenotypic characterization was performed according to Quinn et al. [12], and capsular typing was based on acriflavine [13] and hyaluronidase [14] tests. Additionally, all isolates were submitted to species-specific (*kmt*1 gene) multiplex PCR [15] and to capsular typing A (*hya*D-*hya*C) and D (*dcb*F), as described in Table 3.

Inoculum

The recovery of *P. multocida* type A from the stock was performed by culture on blood agar plates (Blood Agar Base, BD Difco™, 5% sheep's blood) incubated at 37 °C for 18–24 h. A subculture on trypticase soy agar (TSA) plates (Difco™) was incubated at 37 °C for 18–24 h. For challenge, bacterial cultures from the third passage were used. The inoculum was prepared with sterile phosphate-buffered saline (PBS) containing 10e7 colony-forming units (CFU)/mL. Serial dilutions and subsequent counting on TSA plates confirmed the inoculum concentration.

Study design

Eight groups (G1–G8) of eight pigs each were challenged with different strains of *P. multocida* type A. The pigs in the challenged groups (G1-G8) received 3.0 mL (1.5 mL/nostril) of the respective inoculum by slow intranasal

Table 3 Target gene information and primers used for *Pasteurella multocida* type A identification and detection of virulence factors

Gene	Function	Location Gene	N°. Acc.	Primers	DNA-sequences of oligonucleotide primers (5′ – 3′)	Product Size (bp)	Reference
KMT1	Species-specific	213–232	AF016259	KMT1 F	ATCCGCTATTTACCCAGTGG	460	Townsend et al. (2001) [15]
		669–649		KMT1 R	GCTGTAAACGAACTCGCCAC		
hyaD-hyaC	Capsular synthesis	8846–8863	AF067175	CAPA F	TGCCAAAATCGCAGTCAG	1.044	
		9890–9873		CAPA R	TTGCCATCATTGTCAGTG		
dcbF	Capsular synthesis	3142–3165	AF302465.	CAPD F	TTACAAAAGAAAGACTAGG AGCCC	657	
		3789–3766		CAPD R	CATCTACCCACTCAACCAT ATCAG		
fcbD	Capsular synthesis	2881–2896	AF302467	CAPF F	AATCGGAGAACGCAGAAATCAG	851	
		3733–3714		CAPF R	TTCCGCCGTCAATTACTCTG		
pfhA	Adherence	2409–2427	AY035342	PfhA F	AGCTGATCAAGTGGTGAAC	275	Ewers et al. (2006) [10]
		2684–2665		PfhA R	TGGTACATTGGTGAATGGT		
tbpA	Iron acquisition	68–85	Pm0337	TbPA F	TTTG GTT GGA AAC GGT AAA GC	728	Ewers et al. (2006) [10] Modified by Atashpaz et al. (2009) [11]
		487–470		TbPA R	TAA CGT GTA CGG AAA AGC CCC		
hgbB	Iron acquisition	308–328	Pm0337	HgbB F	TCA TTG AGT ACG GCT TGA C	499	Atashpaz et al. (2009) [11]
		1096–1077		HgbB R	CTT ACG TCA GTA ACA CTC G		
toxA	Toxin	1878–1897	AF240778	ToxA F	TTCT TAG ATG AGC GAC AAG G	846	Lichtensteiger et al. (1996) [46] modified by Atashpaz et al. (2009) [11]
		2743–2725		ToxA R	GAA TGC CAC ACC TCT ATA G		

dripping in a sitting position. Animals ($n = 12$) in the control group (G0) received 3.0 mL of sterile PBS (1.5 mL/nostril). Each group was housed in a distinct room.

All 76 pigs were clinically evaluated twice a day (0800–0900 h and 1600–1700 h), starting on the 3rd day before the inoculation and continuing until the fifth day post inoculation (5 dpi). The parameters evaluated were rectal body temperature, dyspnea (with animals lying down) and cough (after five minutes of animal movement during feeding and barn cleaning).

Necropsy

Pigs were euthanized by electrocution, bled and necropsied at 5 dpi. Animals with severe clinical signs were euthanized immediately because of concerns about animal welfare. The lesion features, distribution and severity were recorded at necropsy. The percentage of lung tissue with macroscopic lesions of pneumonia in each lobe was multiplied by each lobe's relative weight [16]. Pleuritis was classified according to the total affected area using the following scores: 1 (1–25%), 2 (26–50%), 3 (51–75%) and 4 (76–100%). Fragments of the lung, trachea, mediastinal lymph node, heart, pericardial sac, liver, kidney and spleen were preserved in 10% buffered formaldehyde for histopathology and immunohistochemistry. Fragments of the same organs and fibrinous exudates of the pleura, pericardium, peritoneum and joints, whenever present, were collected aseptically and transported to the laboratory at 2–8 °C for bacteriological examination.

Histopathology and immunohistochemistry (IHC)

Histopathological assays were performed using routine procedures for hematoxylin and eosin staining. Representative slides of each type of lesion were submitted to *P. multocida* type A detection by IHC assay based on the streptavidin-biotin-peroxidase method (LSAB™ System-HRP kit; Dako Cytomation™) and a hyperimmune polyclonal antibody (anti-*P. multocida* type A) produced in sheep. Briefly, tissue fragments with a thickness of 3–5 µm were fixed on poly-L-lysine-treated slides, dewaxed and hydrated. Next, the tissues on the slides were subjected to the following steps: antigen retrieval from tissues by microwave irradiation for 5 min at 700 W, followed by enzymatic digestion with 0.04% pepsin (pH 7.8) for 10 min at 37 °C; blocking of endogenous peroxidase with H_2O_2; incubation of the sections with anti-*P. multocida* type A primary sheep polyclonal antibody at a dilution of 1:500 for 2 h at 37 °C; incubation with reagents from an LSAB® HRP Kit (Dako Cytomation®) for 30 min at 37 °C; use of 3-amino-9-ethylcarbazole (AEC) for 5 min at 37 °C; and counterstaining with Mayer's hematoxylin for 1 min. PBS (pH 7.4) was used for washes between each step.

A lung fragment from a pig previously inoculated with *P. multocida* type A was used as a positive control. A healthy lung fragment was used as a negative control. The results are expressed according to the intensity of the reaction in the lesion, as follows: (−) absence of immunostaining for *P. multocida* type A; (+) mild focal or multifocal areas of staining (up to 25% of the lesion); (++) moderate focal or multifocal areas of staining (26% to 75% of the lesion); and (+++) marked diffuse staining (greater than 75% of the lesion) [17].

To verify the absence of other primary respiratory pathogens, after challenge and necropsy, IHC of porcine circovirus type 2 (PCV2) [18], influenza virus [19] and *M. hyopneumoniae* was performed in all lung samples [7]. The PCV2 test was also performed in mediastinal lymph nodes.

Pasteurella multocida recovery

Samples were plated immediately after collection on blood agar and MacConkey agar (Difco™) and incubated at 37 °C for 24–48 h under aerobic conditions. A streak of *Staphylococcus aureus* was added to an additional plate and incubated microaerophilically at 37 °C for 24–48 h. The biochemical characterization of the isolates was conducted according to Quinn et al. [12].

Virulence gene profiling

Four virulence-associated genes (VAGs) were assayed by multiplex PCR (Table 3) [11]: *toxA* (a toxin gene), *pfhA* (a gene involved in adhesion), *tbpA* and *hgbB* (genes involved in iron acquisition). DNA was extracted by boiling. The characterization of the target genes and primers and the related references are listed in Table 3. Amplification products were analyzed by gel electrophoresis on a 1.0% agarose gel stained with ethidium bromide and photographed under UV light.

To analyze differences in VAGs and to determine MLST gene relationships, DNA sequencing was performed as follows: 1 ng of DNA was enzymatically fragmented, and libraries were prepared using a Nextera XT DNA Library Prep Kit (Illumina, Inc., San Diego, CA, USA) according to the manufacturer's recommendations. Library size was evaluated on an Agilent 2100 Bioanalyzer (Agilent Technologies, Santa Clara, CA, USA) and quantified by qPCR. Paired-end sequencing (2 × 250 bp) was performed on an Illumina MiSeq (Illumina, Inc., San Diego, CA, USA) at the Functional Genomics Center, ESALQ, University of São Paulo, Piracicaba, SP. Low-quality reads (phred quality score < 25 and length < 180) and adapters were removed using SeqyClean Software (https://github.com/ibest/seqyclean), reads were assembled using Newbler V. 2.9 (ROCHE), and functional annotation was conducted via the RAST Server (http://rast.nmpdr.org/).

Multi-locus sequence typing

The genetic relationships of the eight isolates of *P. multocida* were analyzed by sequence alignment of seven housekeeping genes (*adk, aroA, deoD, gdhA, g6pD, mdh*, and *pgi*) at http://pubmlst.org/pmultocida_multihost. Sequence types and allelic profiles were submitted to the *P. multocida* multi-host MLST database (http://pubmlst.org/pmultocida_multihost/). A neighbor-joining tree was drawn from the concatenated sequences using MEGA 6.0 [20].

Statistics

The frequency of animals presenting clinical signs, gross lesions and *P. multocida* type A positive isolation in the groups was analyzed with Fisher's exact test. The group effect on the lung consolidation area (%) was calculated with a Kruskal-Wallis test, followed by a Wilcoxon test for multiple comparisons of groups. The SAS statistical software package version 9.2 [21] was used.

Results

All animals were negative for respiratory pathogens (*Actinobacillus pleuropneumoniae, Haemophilus parasuis, Bordetella bronchiseptica, M. hyopneumoniae,* PCV2 and influenza virus) when screened before and after inoculation.

Clinical signs

None of the animals presented clinical signs before challenge. Hyperthermia (rectal temperature ≥ 40 °C) and dyspnea were most frequently observed (Table 4). Higher prevalence and severity of clinical signs were observed in groups G1, G3 and G7 ($p \leq 0.001$) than in the other groups, starting at six hours after challenge and persisting until euthanasia. The average rectal temperature ± standard error for the animals did not differ ($p > 0.05$) among these challenged groups: 40.44 °C ± 0.11 (G1), 40.42 °C ± 0.19 (G3) and 40.29 °C ± 0.16 (G7), with peaks above 41 °C in some animals. Some pigs from groups G2, G4 and G5 also showed hyperthermia and dyspnea; however, fewer animals were affected, with average rectal temperatures of 39.79 °C ± 0.20, 39.53 °C ± 0.16 and 39.72 °C ± 0.14, respectively. The average rectal temperatures of groups G0, G6 and G8 remained within normal limits (38.97 °C ± 0.06, 39.01 °C ± 0.04 and 39.01 °C ± 0.05, respectively) and did not differ ($p > 0.05$).

Coughs were sporadic and of low intensity despite significant differences among the groups (p > 0.05). Furthermore, two pigs (one at 1 dpi and the other at 3 dpi) in G7 had internal otitis, as evidenced by the way the pigs held their heads down. Vomiting was another common clinical sign observed in some pigs of groups G1,

Table 4 Clinical signs (%) and pathological lesions (%) in pigs challenged with *Pasteurella multocida* type A

Variables	Groups†									p^*
	G0	G1	G2	G3	G4	G5	G6	G7	G8	
Clinical signs										
Hyperthermia	0.00[b]	100.0[a]	62.50[ab]	100.0[a]	75.00[ab]	75.00[ab]	12.50[b]	100.0[a]	25.00[b]	< 0.0001
Dyspnea	0.00[c]	100.0[a]	37.50[b]	87.50[ab]	0.00[bc]	25.00[bc]	0.00[bc]	100.0[a]	0.00[bc]	< 0.0001
Cough	16.67[b]	50.00[ab]	37.50[ab]	12.50[b]	0.00[b]	37.50[ab]	0.00[b]	87.50[a]	0.00[b]	0.0002
Macroscopic lesions										
Cranioventral lung consolidation**	0.00[c]	62.50[ab]	37,5.00[ab]	87.50[a]	12.50[b]	0.00[bc]	0.00[bc]	75.00[a]	0.00[bc]	< 0.0001
Cranioventral lung consolidation (%)***	0.00 ± 0.00[b]	3.58 ± 1.51[ab]	2.53 ± 1.43[ab]	6.26 ± 2.38[a]	1.30 ± 1.30[b]	0.00 ± 0.00[b]	0.00 ± 0.00[b]	5.01 ± 1.58[a]	0.000 ± 0.00[b]	0.0004
Necrotic nodules	0.00[c]	62.50[a]	37.50[ab]	75.00[a]	0.00[bc]	0.00[bc]	0.00[bc]	37.50[ab]	0.00[bc]	< 0.0001
Diffuse fibrinous pleuritis	0.00[c]	50.00[ab]	0.00[bc]	75.00[a]	0.00[bc]	25.00[abc]	0.00[bc]	50.00[ab]	0.00[bc]	< 0.0001
Mild focal fibrinous pleuritis	0.00	0.00	0.00	0.00	0.00	12.50	0.00	12.50	0.00	0.7074
Diffuse fibrinous pericarditis	0.00[c]	25.00[abc]	25.00[abc]	62.50[a]	0.00[bc]	25.00[abc]	0.00[bc]	37.50[ab]	0.00[bc]	0.0029
Fibrinous peritonitis	0.00[d]	62.50[a]	12.50[bcd]	37.50[ab]	25.00[abc]	50.00[ab]	0.00[cd]	50.00[ab]	0.00[cd]	< 0.0001
Microscopic lesions										
Fibrinonecrotic suppurative/fibrinonecrohaemorrhagic pleuropneumonia	0.00[c]	87.50[a]	50.00[ab]	87.50[a]	0.00[bc]	0.00[bc]	0.00[bc]	75.00[a]	0.00[bc]	< 0.0001
Fibrinopurulent pleuropneumonia	0.00	0.00	0.00	0.00	12.50	0.00	0.00	12.50	0.00	0.7074
Suppurative lymphadenitis	0.00[c]	12.50[bc]	37.50[ab]	75.00[a]	12.50[bc]	12.50[bc]	0.00[bc]	37.50[ab]	0.00[bc]	0.0005

Fever: Rectal temperature ≥ 40.0 °C
*Descriptive level of probability by Fisher's exact test; percentages followed by different letters on the same line differ significantly by Fisher's exact test ($p \leq 0.05$)
**Suppurative bronchopneumonia in the histopathology assay
***Lung consolidation was measured based on the total percentage of the affected pulmonary area. Descriptive level of Kruskal-Wallis probability; averages followed by different letters differ significantly by the Wilcoxon test ($p \leq 0.05$)
†G0 with 12 pigs and G1-G8 with eight pigs per group

G2, G3, G5 and G7 between 1 and 4 dpi. The animals in groups G0 (control), G6 and G8 remained clinically healthy.

Pathology

Because of animal welfare concerns, 19 pigs with severe respiratory clinical signs were euthanized before 5 dpi, as follows: G1 (5/8), G2 (1/8), G3 (6/8), G5 (2/8) and G7 (5/8). All other pigs were euthanized at 5 dpi. The lesions found are described in Table 4. The primary lesions observed according to the frequency and extension were suppurative cranioventral bronchopneumonia, necrosuppurative/necrohemorrhagic fibrinous pleuropneumonia (Fig. 1a), diffuse fibrinous pleuritis (Fig. 1b), fibrinous pericarditis (Fig. 1c), suppurative lymphadenitis and peritonitis (Fig. 1d), which all differed ($p \leq 0.05$) among the groups.

The average pulmonary consolidation, excluding the necrosuppurative/necrohemorrhagic bronchopneumonial App-like lesion area, was highest in G3 (6.26%), followed by G7 (5.01%), G1 (3.58%), G2 (2.53%) and G4 (1.30%). Histologically, the affected areas had suppurative or fibrinosuppurative bronchopneumonia with abundant neutrophils and bacterial colonies in the lumen of the alveoli, bronchi and bronchioles. Necrosuppurative/necrohemorrhagic fibrinous pleuropneumonia was frequent in pigs from groups G1, G2, G3, G4 and G7, characterized by multifocal areas of coagulation necrosis of the lung parenchyma (Fig. 1e) and associated with suppurative inflammatory exudation (Fig. 1f), proteinaceous material, fibrin, neutrophils, bacterial colonies in the alveolar lumen, necrosis of the vessel walls and possibly hemorrhagic multifocal areas. Fewer oat cells were observed surrounding the necrotic areas in some pigs of groups G3, G4 and G7. The visceral pleura and the adjacent interlobular septa were thickened because of the dilation of lymphatic vessels by fibrin, accumulation of degenerate neutrophils and multiple bacterial colonies. Some lymphatics of the interlobular septa and areas of necrosis were distended and obliterated by fibrin thrombi.

Fibrinous pleuritis was frequently observed but varied in severity among the groups ($p < 0.0001$) (Table 4): 41.94% (13/31) of the occurrences were focal, and 58.06% (18/31) were diffuse. Focal pleuritis occurred unilaterally and was always adjacent to lesions in the lung parenchyma. For diffuse pleuritis, 33.33% (6/18) of the occurrences were unilateral, and 66.66% (12/18) were bilateral. Based on the affected area, pleuritis was scored from 1 to 4, with 1 indicating focal areas of pleuritis and 4 indicating diffuse pleuritis. Diffuse fibrinous pleuritis was observed in pigs from groups G1, G3, G5 and G7, usually associated with fibrinous pericarditis. Of these pigs, one pig each from G1, G2 and G3; three from G5 (with diffuse pleuritis); and another from G5 (with focal pleuritis) had no lung lesions. Histologically, serositis was characterized by thickening of the pleura with

accumulation of fibrin, fibroblasts, degenerated neutrophils and multiple bacterial colonies. The pericardial sac was distended by neutrophils and fibrin.

Suppurative lymphadenitis was common except among animals from groups G6 and G8. This lesion was characterized by neutrophils and fibrin and by the distension of the paratrabecular sinus by proteinaceous edema.

Some pigs in groups G1 ($n = 3$), G3 ($n = 4$), G5 ($n = 1$) and G7 ($n = 1$) had peritonitis. Microthrombi in the spleen were observed in one pig in G1 and two pigs in G5. Furthermore, in one animal in each indicated group, necrotic hepatitis (G1, G3 and G7), splenic necrosis (G1, G5 and G7), splenic infarction (G5: Fig. 1g) and lymphoplasmacytic nephritis (G0, G2, G4, G5 and G8) were observed. Internal otitis was confirmed by the suppurative exudate in both pigs from G7 with clinical signs of otitis.

In summary, *Pasteurella multocida* type A strains were classified by pathogenicity scores according to clinical pathological features primarily produced in inoculated animals, as follows: highly pathogenic strains caused persistent clinical signs and severe lesions consisting of necrosuppurative/necrohemorrhagic bronchopneumonia (App-like) and/or diffuse fibrinous pleuritis and/or pericarditis; low pathogenic strains caused mild clinical signs and only focal bronchopneumonia; nonpathogenic strains did not induce clinical signs, and no lesions were observed. The detailed features of the lesions by strain and pig group are presented in Table 5.

Immunohistochemistry

Marked diffuse staining (+++) of *P. multocida* was detected by IHC in the fibrinosuppurative exudate of the pleura and pericardium, in areas of necrosuppurative bronchopneumonia (Fig. 1h), and in the the cytoplasm of the majority of lymphocytic cells (Fig. 1i) but also free in inflammatory exudates. Mild (+) to moderate (++) multifocal staining was observed in the exudate in the lumen of the bronchi and bronchioles and in the interlobular septa in areas of suppurative bronchopneumonia. Moderate (++) *P. multocida* staining was observed in the cytoplasm of the macrophages in the necrotic exudate within the crypts of the tonsils and in macrophages and neutrophils of the mediastinal lymph nodes. *P. multocida* antigen labeling was mild and multifocal (+) in the kidney, liver and spleen macrophages. Moderate and multifocal (++) *P. multocida* antigen labeling was observed in a septic infarction area in the spleen (Fig. 1j). Additionally, mild (+) staining of *P. multocida* was visualized in the lumen of vessels in the lung, heart, mediastinal lymph nodes and spleen of some pigs.

Recovery of *Pasteurella multocida*

The isolation of *P. multocida* type A from tissues differed among groups ($p \leq 0.05$, Table 6), with the highest

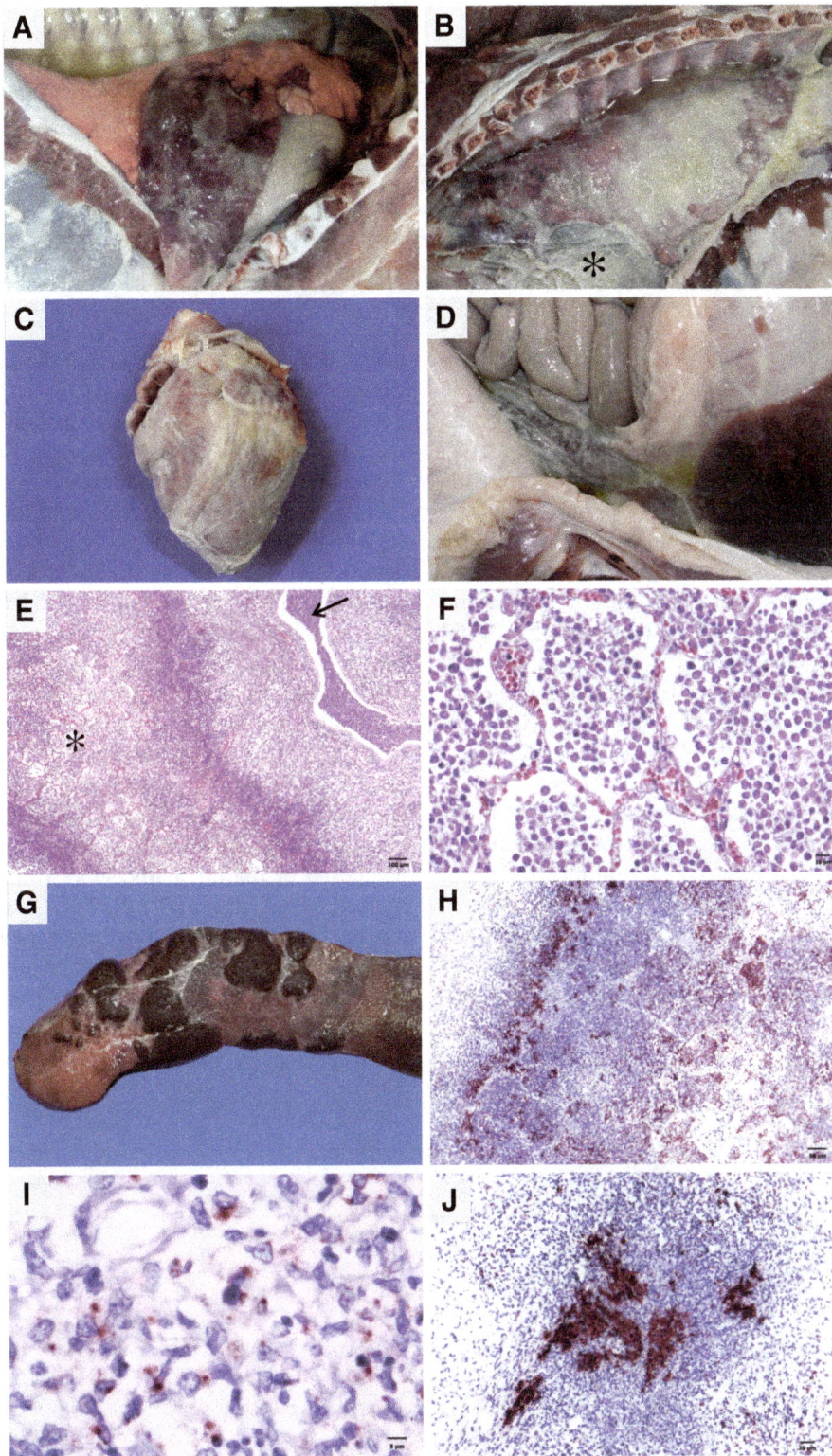

Fig. 1 (See legend on next page.)

(See figure on previous page.)

Fig. 1 Lesions caused by *Pasteurella multocida* type A in experimentally challenged pigs. **a**. Lung, group 2. Focally extensive hemorrhagic pleuropneumonia in the cardiac lobe with fibrin on the pleura. **b**. Thoracic cavity, group 7. Diffuse fibrinous pleuritis and pericarditis (*****). **c**. Heart, group 3. Diffuse fibrinous pericarditis. **d**. Abdominal cavity, group 3. Fibrinous peritonitis. **e**. Lung, group 2. Coagulation necrosis area in the lung parenchyma (*****), surrounded by abundant inflammatory cells, mild proliferation of connective tissue and suppurative exudate in the bronchioles (**thin arrow**). HE. Bar, 100 μm. **f**. Lung, group 2. Abundant (+++) inflammatory exudate, predominantly suppurative, intra-alveolar in a coagulation necrosis area on the lung parenchyma. HE. Bar, 10 μm. **g**. Spleen, group 5. Multiple splenic infarcts with fibrin threads on the capsule. **h**. Lung, group 2. Abundant antigen labeling of *P. multocida* (**red labeling**) in a coagulation necrosis area in the lung and between degenerated inflammatory cells. Bar, 50 μm. **i**. Lung, group 2. Coagulation necrosis area in the lung with *P. multocida* antigen labeling (**red spots**) in the cytoplasm of phagocytic cells. Bar, 5 μm. **j**. Spleen, group 5. Moderate (++) antigen labeling of *P. multocida* (**red labeling**) in a necrotic area. Bar, 20 μm. Immunohistochemistry, streptavidin-biotin-peroxidase method (LSAB™) with 3-amino-9-ethylcarbazole (AEC) and counterstaining with Mayer's hematoxylin

frequency in pigs from G1 (100%), G3 (100%) and G7 (87.5%). The recovery of *P. multocida* type A from the lung, pericardial sac, pleura, trachea, mediastinal lymph nodes and peritoneum differed among groups (p ≤ 0.05), with the highest recovery in the thoracic cavity from tissue lesions in pigs from G1, G2, G3, G4, G5 and G7. *Pasteurella multocida* type A was recovered outside the thoracic cavity in 13 pigs. The sites were the peritoneum cavity, liver, spleen and kidney in animals from G1, G3, G5 and G7; the femoral-tibial-tarsal joint in two animals (G5 and G7); and the purulent exudate of the inner ear of two pigs from G7 with clinical signs of otitis. Bacterial growth was not obtained from animals in groups G0, G6 and G8.

Genotypic characterization

The identity of *P. multocida* was confirmed by PCR detection of the *kmt* gene (species- and type-specific) in all tested isolates. Capsular type A was confirmed by detection of the *hyaD-hyaC* gene in association with a hyaluronidase-positive test and negative acriflavine precipitation. Moreover, the *hgbB* gene was detected in all eight isolates used in the challenge, and the *tbpA* and *toxA* genes were not detected. The *pfhA* gene was detected by PCR exclusively in all the high-pathogenicity isolates.

Consequently, the sequence analysis focused on the region of the *pfhA* gene of all eight isolates. The *pfhA* region of all five highly pathogenic strains consisted of four genes: tpsB1 (1731 bp); *pfhA1* (7842 bp); tpsB2 (1722 bp); and *pfhA2* (11,982 bp). The single low pathogenic strain did not have the tpsB2 and *pfhA2* genes, in addition to presenting a four-base deletion in the beginning of the *pfhA1* gene (at position 892–895 bp) that caused a frameshift and a premature stop codon. The two nonpathogenic isolates also did not have the tpsB2 and *pfhA2* genes and contained a phage DNA insertion of 37 kb located within the *pfhA1* gene (Fig. 2).

MLST profiles and phylogenetic analysis classified the eight isolates into two groups, G1 and G2 (Fig. 3). **G1** contained the five highly pathogenic isolates. **G2** was composed of the low pathogenic strain (G 2.1) and the nonpathogenic strain (G 2.2). The G1 and G.2.1 isolates did not present a corresponding sequence type (ST) in the MLST database for the seven housekeeping genes analyzed. The isolates of the G.2.2 group showed 100% similarity to ST 10.

Table 5 *Pasteurella multocida* type A strains classification by pathogenicity scores according to clinical pathological features observed in eight challenged pigs per group

Strain BRMSA	Group	Pathogenic classification	Lesions			Euthanasia[b]
			N° of pigs	Area[a]	Predominant features	
0496	1	High	8	3.58	Necrosuppurative/necrohemorrhagic bronchopneumonia (App-like lesion) with diffuse fibrinous pleuritis	5
1196	2	High	4	2.53	Necrosuppurative/necrohemorrhagic bronchopneumonia (App-like lesion) with diffuse fibrinous pleuritis	1
1113	3	High	8	6.26	Necrosuppurative/necrohemorrhagic bronchopneumonia (App-like lesion) with diffuse fibrinous pleuritis and pericarditis	6
1197	4	Low	1	1.30	Focal suppurative bronchopneumonia	0
1198	5	High	3	0.0	Diffuse fibrinous pleuritis, pericarditis and peritonitis	2
1199	6	Nonpathogenic	0	0.0	No lesions	0
1200	7	High	7	5.01	Necrosuppurative/necrohemorrhagic bronchopneumonia (App like lesion) with diffuse fibrinous pleuritis and pericarditis	7
1201	8	Nonpathogenic	0	0.0	No lesions	0

[a]Consolidated lung area excluding App-like lesions, %; [b] Number of pigs euthanized before 5 dpi for animal welfare when severe clinical signs were present

Table 6 Frequency of *P. multocida* type A recovery from different organs per group of pigs

Samples	Groups									p^a
	G0	G1	G2	G3	G4	G5	G6	G7	G8	
N° of animals challenged	12	8	8	8	8	8	8	8	8	
Whole Animal	0^d	8^a	3^{bc}	8^a	1^{cd}	3^{bc}	0^{cd}	7^{ab}	0^{cd}	< 0.0001
Lung	0^c	7^a	3^{ab}	7^a	1^{bc}	3^{ab}	0^{bc}	7^a	0^{bc}	< 0.0001
Pericardium	0^b	1^{ab}	0^{ab}	4^a	0^{ab}	2^{ab}	0^{ab}	4^a	0^{ab}	0.0009
Pleura	0^d	5^{ab}	1^{bcd}	7^a	0^{cd}	2^{bcd}	0^{cd}	4^{abc}	0^{cd}	< 0.0001
Trachea	0^b	3^a	1^{ab}	4^a	1^{ab}	2^{ab}	0^{ab}	2^{ab}	0^{ab}	0.0383
Mediastinal lymph node	0^{bc}	5^{ab}	2^b	8^a	0^b	2^b	0^b	3^b	0^b	< 0.0001
Peritoneum	0^b	3^a	0^{ab}	4^a	0^{ab}	1^{ab}	0^{ab}	1^{ab}	0^{ab}	0.0039
Spleen	0	2	0	1	0	1	0	1	0	0.3717
Liver	0	2	0	1	0	1	0	1	0	0.3717
Kidney	0	2	0	1	0	2	0	0	0	0.1188
Joint	0	0	0	0	0	1	0	1	0	0.7074

letters on the same line differ significantly by Fisher's exact test ($p \leq 0.05$)
^{a}Descriptive level of probability by Fisher's exact test; percentages followed by different

Discussion

This study successfully demonstrated that some strains of *P. multocida* type A could induce bronchopneumonia, serositis and septicemia in pigs without interference from other pathogens. Furthermore, two strains were categorized as nonpathogenic. Outbreaks of severe respiratory disease in finishing pigs, characterized by fever, dyspnea, serositis and bronchopneumonia, frequently occur in Brazilian pig production herds. *Pasteurella multocida* type A has been isolated from these outbreaks, associated or not associated with other agents. In some cases, hemorrhagic necrotic foci of pleuropneumonia were found by practitioners in Brazil and named "*A. pleuropneumoniae*-like" because of their similarity to lesions caused by infection with *A. pleuropneumoniae*. Traditionally, *P. multocida* is regarded as a secondary opportunist in the Porcine Respiratory Disease Complex (PRDC) [1–3, 22], and descriptions of cases in which *P. multocida* is suspected to act as a primary agent of lung infection are scarce [4].

Considering the clinical and pathological results obtained with the challenged animals, the isolates were classified into three pathogenic categories: highly pathogenic, low pathogenic and nonpathogenic. The primary observed clinical signs were hyperthermia and dyspnea. Isolates considered nonpathogenic did not primarily induce the disease in healthy pigs; however, these isolates may have an important role in the PRDC [2, 23].

Suppurative/fibrinosuppurative bronchopneumonia, necrosuppurative/necrohemorrhagic pleuropneumonia, pleuritis and pericarditis were the primary observed lesions, similar to the results of other studies of pigs challenged with *P. multocida* type A [4, 24]. In the present study, lung consolidation was not extensive, but *P. multocida* type A was recovered and visualized in low to moderate amounts in the exudates of the bronchi, bronchiolar lumens and interlobular septa. Therefore, *P. multocida* type A is likely not the primary agent in extensive consolidations of lung lesions with mixed infection, as observed in the PRDC [23]. The clinical

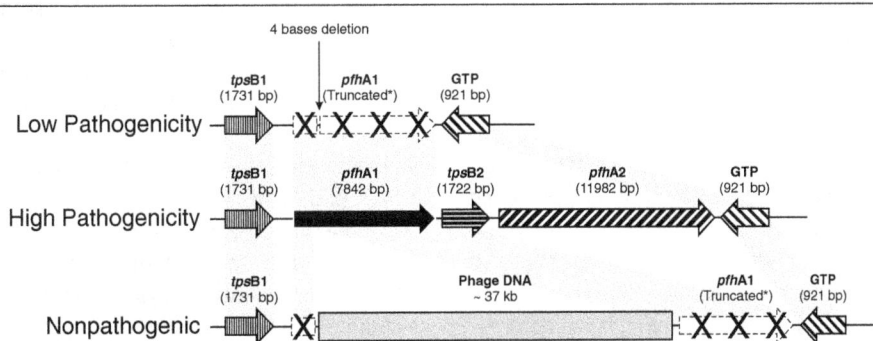

Fig. 2 Schematic representation of the *pfhA* gene region of *P. multocida* type A according to pathogenic classification

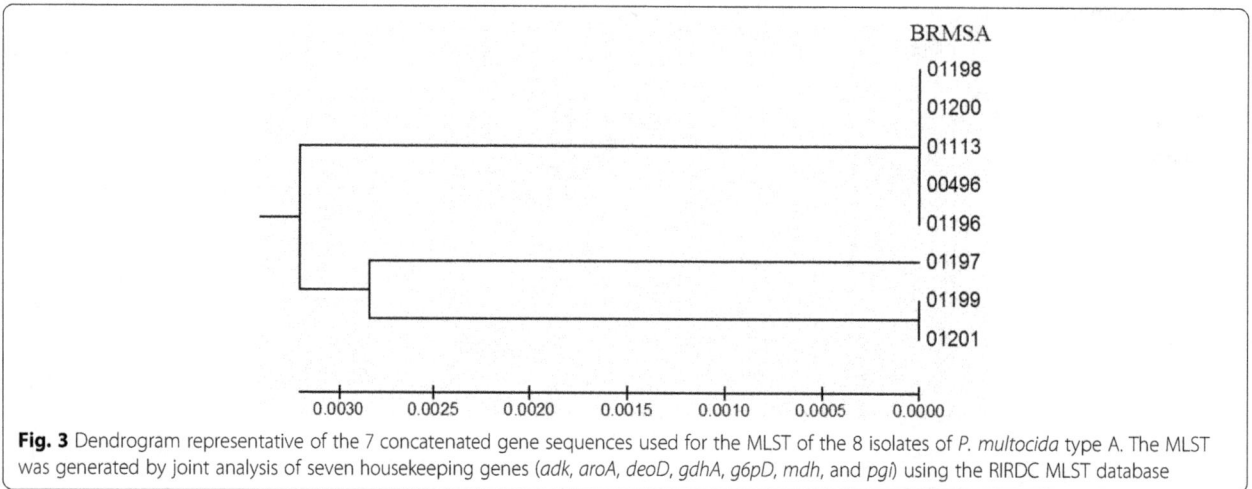

Fig. 3 Dendrogram representative of the 7 concatenated gene sequences used for the MLST of the 8 isolates of *P. multocida* type A. The MLST was generated by joint analysis of seven housekeeping genes (*adk, aroA, deoD, gdhA, g6pD, mdh,* and *pgi*) using the RIRDC MLST database

pathological picture observed in some challenged groups was similar to that of a cattle disease caused by *Mannheimia haemolytica* (family *Pasteurellaceae*) secondary infection triggered by predisposing factors [25].

Some challenged pigs presented peritonitis concurrently with pleuritis and pericarditis, demonstrating bacterial tropism for the serous membranes. *Pasteurella multocida* type A is frequently associated with pleuritis in slaughtered pigs [26]. In this study, severe and diffuse pleuritis and pericarditis were observed in many challenged groups. These findings are important because they suggest that *P. multocida* type A is one of the causes of chronic pleuritis and pericarditis observed at slaughter. Additionally, some pigs only presented fibrinous pleuritis, whether associated with fibrinous pericarditis or not, without lung parenchyma injuries. Such lesions are similar to those caused by *H. parasuis* in Glässer disease [27]. Therefore, in clinical cases of bronchopneumonia and serositis, confirmation of the etiological diagnosis with laboratory tests is essential, particularly in the presence of pulmonary necrotic nodules, pleuritis and pericarditis.

P. multocida type A has been commonly isolated as a secondary pathogen from respiratory lesions caused primarily by *M. hyopneumoniae* or influenza A [1–3]. In 2004, Cappuccio et al. [24] described a new form of severe infection by *P. multocida* type A that caused severe fibrinous and necrohemorrhagic lung lesions in pigs on farms in Argentina. Subsequently, a similar disease was observed in Brazil by Embrapa researchers. Necrosuppurative/necrohemorrhagic pleuropneumonia occurred in some challenged pigs with intense *P. multocida* labeling by IHC in these areas. These lesions were called "*A. pleuropneumoniae*-like" or "App-like" lesions due to their similarity to those produced by *A. pleuropneumoniae* [28]. Notably, as described above, the lesions caused by *P. multocida* type A are similar to those produced by

other agents of the family *Pasteurellaceae*, such as *H. parasuis, A. pleuropneumoniae* and *M. haemolytica.*

Septicemic forms of *P. multocida* infections have been reported to be characteristic of capsular serotype B, affecting birds, buffalo and pigs [29]. However, septicemic forms with capsular serotype A have also been described in pigs [4, 5, 30, 31]. In this study, 13 pigs had a septicemic form. *Pasteurella multocida* type A was isolated and visualized in several parenchymal organs and in serositis (Table 4). The VAGs associated with the pathogenesis of pneumonia and pleuritis caused by *P. multocida* infection are not clear [32]. The lipopolysaccharide of the bacterial cell wall may have an important role in the induction of the inflammatory response of the host [33]. Additionally, the *P. multocida* capsule is clearly involved in the evasion of phagocytosis and complement resistance [34]. However, information related to the invasiveness of *P. multocida* is limited. The mechanisms of mucosal resistance to innate immunity and how these mechanisms cause systemic lesions have not been clearly elucidated.

The genetic diversity among *P. multocida* isolates obtained from cases of pneumonia in pigs has been investigated using different molecular techniques [30, 35, 36]. This study demonstrated differences in *pfhA* PCR results; only highly pathogenic strains were positive. Additionally, the sequence analysis revealed that the PCR target region (*pfhA2*) was absent in the low pathogenic and nonpathogenic isolates. These results support the importance of the multiplex PCR technique [11] for virulence genes and the *pfhA2* gene as a possible marker of high pathogenicity.

The sequence of the *pfhA* region of highly pathogenic strains is composed of four genes (*tpsB1, PfhA1, tpsB2* and *PfhA2*). A similar system including two potential virulence CDs and their accessory genes was previously described by May et al. [37] for the Pm70 strain isolated from fowl cholera. By contrast, as shown in Fig. 2, the low and nonpathogenic strains did not have the genes *tps*B2 and *Pfh*A2. Additionally, a four-base deletion and a 37 kb phage DNA insertion in *pfh*A1 were observed in the low and nonpathogenic strains, respectively.

The *pfh*A gene encodes filamentous hemagglutinin, an adhesin required for bacterial colonization in the upper respiratory system [38]. The PCR results and gene sequencing information demonstrated the absence of *pfh*A2 and a four-base deletion or phage insertion within *pfh*A1. These findings could help explain the reduction or elimination of pathogenic features. Specifically, for the low pathogenic strain, the inactivation of the *pfh*A1 gene by a premature stop codon did not eliminate pathogenicity; thus, other genes are most likely involved in the pathogenic process. Gene inactivation of *P. multocida pfh*A was previously related to colonization ability in the upper respiratory tract in turkey [39] and mouse [40]. The associated *tps*B gene belongs to the TpsB family, which is responsible for transporting sugars (trehalose) to the cell and is therefore related to cellular structure [41].

MLST was previously used to demonstrate clonal differences among *P. multocida* isolates [6, 42]; however, Pors et al. [8] did not find a relationship between MLST results and pulmonary lesions. In this study, MLST differentiated the isolates according to the pathogenic features demonstrated in the experiment. The five highly pathogenic isolates in this analysis originating from 4 different Brazilian states were identical, demonstrating that the highly pathogenic strains are widespread in pig production areas in Brazil. The low pathogenic and nonpathogenic isolates were clustered together in another group with small differences between them. In the MLST analysis, the nonpathogenic isolates were also identical. In addition, only the nonpathogenic isolates were assigned a sequence type (ST10) when submitted to MLST analysis. Of the 17 strains belonging to ST10 deposited in the MLST database, 11 were isolated from pigs, and 8 of these were from pneumonia. By contrast, the high and low pathogenicity isolates were not similar to any strains for the seven housekeeping genes analyzed. These results reinforce our hypothesis that the genetic variability among *P. multocida* type A strains is related to pathogenicity in pigs.

Conclusions

The hypothesis that some *P. multocida* type A strains are primary pathogens and cause disease in pigs without any co-factor was confirmed. The *pfh*A region, consisting of the genes *tps*B1, *tps*B2, *pfh*A1 and *pfh*A2, is related to the pathogenicity of *P. multocida* type A. The highly pathogenic strains produce necrotic bronchopneumonia, fibrin-

ous pleuritis and pericarditis in pigs and can be identified by PCR of the *pfh*A2 gene.

Abbreviations

A. pleuropneumoniae: Actinobacillus pleuropneumoniae; AEC: 3-amino-9-ethylcarbazole; B. bronchiseptica: Bordetella bronchiseptica; BHI: Brain-heart infusion broth; BRMSA: Brasil Microrganismo Suínos e Aves; CFU: Colony-forming units; dpi: day (s) post inoculation; G1-G8: Experimental groups; H. parasuis: Haemophilus parasuis; HP: Highly pathogenic; M. hyopneumoniae: Mycoplasma hyopneumoniae; MLST: Multilocus sequence typing; PBS: Phosphate-buffered saline; PCR: Polymerase chain reaction; PCV2: Porcine circovirus type 2; PmA: Pasteurella multocida Type A; PRDC: Porcine respiratory disease complex; qPCR: Quantitative PCR; RAST: Rapid Annotation using Subsystem Technology; TSA: Trypticase soy agar; VAGs: Virulence-associated genes

Acknowledgments

The authors are grateful to Dr. Márcia Cristina da Silva (Cedisa) and MSc. Suzana Satomi Kuchiishi (Cedisa) for intellectual support; to Altair Althaus, Dejalmo A. da Silva, Franciele Ianiski, Franciana A. Volpato (Embrapa), and Kelen Ascoli (Cedisa) for valuable technical support; to Dr. Valéria Dutra (UFMT), Dr. Luciano Nakazato (UFMT), MSc. Eliana Silva Paladino (UFMG) and to veterinarian Lucas Fernando do Santos (MICROVET®); to others for laboratory support and assistance with sample collection in the states of Mato Grosso, Minas Gerais and Goiás; and to veterinarians Juliana Bassani, Juliana Lazarotto, Lídia Sbaraine Arend, Karine Ludwing Takeuti and Caio C. M. Zaccaro for technical support related to experimental reproduction. RMCG is a recipient of a research fellowship from CNPq.

Funding

This research was supported by the Brazilian Agricultural Research Corporation (Empresa Brasileira de Pesquisa Agropecuária – Embrapa) # 06/2010; InfoSeg Code 35451, Coordination of Improvement of Higher Education Personnel (CAPES) for a scholarship provided to João Xavier de Oliveira Filho and the National Council for Scientific and Technological Development (CNPq) for a research fellowship to Roberto Mauricio Carvalho Guedes. The funders had no role in study design, or the collection, analysis, interpretation of data and writing the manuscript or the decision to submit the article for publication.

Authors' contributions

JXOF performed the experiments, analyzed and interpreted the data, wrote the paper, and revised it critically for important intellectual content; MAZM and RR contributed to laboratory assays (microbial and pathological profiles and molecular assays) and drafting of the manuscript, participated in the experimental challenge and necropsy of the animals, and assisted with the analysis and interpretation of data; JDK and DESNB assisted as intellectual advisors of the work and aided in the analysis and interpretation of the data and drafting of the manuscript; MEC performed the MLST and sequencing analyses and drafted the manuscript; CSK participated in the conception, execution and analysis of the bacteriological assays; RMCG provided support and assistance with sample collection of Pasteurella multocida; AC performed the analysis and interpretation of the statistical data; NM was the general supervisor of the research group, participated in the experimental challenge and necropsy of the animals, and assisted in the analysis and interpretation of the data and drafting of the manuscript. All authors have approved the last revised version of the article for submission and have agreed to be accountable for all aspects of the work to ensure that questions related to the accuracy or integrity of any part of the work are appropriately investigated and resolved.

Consent for publication

Not applicable in these sections.

Competing interests

The authors declare that they have no competing interests.

Author details

[1]Department of Animal Medicine, Universidade Federal do Rio Grande do Sul (UFRGS), Agronomia, Av Bento Gonçalves, 9090, Porto Alegre, Rio Grande do Sul 91540-000, Brazil. [2]Embrapa Suinos e Aves, P.O. Box 121, Concórdia, Santa Catarina 89700-000, Brazil. [3]Preventive Veterinary Medicine Department, Veterinary School, Universidade Federal de Minas Gerais, Belo Horizonte, Brazil.

References

1. Choi YK, Goyal SM, Joo HS. Retrospective analysis of etiologic agents associated with respiratory diseases in pigs. Can Vet J. 2003;44:735–7.
2. Hansen MS, Pors SE, Jensen HE, Bille-Hansen V, Bisgaard M, Flachs EM, Nielsen OL. An investigation of the pathology and pathogens associated with porcine respiratory disease complex in Denmark. J Comp Pathol. 2010; 143:120–31.
3. Pijoan C, Fuentes M. Severe pleuritis associated with certain strains of Pasteurella multocida in swine. J Am Vet Med Assoc. 1987;191:823–6.
4. Ono M, Okada M, Namimatsu T, Fujii S, Mukai T, Sakano T. Septicaemia and arthritis in pigs experimentally infected with Pasteurella multocida capsular serotype a. J Comp Pathol. 2003;129:251–8.
5. Smith IM, Betts AO, Watt RG, Hayward AHS. Experimental infections with Pasteurella multocida (sero-group a) and an adeno- or enterovirus in gnotobiotic piglets. J Comp Pathol. 1973;83:1–12.
6. Ross RF. Pasteurella multocida and its role in porcine pneumonia. Anim Health Res Rev. 2007;7:13–29.
7. Oliveira Filho JX, Morés MAZ, Rebelatto R, Agnol AMD, Plieski CLA, Klein CS, Barcellos DESN, Morés N. Pasteurella multocida type a as the primary agent of pneumonia and septicaemia in pigs. Pesq Vet Bras. 2015;35:716–24.
8. Pors SE, Hansen MS, Christensen H, Jensen HE, Petersen A, Bisgaard M. Genetic diversity and associated pathology of Pasteurella multocida isolated from porcine pneumonia. Vet Microbiol. 2011b;150:354–61.
9. Subaaharan S, Blackall LL, Blackall PJ. Development of a multi-locus sequence typing scheme for avian isolates of Pasteurella multocida. Vet Microbiol. 2010;141:354–61.
10. Ewers C, Lübke-Becker A, Bethe A, Kiebling S, Filter M, Wieler LH. Virulence genotype of Pasteurella multocida strains isolated from different hosts with various disease status. Vet Microbiol. 2006;114:304–17.
11. Atashpaz S, Shayegh J, Hejazi MS. Rapid virulence typing of Pasteurella multocida by multiplex PCR. Res Vet Sci. 2009;87:355–7.
12. Quinn PJ, Markey BK, Leonard FC, Fitzpatrick ES, Fanning S, Hartigen PJ. Pasteurella species, Mannheimia haemolytica and Bibersteinia trehalosi. In: Veterinary microbiology and microbial disease, 27, 2ª edition. Ames, Iowa: Wiley-Blackwell; 2011. p. 300–8.
13. Carter GR, Subronto P. Identification of type D strains of Pasteurella multocida with acriflavine. Am J Vet Res. 1973;34:293–4.
14. Carter GR, Rundell DW. Identification of type a strains of Pasteurella multocida using staphylococcal hyaluronidase. Vet Rec. 1975;87:343.
15. Townsend KM, Boyce JD, Chung JY, Frost AJ, Adler B. Genetic organization of Pasteurella multocida cap loci and development of a multiplex capsular PCR typing system. J Clin Microbiol. 2001;39:924–9.
16. Morrison RB, Hilley HD, Leman AD. Comparison of methods for assessing the prevalence and extent of pneumonia in market weight swine. Can Vet J. 1985;26:381–4.
17. Lorenzo CD, Andrade CP, Machado VSL, Bianchi MV, RolimVM CRAS, Driemeier D. Piglet colibacillosis diagnosis based on multiplex polymerase chain reaction and immunohistochemistry of paraffin-embedded tissues. J Vet Sci. 2018;19:27–33.
18. Ciacci-Zanella JR, Morés N, Simon NL, Oliveira SR, Gava D. Identification of porcine circovirus type 2 by polymerase chain reaction and immunohistochemistry on archived porcine tissues since 1988 in Brazil. Cienc Rural. 2006;36:1480–5.
19. Vincent LL, Janke BH, Paul PS, Halbur PG. A monoclonal-antibody-based immunohistochemical method for the detection of swine influenza virus in formalin-fixed, paraffin-embedded tissues. J Vet Diagn Investig. 1997;9:191–5.
20. Tamura K, Stecher G, Petersonm D, Filipski A, Kumar S. MEGA 6: molecular evolutionary genetics analysis version 60. Mol Biol Evol. 2013;30:2725–9.
21. SAS Institute Inc. SAS/STAT® 9.2 User's Guide. Cary: SAS Institute Inc; 2008.
22. Opriessnig T, Giménez-Lirola LG, Halbur PG. Polymicrobial respiratory disease in pigs. Anim Health Res Rev. 2011;12:133–48.
23. Fablet C, Marois-Créhan C, Simon G, Grasland B, Jestin A, Kobisch M, Madec F, Rose N. Infectious agents associated with respiratory diseases in 125 farrow-to-finish pig herds: a cross-sectional study. Vet Microbiol. 2012;157:152–63.
24. Cappuccio J, Leotta GA, Vigo G, Moredo F, Wolcott MJ, Perfumo CJ. Phenotypic characterization of Pasteurella multocida strains isolated from pigs with bronco and pleuropneumonia. In: Blaha T, Pahlitzsch C, editors. Proceedings of the 18th international pig veterinary society congress. Hamburg: International pig veterinary society; 2004. p. 205.
25. López A. Respiratory system. In: McGavin MD, Zachary JF, editors. Pathologic basis of veterinary disease 4ª edition. St Louis: Mosby; 2007. p. 463–558.
26. Jirawattanapong P, Stockhofe-Zurwieden N, Leengoed LV, Wisselink H, Raymakers R, Cruijsen T, Peet-Schwering CVD, Nielen M, Nes AV. Pleuritis in slaughter pigs: relations between lung lesions and bacteriology in 10 herds with high pleuritis. Res Vet Sci. 2010;88:11–5.
27. Vahle JL, Haynes JS, Andrews JJ. Experimental reproduction of Haemophilus parasuis infection in swine: clinical, bacteriologic, and morphologic findings. J Vet Diagn Investig. 1995;7:476–80.
28. Frey J. The role of RTX toxins in host specificity of animal pathogenic Pasteurellaceae. Vet Microbiol. 2011;153:51–8.
29. Davies RL, MacCorquodale R, Baillie S, Caffrey B. Characterization and comparison of Pasteurella multocida strains associated with porcine pneumonia and atrophic rhinitis. J Med Microbial. 2003;52:59–67.
30. Pijoan C, Morrison RB, Hilley H. Serotyping of Pasteurella multocida isolated from swine lungs collected at slaughter. J Clin Microbiol. 1983;17:1074–6.
31. Pors SE, Hansen MS, Bisgaard M, Jensen HE. Occurrence and associated lesions of Pasteurella multocida in porcine bronchopneumonia. Vet Microbiol. 2011a;150:160–6.
32. Bethe A, Wieler LH, Selbitz H, Ewers C. Genetic diversity of porcine Pasteurella multocida strains from the respiratory tract of healthy and diseased swine. Vet Microbiol. 2009;139:97–105.
33. Fernandez de Henestrosa AR, Badiola I, Saco M, Perez DE, Rozas AM, Campoy S, Barbe J. Importance of the gale gene on the virulence of Pasteurella multocida. FEMS Microbio Lett. 1997;154:311–6.
34. Harper M, Boyce JD, Adler B. The key surface components of Pasteurella multocida: capsule and lipopolysaccharide. Curr Top Microbiol Immunol. 2012;361:39–51.
35. Rubies X, Casal J, Pijoan C. Plasmid and restriction endonuclease patterns in Pasteurella multocida isolated from a swine pyramid. Vet Microbiol. 2002;84:69–78.
36. Zhao G, Pijoan C, Murtaugh MP, Molitor TW. Use of restriction endonuclease analysis and ribotyping to study epidemiology of Pasteurella multocida in closed swine herds. Infect Immun. 1992;60:1401–5.
37. May BJ, Qing Z, Li LL, Paustian ML, Whittam TS, Kapur V. Complete genomic sequence of Pasteurella multocida, Pm70. PNAS. 2001;98:3460–5.
38. Harper M, Boyce JD, Adler B. Pasteurella multocida pathogenesis: 125 years after Pasteur Federation of European Microbiological Societies. FEMS Microbiol Lett. 2006;265:1–10.
39. Tatum FM, Yersin AG, Briggs RE. Construction and virulence of a Pasteurella multocida fhaB2 mutant in turkeys. Microb Pathog. 2005;39:9–17.
40. Fuller TE, Kennedy MJ, Lowery DE. Identification of Pasteurella multocida virulence genes in a septicemic mouse model using signature-tagged mutagenesis. Microb Pathog. 2000;29:25–38.
41. Chen Q, Haddad GG. Role of trehalose phosphate synthase and trehalose during hypoxia: from flies to mammals. J Exp Biol. 2004;207:3125–9.
42. Hotchkiss EJ, Hodgson JC, Lainson FA, Zadoks RN. Multilocus sequence

typing of a global collection of Pasteurella multocida isolates from cattle and other host species demonstrates niche association. BMC Microbiol. 2011;11:115.

43. Yamaguti M, Muller EE, Piffer AI, Kich JD, Klein CS, Kuchiishi SS. Detection of *Mycoplasma hyopneumoniae* by polymerase chain reaction in swine presenting respiratory problems. Braz J Microbiol. 2008;39:471–47.

44. Souza KK, Klein CS, Kich JD, Coldebella A, Alberton GC. Polymerase chain reaction (PCR) based on the cpx gene for detection of *Actinobacillus pleuropneumoniae* in natural and experimentally infected pigs. Cienc Rural. 2008;38:1954–60.

45. Redondo VA, Méndez JN, Blanco GD, Boronat NL, Martín CBG, Ferri EFR. Typing of *Haemophilus parasuis* strain by PCR-RFLP analyses of the *tbp*A gene. Vet Microbiol. 2003;92:253–62.

46. Lichtensteiger C, Steenbergen SM, Lee RM, Polson DD, Vimr ER. Direct PCR analysis for toxigenic *Pasteurella multocida*. J Clin Microbiol. 1996;34(12):3035–9.

22

Pathologic and biochemical characterization of PrP^{Sc} from elk with *PRNP* polymorphisms at codon 132 after experimental infection with the chronic wasting disease agent

S. Jo Moore[1], Catherine E. Vrentas[1], Soyoun Hwang[1], M. Heather West Greenlee[2], Eric M. Nicholson[1] and Justin J. Greenlee[1]* (iD)

Abstract

Background: The Rocky Mountain elk (*Cervus elaphus nelsoni*) prion protein gene (*PRNP*) is polymorphic at codon 132, with leucine (L132) and methionine (M132) allelic variants present in the population. In elk experimentally inoculated with the chronic wasting disease (CWD) agent, different incubation periods are associated with *PRNP* genotype: LL132 elk survive the longest, LM132 elk are intermediate, and MM132 elk the shortest. The purpose of this study was to investigate potential mechanisms underlying variations in incubation period in elk of different prion protein genotypes. Elk calves of three *PRNP* genotypes (*n* = 2 MM132, *n* = 2 LM132, *n* = 4 LL132) were orally inoculated with brain homogenate from elk clinically affected with CWD.

Results: Elk with longer incubation periods accumulated relatively less PrP^{Sc} in the brain than elk with shorter incubation periods. PrP^{Sc} accumulation in LM132 and MM132 elk was primarily neuropil-associated while glial-associated immunoreactivity was prominent in LL132 elk. The fibril stability of PrP^{Sc} from MM132 and LM132 elk were similar to each other and less stable than that from LL132 elk. Real-time quaking induced conversion assays (RT-QuIC) revealed differences in the ability of PrP^{Sc} seed from elk of different genotypes to convert recombinant 132 M or 132 L substrate.

Conclusions: This study provides further evidence of the importance of *PRNP* genotype in the pathogenesis of CWD of elk. The longer incubation periods observed in LL132 elk are associated with PrP^{Sc} that is more stable and relatively less abundant at the time of clinical disease. The biochemical properties of PrP^{Sc} from MM132 and LM132 elk are similar to each other and different to PrP^{Sc} from LL132 elk. The shorter incubation periods in MM132 compared to LM132 elk may be the result of genotype-dependent differences in the efficiency of propagation of PrP^{Sc} moieties present in the inoculum. A better understanding of the mechanisms by which the polymorphisms at codon 132 in elk *PRNP* influence disease pathogenesis will help to improve control of CWD in captive and free-ranging elk populations.

Keywords: Chronic wasting disease, Conformational stability, Elk, RT-QuIC, Prion protein

* Correspondence: Justin.Greenlee@ARS.USDA.GOV
[1]USDA, Agricultural Research Service, National Animal Disease Center, Virus and Prion Research Unit, Ames, USA
Full list of author information is available at the end of the article

Background

Chronic wasting disease (CWD) is a transmissible spongiform encephalopathy (TSE) that affects a number of cervid species including elk, moose, mule deer, white-tailed deer and reindeer. The TSE's are a group of neuro-degenerative diseases that are characterized by the accumulation of disease-associated prion protein (PrPSc) in the nervous system and other body tissues. In cervids, CWD infection is associated with clinical signs including behavioral abnormalities, excess salivation, emaciation, and eventually death [49].

The host prion protein (PrP) amino acid sequence that is encoded by the prion protein gene (*PRNP*) influences the susceptibility of both humans and animals to TSE's. Rocky Mountain elk (*Cervus elaphus nelsoni*) are polymorphic at *PRNP* codon 132, encoding either methionine (M) or leucine (L) [30]. The elk *PRNP* codon 132 polymorphism is homologous to the human *PRNP* codon 129 polymorphism that encodes either methionine (M) or valine (V) [39, 40]. In TSE-affected humans, the MM129 genotype is associated with susceptibility to kuru [23] and variant Creutzfeldt-Jakob disease (vCJD) [38]. Some studies have found that elk expressing prion protein homozygous for methionine at codon 132 (hereafter referred to as MM132 elk) are over-represented among CWD-affected elk [11, 12, 31, 41], while another study concluded that elk of all 3 genotypes (MM132, LM132, LL132) show equivalent susceptibility [36]. In experimental studies, LL132 elk orally inoculated with CWD have incubation periods approximately 1.5 times longer than LM132 elk, and 3 times longer than MM132 elk [14, 28]. A better understanding of the biological effects of polymorphisms at elk *PRNP* codon 132 may help to clarify the role of this locus in the spread of CWD in North American elk populations.

Here, we provide further histopathologic characterization of experimental CWD infection in MM132, LM132 [14] and LL132 [28] elk. We examine the intersection of host genotype, incubation period, PrPSc fibril stability, and amyloid formation rate and demonstrate that genotype-dependent differences in PrPSc stability and amyloid formation rate may contribute to the observed variation in incubation periods of elk of different genotypes. These results may help us to better understand the influence of the *PRNP* 129 polymorphism in human prion diseases.

Methods

Ethics statement

This experiment was carried out in accordance with the Guide for the Care and Use of Laboratory Animals (Institute of Laboratory Animal Resources, National Academy of Sciences, Washington, DC) and the Guide for the Care and Use of Agricultural Animals in Research and Teaching (Federation of Animal Science Societies, Champaign, IL). The Institutional Animal Care and Use Committee at the National Animal Disease Center reviewed and approved the animal use protocol (protocol number: 3833).

Inoculum preparation and animal procedures

The source, genotyping, husbandry and oral inoculation of the eight elk in this study has been described previously [14]. Briefly, elk were obtained from a captive elk game farm on which 79 cases of CWD were diagnosed between 1997 and 2001. All CWD-positive elk were of the MM132 or LM132 genotypes; no cases were found in LL132 elk [28]. MM132 and LM132 elk calves were sourced from the 2000 birth cohort of 1 of the 3 premises operated by the captive elk game farm; LL132 elk calves were sourced from the 2001 birth cohort of a different premises to the MM132 and LM132 calves. Genotype analysis was conducted on nucleic acid extracted from live animal blood samples as described previously [8]. The inoculum was prepared from pooled brain material from one MM132 and one LM132 elk (equal parts MM132 and LM132 donor tissue), both of which had showed clinical signs of CWD. At 8 months of age four LL132 elk, two LM132 elk and two MM132 elk were inoculated orally with 3 mL of inoculum daily for five consecutive days (total dose equivalent to 15 g of pooled brain) [14, 28]. Elk were housed in a biosafety level-2 isolation barn at the National Animal Disease Center (Ames, IA). This barn had not previously housed CWD-infected animals and entry and exit procedures were in place to eliminate potential cross-contamination from any source. Health was monitored twice daily. Sentinel LL132 animals were not included in the study design.

Animals were necropsied after being found dead, or euthanized upon showing clinical signs or at the conclusion of the experiment at 64 months postinoculation (MPI). Two sets of tissue samples were collected. One set of tissues included representative sections of: brain, eye (retina), optic nerve, sciatic nerve, trigeminal ganglion, peripheral nerves (optic, sciatic), lymph nodes (retropharyngeal, mesenteric, popliteal, prescapular), tonsils (palatine, pharyngeal), 3rd eyelid, foregut (esophagus, reticulum, omasum, rumen, abomasum), jejunum, ileum, recto-anal mucosa-associated lymphoid tissue (RAMALT), salivary gland, liver, pancreas, kidney, urinary bladder, spleen, adrenal, pituitary, thyroid, skeletal muscles (diaphragm, biceps femoris, masseter, psoas major, triceps), heart muscle, tongue, turbinate, lung, trachea, skin. These tissues were fixed in 10% buffered formalin, embedded in paraffin wax, and sectioned at 5 μm for microscopy examination after hematoxylin and eosin staining. The second set of tissues, comprising subsamples of all tissues collected into formalin, was frozen.

Immunohistochemistry

All paraffin-embedded tissues were immunostained by an automated immunohistochemical method for detection of PrP^{Sc} as described previously [9] using the anti-PrP monoclonal antibody F99/96.7.1 [29].

Antigen-capture enzyme immunoassay (EIA)

The IDEXX HerdChek BSE-Scrapie Ag EIA plate (Westbrook, ME) was used with modifications for the EIA-based fibril stability assay and the determination of PrP^{Sc} levels. Brain samples from elk were recovered from archived frozen brainstem stored at either $-20\ °C$ or $-80\ °C$. Brainstem samples were mixed with 1X PBS (phosphate-buffered saline, lacking calcium and magnesium) and homogenized in a bead beater.

EIA-based fibril stability assay

PrP^{Sc} fibril stability was determined using an EIA-based assay as described previously ([9]. This assay is a protease-free method to monitor PrP^{Sc} unfolding that exposes the epitopes for the antibodies used in the IDEXX assay. The capture surface of the IDEXX EIA is a proprietary ligand that is specific for misfolded protein with detection of bound protein by a PrP specific antibody, and does not require protease digestion to distinguish PrP^{Sc} from PrP^{C}. Briefly, dilutions of elk brain samples were incubated at concentrations of guanidine hydrochloride (GdnHCl) over a range from 0.25 M to 4.0 M. Neither brainstem samples nor intact brain were available for MM132 elk #2 so spinal cord was used for a comparison of elk #2 and elk #1; sections of gray matter from the cervical spinal cord were excised and homogenized as for the brainstem samples. The relative amount of PrP^{Sc} remaining was assessed by the EIA optical density (OD$_{450}$) after dilution of treated brain homogenates to a final [GdnHCl] of 0.25 M and application to the IDEXX plate. The amount of PrP^{Sc} remaining was then plotted against GdnHCl concentration. The midpoint of the curve, or [GdnHCl]$_{1/2}$, is defined as the concentration of GdnHCl at which the PrP^{Sc} signal was reduced by half of the signal at 0.25 M GdnHCl; PrP^{Sc} with a smaller [GdnHCl]$_{1/2}$ is less stable. As described previously [44], due to variations in the upper baseline shape, the Smooth Line function in Microsoft Excel was used to connect data points in each curve and visualize the midpoint.

Calculation of amount of PrP^{Sc} versus incubation period

To determine the relative amount of PrP^{Sc} in brain from elk at clinical disease, 1% w/v brain homogenates were serially diluted in 1X PBS and tested using the EIA assay and diluted until the OD$_{450}$ readings were in the linear range of detection. To provide a normalization metric across multiple samples, the 1% (w/v) homogenate was

assigned a brain unit equivalent (BU) value of 100 and equivalent BU's were calculated for each dilution, i.e. 1:2 dilution = 50 BU, 1:4 dilution = 25 BU. For each sample, the EIA OD reading in the linear range (minus the negative control value) was divided by the BU of the dilution at which the linear range OD was measured, to generate an OD/BU value. We then calculated the ratio of the OD/BU values for each sample compared to the sample with the lowest OD/BU value. Ratio values were plotted against incubation period.

Recombinant prion protein production and purification

E. coli (BL21(λDE3)) was transformed with the pET28a vector containing the elk PrP gene corresponding to mature length PrP (amino acids 23–231, GenBank accession number AAC12860.2), and elk recombinant PrP was expressed and purified as described for bovine PrP [17, 46]. The concentration of filtered protein eluent was determined by UV absorbance at 280 nm using an extinction coefficient of 59,485 M^{-1} cm^{-1} as calculated for mature length elk prion protein.

Real-time quaking induced conversion (RT-QuIC) protocol

RT-QuIC was performed on 10% (w/v) brainstem homogenized in PBS from elk #1 (MM132), elk #4 (LM132) and elk #7 (LL132) as described previously [17]. The reaction mix was composed of 10 mM phosphate buffer (pH 7.4), 400 mM NaCl, 0.1 mg/ml recombinant mature length elk prion protein (132 L, [23–231]; 132 M, [23–231]), 10 μM thioflavin T (ThT), 1 mM ethylenediaminetetraacetic acid tetrasodium salt (EDTA). The positive threshold was calculated as the mean value of normal elk brain homogenates plus 10 standard deviations. Previously described criteria were applied for classification of positive samples of RT-QuIC [5, 32, 34].

Results

Differences in incubation period were associated with polymorphisms at *PRNP* codon 132

At approximately 23 MPI MM132 elk (animals #1 and #2) developed loss of appetite and body condition. Both elk rapidly became unable to stand without assistance and were euthanized. At 38 (#3) and 40 (#4) MPI respectively, LM132 elk developed similar clinical signs and were euthanized (average incubation period = 39 MPI) (Table 1). The first LL132 elk (#5) to succumb to CWD was found dead at 59 MPI. This elk had previously been noted to be smaller and thinner than the other LL132 elk. During month 63 post-inoculation elk #6 developed muscle fasciculations, staggering, tremor, anorexia, mental dullness, head pressing and loss of bladder control, and was euthanized. The two remaining elk (#7 and #8) were euthanized at 64 MPI after displaying early signs of clinical disease, including subtle

Table 1 Animal information and results for study elk

Animal number	1	2	3	4	5	6	7	8
Genotype codon 132	MM	MM	LM	LM	LL	LL	LL	LL
Incubation period (MPI)	23	23	38	40	60	63	64	64
Clinical presentation	LBC, Rec	LBC, Rec	LBC, ataxia	LBC	LBC	Neuro	FD	LBC
Tissue results								
Brain	+/+	+/+	+/+	+/+	+/+	+/+	+/+	+/+
Retina	+	+	+	+	+	+	+	+
Peripheral NS	+	+	+	–	+	+	–	+
Lymphoid head	+	+	+	+	+	+	+	+
Lymphoid other	+	+	+	+	+	+	+	n/a
Intestines	+	+	+	+	–	+	+	+
Spleen	+	+	+	–	+	–	–	+
Pituitary	n/a	n/a	+	+	n/a	+	–	n/a
Foregut	n/a	–	–	+	–	–	–	+
Adrenal	n/a	+	–	–	n/a	–	+	n/a

M methionine, L leucine, MPI months post inoculation, LBC Loss of body condition, Rec recumbency, Neuro neurological signs (for more detail see Results), FD found dead. Tissue results: brain, vacuolation/PrPSc; other tissues, PrPSc; n/a, tissue not available for examination

behavior changes, mild loss of body condition, and roughened hair coat (Table 1). The average incubation period for the four LL132 elk was 62.8 MPI.

Spongiform change was more prominent in the gray matter in MM132 and LM132 elk, while in LL132 elk the white matter was more severely affected

To investigate the patterns of spongiform change in the brain, hematoxylin and eosin stained coronal sections of brain and spinal cord were examined by light microscopy. Pathologic changes in MM132 and LM132 elk have been described previously [14]. Microscopic lesions of spongiform encephalopathy were present in all elk. In LM132 and MM132 elk, microcavitation of the gray matter was more prevalent than intraneuronal vacuolation and neuronal degeneration, and there was mild astrocytosis [14]. In all LM132 and MM132 elk, moderate to severe spongiform change was present in the dorsal motor nucleus of the vagus nerve (Fig. 1a) and surrounding nuclei. In LL132 elk, vacuolation of white matter tracts (Fig. 1b) was more prevalent than microcavitation of the gray matter.

In summary, microcavitation of gray and white matter was observed in all elk. Spongiform change was more prominent in the gray matter of LM132 and MM132 elk and more prominent in the white matter of LL132 elk.

PrPSc accumulation in LM132 and MM132 elk was primarily neuropil-associated while intra-glial immunoreactivity was prominent in LL132 elk

To investigate the patterns of PrPSc deposition in the brain, immunolabeled sections of brain, spinal cord, and

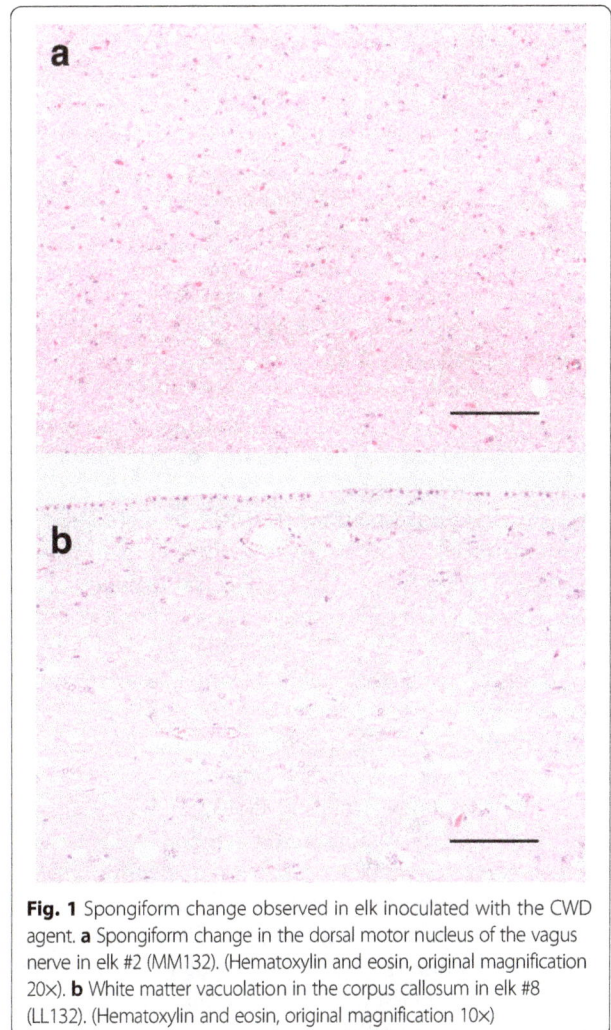

Fig. 1 Spongiform change observed in elk inoculated with the CWD agent. a Spongiform change in the dorsal motor nucleus of the vagus nerve in elk #2 (MM132). (Hematoxylin and eosin, original magnification 20×). b White matter vacuolation in the corpus callosum in elk #8 (LL132). (Hematoxylin and eosin, original magnification 10×)

peripheral tissues were examined by light microscopy. Subjectively, the total amount of PrPSc immunoreactivity was greater in MM132 and LM132 elk compared to LL132 elk. In LM132 and MM132 elk, PrP^{Sc} immunoreactivity in the brain appeared as coarse granular material that was scattered throughout the neuropil. Perineuronal immunolabeling was common while intraneuronal immunolabeling was rare [14].

In LL132 elk, coarse granular and perineuronal immunolabeling were common, as was intraneuronal immunolabeling (Fig. 2a). In addition, there was granular to punctate immunolabeling that was often associated with astrocytes. This astrocyte-associated immunolabeling was most prominent in white matter (Fig. 2b) but also was observed in gray matter (Fig. 2c).

In elk of all genotypes, PrP^{Sc} was abundant in the lymphoid follicles of the palatine tonsil, retropharyngeal lymph node and gut-associated lymphoid tissue. The skeletal muscles (M. biceps femoris, M. masseter, M. psoas major, M. triceps), diaphragm, kidney, urinary bladder, nose skin, turbinate, trachea, lung, tongue, liver, pancreas, salivary gland, and thyroid were negative in all samples examined.

PrP^{Sc} immunoreactivity was widespread in the central nervous system and peripheral lymphoid tissues of all elk. Intraneuronal immunolabeling was less prominent in LM132 and MM132 elk compared to LL132 elk. Glial-associated immunolabeling observed in LL132 elk was not seen in LM132 or MM132 elk.

PrP^{Sc} fibrils from LL132 elk are more stable than fibrils from LM132 and MM132 elk

To determine whether there is an association between fibril stability of PrP^{Sc} and incubation period in CWD-affected elk, we assessed the stability of PrP^{Sc} using an EIA-based stability assay.

When the fibril stability of PrP^{Sc} in homogenized brainstem of elk of each genotype was measured, two clusters of curves were evident (Fig. 3a). Samples from MM132 and LM132 elk exhibited lower fibril stability, with a [GdnHCl]$_{1/2}$ of ≈2.75, while samples from LL132 elk exhibited higher fibril stability, with a [GdnHCl]$_{1/2}$ of ≈3.2–3.3. When fibril stability data from samples from MM132 and LM132 elk are combined and compared to LL132 elk samples (Fig. 3b), average values of LL132 versus M132-containing groups (MM132 and LM132) exhibited statistically significant differences at 2.5, 3, and 3.5 M GdnHCl ($p < 0.004$, t-test with unequal variances). Since unfixed brainstem tissue was unavailable for the second MM132 elk (elk #2) spinal cord homogenate was used to determine the fibril stability of PrP^{Sc} from this elk. The stability of PrP^{Sc} from the elk #2 spinal cord sample was similar to PrP^{Sc} from brainstem homogenate

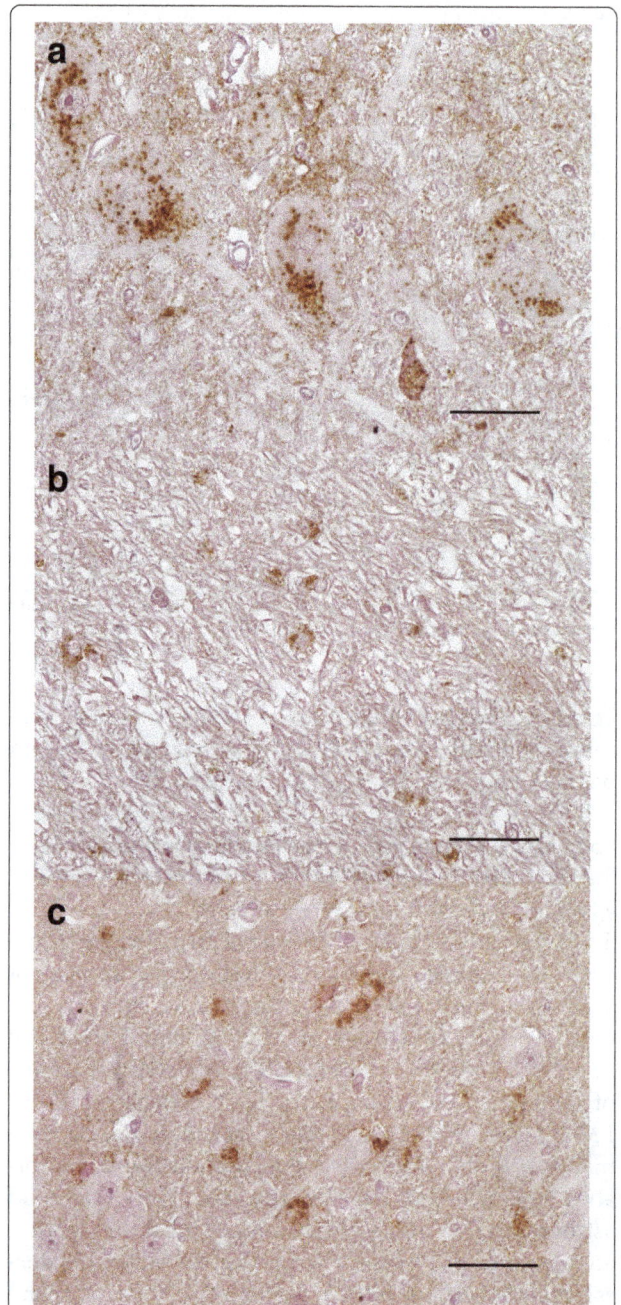

Fig. 2 Spongiform change and patterns of PrP^{Sc} immunoreactivity observed in elk inoculated with the CWD agent. **a** Intraneuronal immunoreactivity in the hypoglossal nucleus in elk #5 (LL132) elk. **b** Glial associated immunoreactivity in the cerebellar white matter of elk #5 (LL132). **c** Glial associated immunoreactivity in the lateral geniculate nucleus of elk #5 (LL132). **a-c** immunostained using monoclonal anti-PrP antibody F99/96.7.1, original magnification 40×

from the other MM132 elk (#1) in the study (data not shown).

In summary, PrP^{Sc} from samples from MM132 and LM132 elk that have short and intermediate incubation

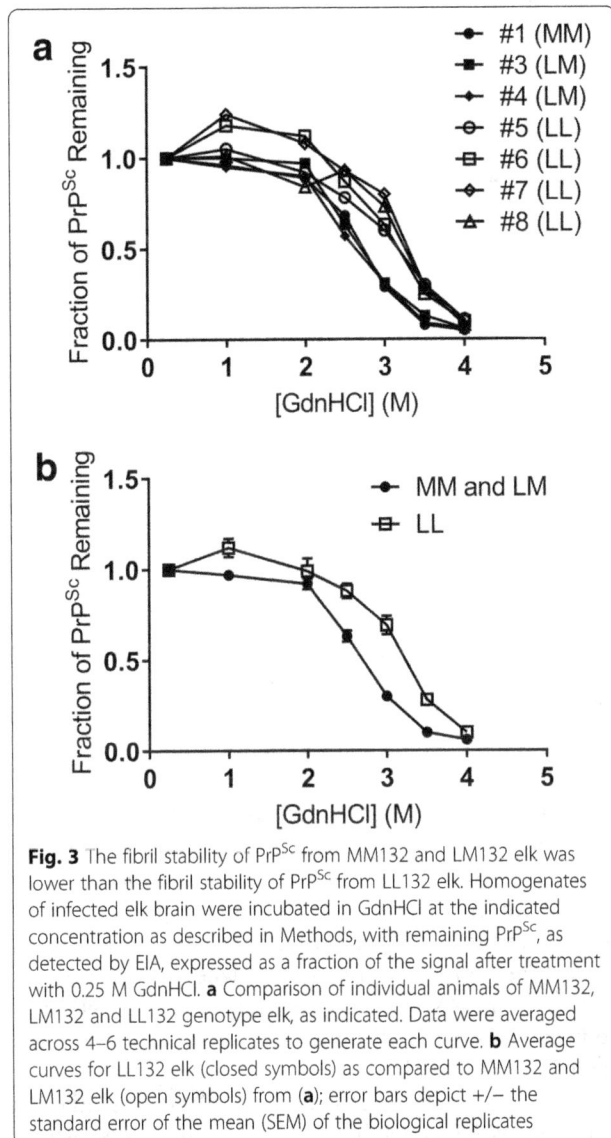

a (y-axis: Fraction of PrP^{Sc} Remaining; x-axis: [GdnHCl] (M))

Legend:
- #1 (MM)
- #3 (LM)
- #4 (LM)
- #5 (LL)
- #6 (LL)
- #7 (LL)
- #8 (LL)

b (y-axis: Fraction of PrP^{Sc} Remaining; x-axis: [GdnHCl] (M))

Legend:
- MM and LM
- LL

Fig. 3 The fibril stability of PrP^{Sc} from MM132 and LM132 elk was lower than the fibril stability of PrP^{Sc} from LL132 elk. Homogenates of infected elk brain were incubated in GdnHCl at the indicated concentration as described in Methods, with remaining PrP^{Sc}, as detected by EIA, expressed as a fraction of the signal after treatment with 0.25 M GdnHCl. **a** Comparison of individual animals of MM132, LM132 and LL132 genotype elk, as indicated. Data were averaged across 4–6 technical replicates to generate each curve. **b** Average curves for LL132 elk (closed symbols) as compared to MM132 and LM132 elk (open symbols) from (**a**); error bars depict +/− the standard error of the mean (SEM) of the biological replicates

periods, respectively, was less stable than PrP^{Sc} from samples from LL132 elk that have the longest incubation periods.

Relative amount of PrP^{Sc} in comparison to incubation period in elk

To investigate the relationship between the incubation period and relative amount of PrP^{Sc} accumulation in the brain, the amount of PrP^{Sc} in brain homogenates was quantified using EIA.

The relative amount of PrP^{Sc} in the brain was lowest for LL132 elk, intermediate for LM132 elk, and highest for MM132 elk. When the relative amount of PrP^{Sc} in the brain was plotted against elk incubation period, a strong negative correlation between these two variables was apparent (Fig. 4).

Real-time quaking induced conversion assays seeded with samples from LM132 and MM132 elk produced shorter lags times in 132 M substrate and longer lag times in 132 L substrate

To investigate if RT-QuIC can be used to detect differences in either conversion efficiency of the substrate or the prion seeding activity from CWD infected elk brain of different genotypes, we used infected and normal elk brain homogenates as seed for mature length recombinant 132 L or 132 M elk prion protein substrates. To allow for comparison between substrates, all assays were performed in the same reaction conditions as described in the Materials and Methods.

Using the 132 L substrate (Fig. 5a) and 132 M substrate (Fig. 5b) an increase in Thioflavin-T fluorescence, indicating the presence of misfolded prion protein, was observed in each quadruplicate reaction seeded with 10^{-2} dilution of normalized elk brain homogenate, but no increase in fluorescence was observed in reactions seeded with normal brain homogenates. The lag times in assays using the 132 L substrate were similar for seeds from elk of all three genotypes (LM132 = 21 h, MM132 = 23 h, LL132 = 20.5 h). For LM132 and MM132 seeds, the lag times in assays using 132 M substrate (LM132 = 12 h, MM132 = 12.5 h) were shorter than the lag times in assays using 132 L substrate (LM132 = 21 h, MM132 = 23 h). The lag time for the LL132 seed in 132 L substrate (19 h) was similar to the lag time in 132 M substrate (20.5 h).

Discussion

We demonstrate that the shorter incubation periods of elk that are homozygous for methionine at *PRNP* codon 132 (MM132) or heterozygous for leucine and methionine (LM132) elk are associated with PrP^{Sc} that is less stable than PrP^{Sc} from elk that are homozygous for leucine (LL132), which have the longest incubation periods. Subjectively, the amount of PrP^{Sc} immunoreactivity in the brain was similar across elk of all genotypes using IHC. However, serial dilution studies using EIA revealed that the brains of LL132 elk contain relatively lower amounts of PrP^{Sc} than LM132 and MM132 elk. Although the interpretation of results from this study is limited by the small number of elk of each genotype that were available for inoculation, this study nevertheless provides valuable baseline data on the relationship between *PRNP* codon 132 genotype and disease pathogenesis in elk with chronic wasting disease.

We observed a strong negative association between incubation period and the relative amount of PrP^{Sc} in the brain in elk of different genotypes, i.e. elk with longer incubation periods accumulate less PrP^{Sc}. Differences in the relative amount of PrP^{Sc} in the brain were detected using EIA on frozen brain tissue and IHC on formalin-

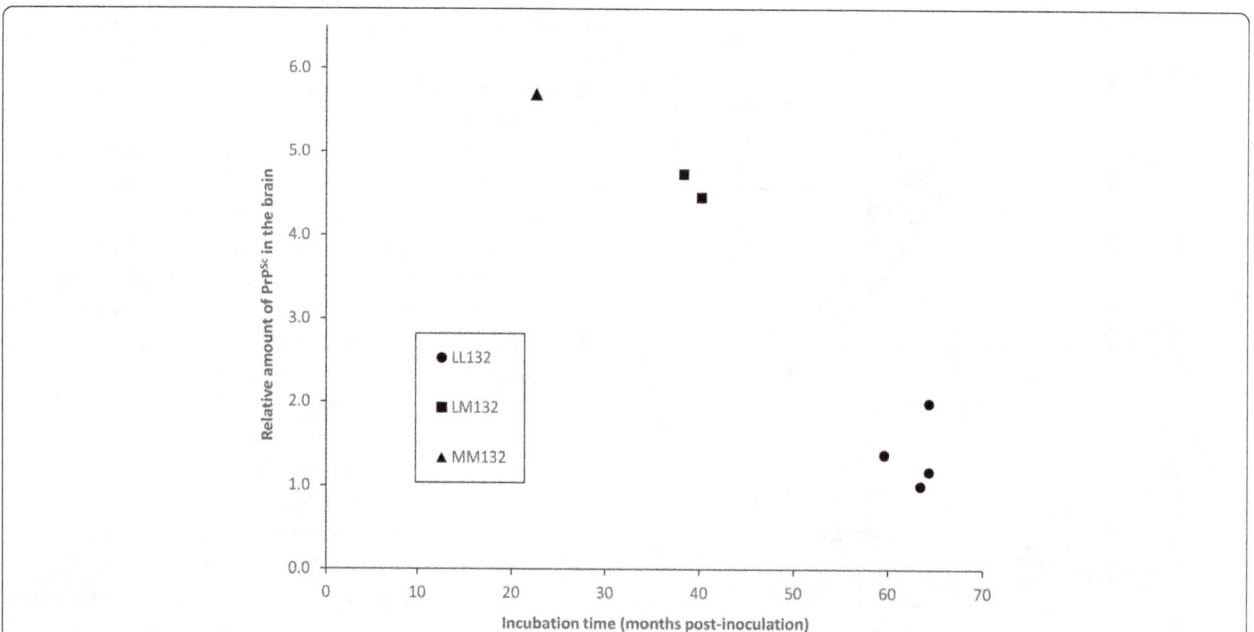

Fig. 4 The relative amount of PrP^{Sc} in the brainstem (obex) is strongly associated with incubation period. The amount of PrP^{Sc} in the brain was calculated using optical density readings from an antigen-capture enzyme immunoassay (EIA). The relative amount of PrP^{Sc} in the brain of the elk with the lowest EIA result in the linear range was designated a baseline value of 1.0. Results for other elk are expressed as a ratio relative to the baseline elk. Frozen obex was not available for elk #2 (MM132) so this animal is not included in the figure

fixed paraffin-embedded brain tissue. This suggests that MM132 elk may be more permissive to PrP^{Sc} accumulation than LM132 elk. This observation is supported by a previous study in transgenic mice that showed that the L132 polymorphism severely restricts propagation of CWD prions [7]. Since PrP^{Sc} from MM132 and LM132 elk show similar fibril stability profiles and RT-QuIC conversion profiles using recombinant 132 L and 132 M elk prion protein, one explanation for the rapid PrP^{Sc} accumulation in MM132 elk may be a potential difference in the effective concentration of PrP^{C-132M}. In heterozygous sheep, both allelic variants of PrP^{C} are present in

equal amounts [27]. It is assumed that this relationship is similar in heterozygous elk, which means that the amount of PrP^{C-132M} in MM132 elk is twice that of LM132 elk. In transgenic mice higher expression levels of PrP^{C} result in reduced incubation times (reviewed in [47]). Therefore, the relatively higher proportion of PrP^{C-132M} in MM132 elk compared to LM132 elk may contribute to the relatively shorter incubation times observed in MM132 elk.

In sheep, conversion of PrP^{C} to PrP^{Sc} is more efficient when the *PRNP* genotype of the inoculum and substrate are the same [2, 3, 21]. Furthermore, in heterozygous

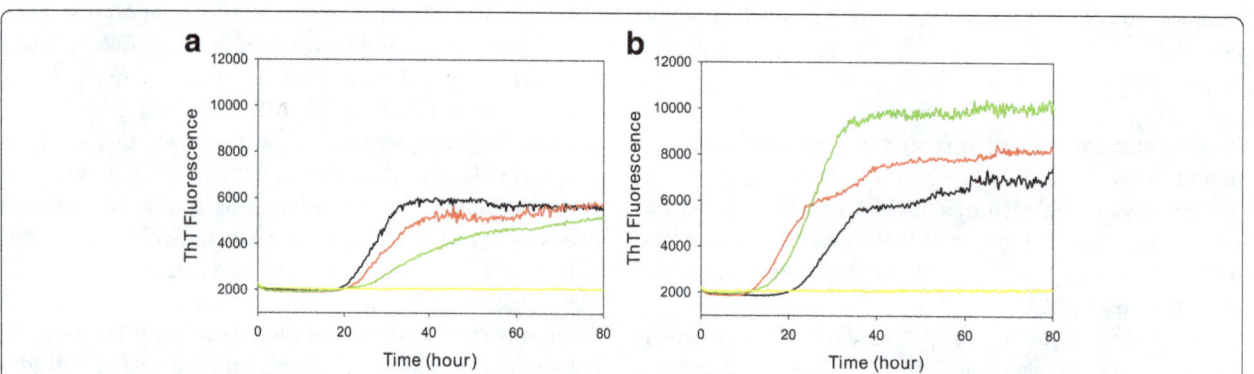

Fig. 5 RT-QuIC detection of seeding activity in elk brain samples using mature length recombinant elk prion protein 132 L (**a**) and 132 M (**b**) substrates. RT-QuIC assays seeded with MM132 (green), LM132 (red), LL132 (black) or negative seed (yellow) are shown. RT-QuIC reaction mixtures were seeded with 10^{-2} dilutions of normalized brain homogenate. A final 400 mM NaCl was used with each substrate. Data are presented as mean ThT fluorescence of quadruplicate reactions

animals there is preferential conversion of the PrP^C moiety of the allele associated with a higher susceptibility to disease [18, 27]. Since the biological behavior of scrapie prions in sheep and CWD prions in cervids are similar, it seems reasonable to assume that the conversion efficiency of elk CWD prions has a sequence dependence similar to sheep scrapie prions. The brain homogenate used to inoculate the elk was prepared from pooled brain material from one MM132 and one LM132 elk. Titration of brain homogenate was not performed prior to pooling. Based on observations in sheep [18, 27] it is probable that the PrP^{Sc} in the LM132 brain was predominantly PrP$^{Sc-132M}$ and therefore that the pooled brain homogenate contained mostly PrP$^{Sc-132M}$. This PrP$^{Sc-132M}$ would propagate more efficiently in elk expressing PrP^{C-132M} than those expressing PrP^{C-132L} or a mixture of PrP^{C-132M} and PrP^{C-132L}. Experimental challenge of elk of each genotype with brain homogenates from homozygous and heterozygous donors may help to elucidate the relative contribution of donor and recipient *PRNP* genotypes to incubation time in CWD-affected elk.

If relative incubation period reflects the relative permissibility of elk of different *PRNP* genotypes to PrP^{Sc} accumulation and by extension, their susceptibility to disease, our findings support previous CWD surveys that have shown that MM132 elk are most susceptible to CWD, the susceptibility of LM132 elk is intermediate, and LL132 elk are least susceptible to CWD [31, 41]. These findings suggest that genetic selection for the L132 allele has the potential to reduce the impact of CWD in captive and free-ranging elk populations, although it should be kept in mind that the protective effects of the L132 allele against CWD prions are not absolute [4, 7]. The elk breeding facility from which the elk calves for this experiment were obtained was known to have a high prevalence of CWD [14] so infection of elk calves with CWD prior to being moved to the quarantine facility at 8 months of age cannot be ruled out. However, since incubation periods for elk within each genotype group were similar to each other and different to elk of different genotypes, it appears that potential infection at the breeding facility did not influence the outcome of experimental infection at the quarantine facility in this study.

We have shown that the fibril stability of PrP^{Sc} from elk with shorter incubation periods (i.e. MM132 and LM132) is lower, while PrP^{Sc} fibrils from elk with longer incubation periods (LL132) are more stable. These observations are in agreement with previous observations in mice challenged with synthetic [24] and mouse-adapted [1, 25] prion strains, and in sheep challenged with different scrapie isolates [45]. It is hypothesized that lower fibril stability leads to increased PrP^{Sc} fibril fragmentation that facilitates the conversion of PrP^C to

PrP^{Sc} and results in faster replication of PrP^{Sc} and reduced incubation periods [42, 51]. However, an inverse relationship between incubation period and fibril stability – that is, PrP^{Sc} from animals with shorter incubation periods is more stable – has been observed in Syrian hamsters challenged with hamster adapted scrapie or transmissible mink encephalopathy strains [35], sheep with naturally occurring classical or Nor98 scrapie [37, 48], and cattle challenged with classical or atypical (H-type) bovine spongiform encephalopathy [44]. These variable relationships between incubation period and fibril stability suggest that factors other than, or in addition to, fibril stability of PrP^{Sc} can influence incubation periods.

Western blot analyses of brain samples from elk in this study have been published previously [14, 28]. The three characteristic bands of the proteinase-resistant core of PrP^{Sc} were observed in all elk and samples from MM132 and LM132 elk showed similar migration profiles, glycoform ratios, and N-terminal cleavage sites [14, 28]. However, samples from LL132 elk showed a significantly lower mean apparent molecular mass compared to MM132 and LM132 elk; this was associated with cleavage near residues 98–113 [28], as compared to cleavage at residues 78 and 82 in MM132 elk [50]. Therefore, similar to fibril stability and amyloid formation rate, western blot phenotype does appear to be a strongly associated with differences in incubation periods in MM132 and LM132 elk.

Until now, RT-QuIC applications in cervids have mainly focused on detection of small amounts of prions in fluids and tissues relevant to pre-clinical diagnosis of disease or disease transmission: urine [15, 20], feces [4, 20], saliva [15, 16], blood [6], cerebrospinal fluid [13], rectal biopsy and nasal brush samples [11, 12]. RT-QuIC has also been utilized for the discrimination of subtypes of bovine spongiform encephalopathy (BSE) [17, 26, 33].

To investigate if conversion efficiency of PrP^{Sc} influences incubation period, real-time quaking induced conversion (RT-QuIC) was performed using recombinant mature length elk prion protein (132 L and 132 M) seeded with brain homogenates from one elk of each genotype. These experiments revealed differences in the ability of PrP^{Sc} seed from CWD-infected elk of different genotypes to convert recombinant elk prion substrate. The MM132 or LM132 seeds convert 132 M substrate protein readily, whereas LL132 seed is much slower to do so. In contrast, all seeds convert 132 L substrate protein although the LL132 seed exhibited the fastest conversion. This conversion data suggests two potential hypotheses: (a) there are two distinct and stably propagating conformations of elk PrP^{Sc} present, one that is adopted more readily by 132 M protein and one that is adopted more readily by 132 L protein; or (b) the differences in conversion rate (both in the animal and in RT-QuIC) are the result of genotype mismatches between seed PrP^{Sc} and substrate. The similar lag phases observed with MM132 and LM132 seed are consistent with previously reported RT-QuIC analyses [10] and the fibril stability results reported here, and may provide further evidence that the LM132 seed contains a relatively large proportion of PrP$^{Sc-132M}$. The results of the stability assay also provide evidence that there are two conformations with distinct molecular properties, but future investigations are needed to explore this question. Inoculation of both the MM132 and LL132 seeds into transgenic mice carrying the elk prion gene will be useful in assessing differences in PrP^{Sc} fibril stability and incubation times upon serial passage into mice of a single *PRNP* genotype.

PrP^{Sc} from CWD-infected LL132 elk shares a number of immunohistochemical features with the ovine scrapie strain CH1641, namely a loss of the epitope for the anti-PrP monoclonal antibody P4 that binds PrP residues 93–99 [43], and reduced but detectable immunoreactivity with the monoclonal antibody 8G8 (that binds residues 98–113 [22]) [19, 28]. The phenotype of PrP^{Sc} accumulation in the brain of sheep with CH1641 is characterized by prominent intracellular immunoreactivity in neurons and glial cells, and relatively little extracellular immunoreactivity [19]. Intraneuronal PrP^{Sc} accumulation is rare in MM132 and LM132 elk with CWD [14] but was commonly observed in the LL132 elk in this study. Furthermore, glial-associated immunolabeling was prominent in LL132 elk and not observed in MM132 or LM132 elk.

Conclusions

This study provides further evidence of the importance of *PRNP* genotype in the pathogenesis of CWD of elk. We have shown that the biochemical properties of PrP^{Sc} from MM132 and LM132 elk are similar to each other and different to PrP^{Sc} from LL132 elk. The shorter incubation periods in MM132 compared to LM132 elk may be the result of genotype-dependent differences in the efficiency of propagation of PrP^{Sc} moieties present in the inoculum. Further work is needed to develop a better understanding of the underlying mechanisms by which the polymorphisms at codon 132 in elk *PRNP* influence disease pathogenesis, with a view to improving control of CWD in captive and free-ranging elk populations.

Abbreviations

CWD: Chronic wasting disease; EIA: Antigen-capture enzyme immunoassay; MPI: Months postinoculation; *PRNP*: Prion protein gene; PrP^C: Cellular prion protein, not associated with disease; PrP^{Sc}: Disease-associated prion protein; RAMALT: Recto-anal lymphoid tissue; RT-QuIC: Real-time quaking induced conversion; TSE: Transmissible spongiform encephalopathy; vCJD: variant Creutzfeldt-Jakob disease

Acknowledgements

We would like to thank Trudy Tatum for optimizing and performing the EIA assays, and Joe Lesan, Leisa Mandell, Kevin Hassall and Semakelang Lebepe-Mazur for excellent technical support.

Funding

This research was funded in its entirety by congressionally appropriated funds to the United States Department of Agriculture, Agricultural Research Service. The funders of the work did not influence study design, data collection and analysis, decision to publish, or the preparation of the manuscript.

Disclaimer

Mention of trade names or commercial products in this publication is solely for the purpose of providing specific information and does not imply recommendation or endorsement by the U.S. Department of Agriculture. USDA is an equal opportunity provider and employer.

Authors' contributions

SJM drafted the manuscript and performed the microscopic examinations. CEV performed fibril stability assays and assisted with the drafting of the manuscript. SH performed the RT-QuIC experiments and assisted with the drafting of the manuscript. MHWG contributed to data analysis and critically revised the manuscript. JJG and EN designed the study, supervised the work, and critically revised the manuscript. All authors read and approved the final manuscript.

Consent for publication

Not applicable.

Competing interests

The authors declare that they have no competing interests.

Author details

[1]USDA, Agricultural Research Service, National Animal Disease Center, Virus and Prion Research Unit, Ames, USA. [2]Department of Biomedical Sciences, College of Veterinary Medicine, Iowa State University, Ames, USA.

References

1. Bett C, Joshi-Barr S, Lucero M, Trejo M, Liberski P, Kelly JW, Masliah E, Sigurdson CJ. Biochemical properties of highly neuroinvasive prion strains. PLoS Pathog. 2012;8(2):e1002522.
2. Bossers A, Belt P, Raymond GJ, Caughey B, de Vries R, Smits MA. Scrapie susceptibility-linked polymorphisms modulate the *in vitro* conversion of sheep prion protein to protease-resistant forms. Proc Natl Acad Sci U S A. 1997;94(10):4931–6.
3. Bossers A, de Vries R, Smits MA. Susceptibility of sheep for scrapie as assessed by *in vitro* conversion of nine naturally occurring variants of PrP. J Virol. 2000;74(3):1407–14.
4. Cheng YC, Hannaoui S, John TR, Dudas S, Czub S, Gilch S. Early and non-invasive detection of chronic wasting disease prions in elk feces by real-time quaking induced conversion. PLoS One. 2016;11(11):e0166187.
5. Dassanayake RP, Orru CD, Hughson AG, Caughey B, Graca T, Zhuang D, Madsen-Bouterse SA, Knowles DP, Schneider DA. Sensitive and specific detection of classical scrapie prions in the brains of goats by real-time

quaking-induced conversion. J Gen Virol. 2016;97(3):803–12.

6. Elder AM, Henderson DM, Nalls AV, Wilham JM, Caughey BW, Hoover EA, Kincaid AE, Bartz JC, Mathiason CK. In vitro detection of prionemia in TSE-infected cervids and hamsters. PLoS One. 2013;8(11):e80203.

7. Green KM, Browning SR, Seward TS, Jewell JE, Ross DL, Green MA, Williams ES, Hoover EA, Telling GC. The elk PRNP codon 132 polymorphism controls cervid and scrapie prion propagation. J Gen Virol. 2008;89(Pt 2):598–608.

8. Greenlee JJ, Smith JD, Kunkle RA. White-tailed deer are susceptible to the agent of sheep scrapie by intracerebral inoculation. Vet Res. 2011;42(1):107.

9. Greenlee JJ, Smith JD, West Greenlee MH, Nicholson EM. Clinical and pathologic features of H-type bovine spongiform encephalopathy associated with E211K prion protein polymorphism. PLoS One. 2012;7(6): e38678.

10. Haley NJ, Rielinger R, Davenport KA, O'Rourke K, Mitchell G, Richt JA. Estimating chronic wasting disease susceptibility in cervids using real-time quaking-induced conversion. J Gen Virol. 2017;98(11):2882–92.

11. Haley NJ, Siepker C, Hoon-Hanks LL, Mitchell G, Walter WD, Manca M, Monello RJ, Powers JG, Wild MA, Hoover EA, Caughey B, Richt JA. Seeded amplification of chronic wasting disease prions in nasal brushings and recto-anal mucosa-associated lymphoid tissues from elk by real-time quaking-induced conversion. J Clin Microbiol. 2016;54(4):1117–26.

12. Haley NJ, Siepker C, Walter WD, Thomsen BV, Greenlee JJ, Lehmkuhl AD, Richt JA. Antemortem detection of chronic wasting disease prions in nasal brush collections and rectal biopsy specimens from white-tailed deer by real-time quaking-induced conversion. J Clin Microbiol. 2016;54(4):1108–16.

13. Haley NJ, Van de Motter A, Carver S, Henderson D, Davenport K, Seelig DM, Mathiason C, Hoover E. Prion-seeding activity in cerebrospinal fluid of deer with chronic wasting disease. PLoS One. 2013;8(11):e81488.

14. Hamir AN, Gidlewski T, Spraker TR, Miller JM, Creekmore L, Crocheck M, Cline T, O'Rourke KI. Preliminary observations of genetic susceptibility of elk (Cervus elaphus nelsoni) to chronic wasting disease by experimental oral inoculation. J Vet Diagn Investig. 2006;18(1):110–4.

15. Henderson DM, Davenport KA, Haley NJ, Denkers ND, Mathiason CK, Hoover EA. Quantitative assessment of prion infectivity in tissues and body fluids by real-time quaking-induced conversion. J Gen Virol. 2015;96(Pt 1):210–9.

16. Henderson DM, Manca M, Haley NJ, Denkers ND, Nalls AV, Mathiason CK, Caughey B, Hoover EA. Rapid antemortem detection of CWD prions in deer saliva. PLoS One. 2013;8(9):e74377.

17. Hwang S, Greenlee JJ, Nicholson EM. Use of bovine recombinant prion protein and real-time quaking-induced conversion to detect cattle transmissible mink encephalopathy prions and discriminate classical and atypical L- and H-type bovine spongiform encephalopathy. PLoS One. 2017; 12(2):e0172391.

18. Jacobs JG, Bossers A, Rezaei H, van Keulen LJ, McCutcheon S, Sklaviadis T, Lantier I, Berthon P, Lantier F, van Zijderveld FG, Langeveld JP. Proteinase K-resistant material in ARR/VRQ sheep brain affected with classical scrapie is composed mainly of VRQ prion protein. J Virol. 2011;85(23):12537–46.

19. Jeffrey M, Gonzalez L, Chong A, Foster J, Goldmann W, Hunter N, Martin S. Ovine infection with the agents of scrapie (CH1641 isolate) and bovine spongiform encephalopathy: immunochemical similarities can be resolved by immunohistochemistry. J Comp Pathol. 2006;134(1):17–29.

20. John TR, Schatzl HM, Gilch S. Early detection of chronic wasting disease prions in urine of pre-symptomatic deer by real-time quaking-induced conversion assay. Prion. 2013;7(3):253–8.

21. Kirby L, Goldmann W, Houston F, Gill AC, Manson JC. A novel, resistance-linked ovine PrP variant and its equivalent mouse variant modulate the in vitro cell-free conversion of rPrP to PrP(res). J Gen Virol. 2006;87(Pt 12): 3747–51.

22. Krasemann S, Groschup MH, Harmeyer S, Hunsmann G, Bodemer W. Generation of monoclonal antibodies against human prion proteins in PrP$^{0/0}$ mice. Mol Med. 1996;2(6):725–34.

23. Lee HS, Brown P, Cervenakova L, Garruto RM, Alpers MP, Gajdusek DC, Goldfarb LG. Increased susceptibility to kuru of carriers of the PRNP 129 methionine/methionine genotype. J Infect Dis. 2001;183(2):192–6.

24. Legname G, Nguyen HO, Baskakov IV, Cohen FE, Dearmond SJ, Prusiner SB. Strain-specified characteristics of mouse synthetic prions. Proc Natl Acad Sci U S A. 2005;102(6):2168–73.

25. Legname G, Nguyen HO, Peretz D, Cohen FE, DeArmond SJ, Prusiner SB. Continuum of prion protein structures enciphers a multitude of prion isolate-specified phenotypes. Proc Natl Acad Sci U S A. 2006;103(50):19105–10.

26. Masujin K, Orru CD, Miyazawa K, Groveman BR, Raymond LD, Hughson AG, Caughey B. Detection of atypical H-type bovine spongiform encephalopathy and discrimination of bovine prion strains by real-time quaking-induced conversion. J Clin Microbiol. 2016;54(3):676–86.

27. Morel N, Andreoletti O, Grassi J, Clement G. Absolute and relative quantification of sheep brain prion protein (PrP) allelic variants by matrix-assisted laser desorption/ionisation time-of-flight mass spectrometry. Rapid Commun Mass Spectrom. 2007;21(24):4093–100.

28. O'Rourke K, Spraker T, Zhuang D, Greenlee J, Gidlewski T, Hamir A. Elk with a long incubation prion disease phenotype have a unique PrP^d profile. Cell Mol Dev Neurosci. 2007;18(18):1935–8.

29. O'Rourke KI, Baszler TV, Besser TE, Miller JM, Cutlip RC, Wells GA, Ryder SJ, Parish SM, Hamir AN, Cockett NE, Jenny A, Knowles DP. Preclinical diagnosis of scrapie by immunohistochemistry of third eyelid lymphoid tissue. J Clin Microbiol. 2000;38(9):3254–9.

30. O'Rourke KI, Baszler TV, Miller JM, Spraker TR, Sadler-Riggleman I, Knowles DP. Monoclonal antibody F89/160.1.5 defines a conserved epitope on the ruminant prion protein. J Clin Microbiol. 1998;36(6):1750–5.

31. O'Rourke KI, Besser TE, Miller MW, Cline TF, Spraker TR, Jenny AL, Wild MA, Zebarth GL, Williams ES. PrP genotypes of captive and free-ranging Rocky Mountain elk (Cervus elaphus nelsoni) with chronic wasting disease. J Gen Virol. 1999;80(Pt 10):2765–9.

32. Orru CD, Bongianni M, Tonoli G, Ferrari S, Hughson AG, Groveman BR, Fiorini M, Pocchiari M, Monaco S, Caughey B, Zanusso G. A test for Creutzfeldt-Jakob disease using nasal brushings. N Engl J Med. 2014;371(6): 519–29.

33. Orru CD, Favole A, Corona C, Mazza M, Manca M, Groveman BR, Hughson AG, Acutis PL, Caramelli M, Zanusso G, Casalone C, Caughey B. Detection and discrimination of classical and atypical L-type bovine spongiform encephalopathy by real-time quaking-induced conversion. J Clin Microbiol. 2015;53(4):1115–20.

34. Orru CD, Groveman BR, Hughson AG, Zanusso G, Coulthart MB, Caughey B. Rapid and sensitive RT-QuIC detection of human Creutzfeldt-Jakob disease using cerebrospinal fluid. MBio. 2015;6(1) https://doi.org/10.1128/mBio. 02451-14.

35. Peretz D, Williamson RA, Legname G, Matsunaga Y, Vergara J, Burton DR, DeArmond SJ, Prusiner SB, Scott MR. A change in the conformation of prions accompanies the emergence of a new prion strain. Neuron. 2002; 34(6):921–32.

36. Perucchini M, Griffin K, Miller MW, Goldmann W. PrP genotypes of free-ranging wapiti (Cervus elaphus nelsoni) with chronic wasting disease. J Gen Virol. 2008;89(Pt 5):1324–8.

37. Pirisinu L, Di Bari M, Marcon S, Vaccari G, D'Agostino C, Fazzi P, Esposito E, Galeno R, Langeveld J, Agrimi U, Nonno R. A new method for the characterization of strain-specific conformational stability of protease-sensitive and protease-resistant PrP. PLoS One. 2010;5(9):e12723.

38. Saba R, Booth SA. The genetics of susceptibility to variant Creutzfeldt-Jakob disease. Public Health Genomics. 2013;16(1–2):17–24.

39. Schätzl HM, Da Costa M, Taylor L, Cohen FE, Prusiner SB. Prion protein gene variation among primates. J Mol Biol. 1997;265(2):257.

40. Schätzl HM, Wopfner F, Gilch S, von Brunn A, Jager G. Is codon 129 of prion protein polymorphic in human beings but not in animals? Lancet. 1997; 349(9065):1603–4.

41. Spraker TR, Balachandran A, Zhuang D, O'Rourke KI. Variable patterns of distribution of PrP(CWD) in the obex and cranial lymphoid tissues of Rocky Mountain elk (Cervus elaphus nelsoni) with subclinical chronic wasting disease. Vet Rec. 2004;155(10):295–302.

42. Sun Y, Makarava N, Lee CI, Laksanalamai P, Robb FT, Baskakov IV. Conformational stability of PrP amyloid fibrils controls their smallest possible fragment size. J Mol Biol. 2008;376(4):1155–67.

43. Thuring CM, Erkens JH, Jacobs JG, Bossers A, Van Keulen LJ, Garssen GJ, Van Zijderveld FG, Ryder SJ, Groschup MH, Sweeney T, Langeveld JP. Discrimination between scrapie and bovine spongiform encephalopathy in sheep by molecular size, immunoreactivity, and glycoprofile of prion protein. J Clin Microbiol. 2004;42(3):972–80.

44. Vrentas CE, Greenlee JJ, Baron T, Caramelli M, Czub S, Nicholson EM. Stability properties of PrP(Sc) from cattle with experimental transmissible spongiform encephalopathies: use of a rapid whole homogenate, protease-free assay. BMC Vet Res. 2013;9:167.

45. Vrentas CE, Greenlee JJ, Tatum TL, Nicholson EM. Relationships between PrP^{Sc} stability and incubation time for United States scrapie isolates in a

natural host system. PLoS One. 2012;7(8):e43060.

46. Vrentas CE, Onstot S, Nicholson EM. A comparative analysis of rapid methods for purification and refolding of recombinant bovine prion protein. Protein Expr Purif. 2012;82(2):380–8.

47. Watts JC, Prusiner SB. Mouse models for studying the formation and propagation of prions. J Biol Chem. 2014;289(29):19841–9.

48. Wemheuer WM, Benestad SL, Wrede A, Schulze-Sturm U, Wemheuer WE, Hahmann U, Gawinecka J, Schutz E, Zerr I, Brenig B, Bratberg B, Andreoletti O, Schulz-Schaeffer WJ. Similarities between forms of sheep scrapie and Creutzfeldt-Jakob disease are encoded by distinct prion types. Am J Pathol. 2009;175(6):2566–73.

49. Williams ES, Young S. Spongiform encephalopathy of Rocky Mountain elk. J Wildl Dis. 1982;18(4):465–71.

50. Xie Z, O'Rourke KI, Dong Z, Jenny AL, Langenberg JA, Belay ED, Schonberger LB, Petersen RB, Zou W, Kong Q, Gambetti P, Chen SG. Chronic wasting disease of elk and deer and Creutzfeldt-Jakob disease: comparative analysis of the scrapie prion protein. J Biol Chem. 2006;281(7):4199–206.

51. Zampieri M, Legname G, Altafini C. Investigating the conformational stability of prion strains through a kinetic replication model. PLoS Comput Biol. 2009;5(7):e1000420.

23

First report on nasal myiasis in an alpaca *"Vicugna pacos"*

Teresa Maria Punsmann*[iD], Lucie Marie Grimm, Carolin Reckmann, Cornelia Schwennen, Matthias Gerhard Wagener and Martin Ganter

Abstract

Background: An infestation of bot fly larvae causes myiasis which is known to cause respiratory symptoms in ruminants. There are reports of bot fly larvae in llamas, but to our knowledge there are no previous reports of nasal myiasis due to bot flies in alpacas (*"Vicugna pacos"*).

Case presentation: The following case report describes a neutered male alpaca showing sneezing and mild nasal discharge. Endoscopic examination of the upper respiratory tract revealed bot fly larvae in one nostril. After treatment with doramectin, there was no evidence of living bot fly larvae visible in the nostril.

Conclusion: Bot fly larvae should be considered as a potential cause of respiratory symptoms in alpacas. In the present case, a treatment with doramectin was successful.

Keywords: Alpaca, New world camelids, Bot flies, Treatment, Doramectin, Germany

Background

In New World camelids bot flies play a role causing parasite-induced respiratory symptoms [1]. However, case reports of myiasis due to bot flies in New World camelids are rare. All reports published to date deal with nasal bots in llamas. There are, in total, four described cases of bot fly larvae in llamas in the United States and South America [2–4]. The animals were presented because of respiratory symptoms like sneezing and nasal discharge, which were not responsive to antibiotic treatment. In cases where the causative species could be isolated, *Oestrus ovis* (sheep and goat bot fly) [3] and *Cephenemyia* spp. (deer bot flies) were identified [4]. In two cases, the species remained unknown [2].

Oestrus ovis is a common parasite in sheep and goats. The adult fly shoots larvae onto the area around the nostrils of the affected animals, whence the larvae move into the nasal cavity where they become mature. When they become the third instar larvae they fall to the ground and pupate in the environment [1]. *Cephenemyia* spp. larvae are shot by the flies directly into the nasal cavity where they remain until they reach the third larval

stage. The third instar larvae is sneezed out into the environment where they pupate [1].

Cephenemyia spp. lead to worse reactions in New World camelids than in deer. In the nasal meatus a granulomatous swelling evolves [1, 4].

Knowledge about the life cycle of bot flies in llamas and alpacas is insufficient and further investigations are needed.

In Old World camelids myiasis can be caused by *Cephalopina titillator* [5]. Infections of New World camelids with this species have not been described.

As there are only few described cases of myiasis caused by bot flies in New World camelids recommendations for treatment are rare. In one llama [3] bot fly larvae were identified during necropsy after the animal had died due to haemorrhagic pneumonia. Therefore, no specific treatment was provided. The other affected animals were treated with ivermectin 0.2 mg/kg. In one llama the treatment had to be repeated and combined with local ivermectin administration in order to kill the larvae [2]. One llama, which had been successfully treated subcutaneously with ivermectin, died shortly afterwards due to unknown reasons [2]. To date a treatment with doramectin against bot fly larvae in New World camelids has not been described, while in sheep

* Correspondence: teresa.maria.punsmann@tiho-hannover.de
Clinic for Swine, Small Ruminants and Forensic Medicine, University of Veterinary Medicine Hannover, Foundation, Hannover, Germany

it is described as an effective drug against *Oestrus ovis* at a dosage of 200 µg/kg [6].

This case report gives the first clinical description of bot flies in an alpaca.

Case description

A five-year-old neutered male huacaya-alpaca showing sneezing for three weeks was presented to the Clinic for Swine, Small Ruminants and Forensic Medicine, University of Veterinary Medicine Hannover, Foundation, Germany. The alpaca was privately owned and kept on pasture together with four female alpacas. The sneezing was noticed for the first time by the owner about two to three weeks before presenting the animal to the clinic. He reported sneezing fits lasting up to two hours. Apart from that, the general condition of the animal was good. The four female alpacas did not show any symptoms to the author's knowledge.

The alpaca had serous, clear nasal discharge coming out of both nostrils. During examination sneezing could be triggered by applying pressure to the bridge of the nose. The distending of the nostrils indicated that breathing was impeded (Fig. 1). Auscultation of the lung revealed physiologically mild respiratory sounds on both sides.

The analysis of blood samples and faeces showed mild anaemia, granulocytosis and lymphopenia (Table 1). Eosinophils were not increased above the upper reference limits [7]. Clinical chemistry revealed slight hyperproteinaemia, hyperalbuminaemia, hypercalcaemia and hypophosphataemia (Table 1). In the faecal sample a very low number of gastrointestinal nematode eggs was found.

Endoscopic examination of the nose was carried out. Due to the tension of the alpaca, the examination was conducted under general anaesthesia (0.4 mg/kg xylazine [Xylavet 20 mg/ml®, CP-Pharma, Burgdorf, Germany], 4 mg/kg ketamine [Ketamidor 100 mg/ml®, WDT,

Table 1 Haematology and clinical chemistry of the alpaca

	Unit	Reference	Patient
Haematology			
Haemoglobin	g/L	127–166	124
PCV	L/L	0.29–0.37	0.28
MCHC	g/L	414–459	443
Leucozytes	G/L	9.8–15.8	14.9
Neutrophils	G/L	4.5–9.3	10.9
Band neutrophils	G/L	0–0.1	0.07
Lymphocytes	G/L	1.7–4.5	1.1
Monocytes	G/L	0.1–0.7	0.4
Eosinophils	G/L	1–3.6	2.2
Basophils	G/L	0–0.3	0.2
Neutrophils	%	44–70.5	73
Band neutrophils	%	0–1	0.5
Lymphocytes	%	15.2–31	7.5
Monocytes	%	2–5.5	2.5
Eosinophils	%	8–27	15
Basophils	%	0–2	1.5
Clinical chemistry			
Total protein	g/L	59.9–69.1	74.3
Albumin	g/L	31.3–38.6	46.7
Creatinine	µmol/L	97–167	142
Urea	mmol/L	5.2–9.7	4.9
Calcium	mmol/L	2.2–2.5	2.7
Phosphorus	mmol/L	1.6–3	1.5

References from [7]. Only small deviations from reference range were found in the alpaca affected by bot fly larvae

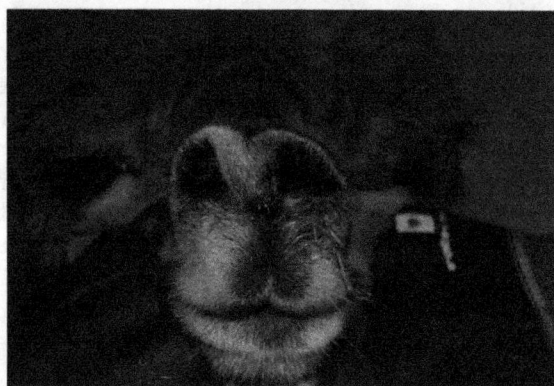

Fig. 1 The affected alpaca showing serous nasal discharge and impeded breathing

Garbsen, Germany]) [1], [8] and local anaesthesia of the nostrils (Procainhydrochlorid, Epinephrin [Isocain ad us. vet.®, Selectavet, Dr. Otto Fischer GmbH, Weyarn/ Holzolling, Germany]). The endoscope was inserted approximately 15 cm into the right ventral nasal meatus. At this position a soft tissue mass originating from the nasal mucosa was observed. There were no signs of an acute inflammation at this location. The mass filled out about a third of the lumen of the meatus and at least four living larvae were revealed in this tissue (Fig. 2). No larvae could be removed due to technical reasons. Examination of the left nostril was not carried out because bleeding and noticeable mucosal irritation occurred while examining the right nostril. Under general anaesthesia radiographs of the head were taken. No abnormal radiopaque structures could be found on the radiographs.

The alpaca was treated subcutaneously with doramectin by a dose of 0.2 mg/kg (Dectomax®, Lilly Deutschland GmbH, Elanco Animal Health, Bad Homburg, Germany).

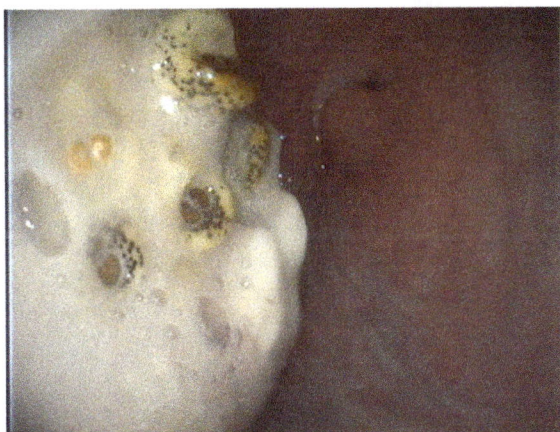

Fig. 2 Endoscopic picture of the right ventral meatus from the affected alpaca before treatment. A soft tissue mass with moving larvae was found

Five days after treatment, sneezing could not be triggered any more by pressing on the bridge of the nose. Six days after treatment another endoscopic examination under local anaesthesia (Isocain ad us. vet.®) was carried out. Compared to the first examination, the soft tissue mass had notably decreased; there were no more larvae visible within the mass (Fig. 3).

In the endoscopy before the treatment with doramectin no larvae could be removed and, in addition, no larvae were sneezed out, so species of the bots could not be determined.

Discussion

To the authors' knowledge the present case is the first report of respiratory symptoms due to bot fly larvae in an alpaca. To date it is mentioned, that *Oestrus ovis* and

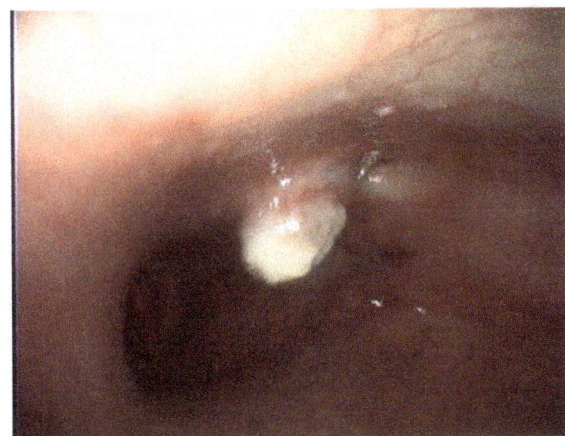

Fig. 3 Endoscopic picture of the right ventral meatus from the affected alpaca after treatment. The soft tissue mass has decreased and no more larvae were found

Cephenemyia spp. are ectoparasites alpacas are exposed to [9], but no clinical symptoms are outlined. Additionally, it is the first published successful treatment of bot flies in New World camelids using doramectin.

In order to determine the causative species which has caused the alterations of the mucosa we tried to remove the larvae endoscopically. The larvae could not be gripped successful and additionally bleeding and swelling of the mucosa occurred. In some of the reported cases respiratory distress leading to a tracheotomy was caused by trying to remove larvae from the nostrils [2, 4]. To avoid such a serious intervention the attempt to remove the larvae was interrupted. Moreover, no larvae were found in the stable, so the species could not be identified. Both bot fly species which have been found in llamas (*Cephenemyia* spp. and *Oestrus ovis*) occur in Germany. The Camel nasal bot fly (*Cephalopina titillator*) occurs in large parts of Africa, Asia, Australia and the Middle East. Central Europe is not the natural habitat of this species [10]. An indication as to the identity of the causative bot fly species may be seen in the fact that the neutered male alpaca did not have any contact to sheep, but as it was kept on pasture with contact to deer, the end host of *Cephenemyia* spp.. Another hint to the causal species in the present case is the severe swelling within the nostril. It is known that *Cephenemyia* spp. in New World camelids cause a severe reaction, with noticeable swelling and granulation tissue [1, 4]. If it was *Oestrus ovis* the button in the posterior spiracular plate would be located in the center of the plate [10, 11]. In the photographs taken during endoscopy the buttons seem to be located at the medial border of the plate. This finding supports the suspicion, that the bot fly causing the myiasis could be *Cephenemyia* spp..

The small deviations from the reference range found in the haematology and clinical chemistry are not associated with the occurrence of bot fly larvae according to the current state of knowledge.

The formerly described cases of bot flies fly larvae in llamas were treated with ivermectin [2, 4], but this treatment was not successful after one administration in all cases. As alternative therapy we decided to use doramectin, as doramectin is an effective drug against myiasis due to bot flies in sheep. In sheep a dosage of 200 µg/kg has a sufficient effect on *Oestrus ovis* [6]. As such a dosage has no negative effects on alpacas [1] the alpaca in the present case was treated subcutaneously with doramectin 200 µg/kg. A single treatment was successful, the sneezing stopped, no larvae could be found within the nostril and the swelling decreased.

Conclusion

This case report describes the first clinical finding of myiasis caused by bot flies in an alpaca. Additionally it is the first description of a successful treatment with doramectin. Bot fly larvae should be perceived as a differential diagnosis when an alpaca is presented with nonspecific respiratory symptoms, especially sneezing.

Acknowledgements
We would like to thank our animal keepers Tanja Bode and Thorsten Waßmann for helping during treatment and examination of the alpaca and our laboratory staff for their prompt and reliable work. Furthermore we would like to thank Frances Sherwood-Brock, English editorial office, University of Veterinary Medicine Hannover, Foundation, Germany, for proofreading the manuscript.

Funding
Not applicable.

Authors' contributions
TP, LG, CS, MW and MG dealt with the case. TP drafted the manuscript. CR was involved in drafting the manuscript and revised it critically. All authors reviewed and approved the final manuscript.

Consent for publication
The owner of the alpaca gave written consent for publication.

Competing interests
The authors declare that they have no competing interests.

References
1. Fowler ME. Medicine and surgery of camelids. 3 ed. Wiley-Blackwell, 2010.
2. Belknap EB. Medical problems of llamas. The Veterinary clinics of North America: Food animal practice. 1994;10(2):291–307.
3. Gomez-Puerta LA, Alroy KA, Ticona DS, Lopez-Urbina MT, Gonzalez AE. A case of nasal myiasis due to Oestrus ovis (Diptera: Oestridae) in a llama (Lama glama). Rev Bras Parasitol Vet. 2013;22(4):608–10.
4. Mattoon JS, Gerros TC, Parker JE, Carter CA, LaMarche RM. Upper airway obstruction in a llama caused by aberrant nasopharyngeal bots (Cephenemyia sp.). Vet Radiol Ultrasound. 1997;38(5):384–6.
5. Oryan A, Valinezhad A, Moraveji M. Prevalence and pathology of camel nasal myiasis in eastern areas of Iran. Trop Biomed. 2008;25(1):30–6.
6. Dorchies P, Jacquiet P, Bergeaud J, Duranton C, Prévot F, Alzieu J, et al. Efficacy of doramectin injectable against Oestrus ovis and gastrointestinal nematodes in sheep in the southwestern region of France. Vet Parasitol. 2001;96(2):147–54.
7. Hengrave Burri I, Tschudi P, Martig J, Liesegang A, Meylan M. Neuweltkameliden in der Schweiz. II. Referenzwerte für hämatologische und blutchemische Parameter. Schweiz Arch Tierheilkd. 2005;147(8):335–43.
8. Gauly MV, Jane Cebra Christopher. Neuweltkameliden. Enke Stuttgart, 2011.
9. Bornstein S. (2010). Important ectoparasites of alpaca (Vicugna pacos). Acta Vet Scand. 2010;52(1):S17.
10. Taylor MA, Coop RL, Wall RL. Veterinary parasitology. 4th ed: Wiley Blackwell; 2016.
11. An Introduction to Medical Entomology. Key to 3rd stage larvae causing myiasis. http://www.faculty.ucr.edu/~legneref/medical/myiasisflieskey.htm. Accessed 17.10.2018.

24

Pathological changes and bacteriological assessments in the urinary tract of pregnant goats experimentally infected with *Brucella melitensis*

M. Mazlina[1,2], S. Khairani-Bejo[2], H. Hazilawati[2], T. Tiagarahan[3], N. N. Shaqinah[1] and M. Zamri-Saad[1,4*] (iD)

Abstract

Background: This study was conducted to investigate the pathological changes and distribution of *B. melitensis* in the urinary tract of pregnant goats following acute experimental infection. Six Jamnapari crossbred does in their third trimester of pregnancy were randomly assigned into two groups; Group 1 was uninfected control and Group 2 was inoculated conjunctival with 0.1 mL of the inoculums containing 10^9 cfu/mL of live *B. melitensis*. All does were sacrificed 30 days post-inoculation before the kidney, ureter, urinary bladder, urethra and vaginal swab were collected for isolation of *B. melitensis*. The same tissue samples were fixed in 10% neutral buffered formalin for hematoxylin and eosin, and immunoperoxidase staining.

Results: None of the goats showed clinical signs or gross lesions. The most consistent histopathology finding was the infiltration of mononuclear cells, chiefly the macrophages with few lymphocytes and occasionally neutrophils in all organs along the urinary tract of the infected goats of Group 2. Other histopathology findings included mild necrosis of the epithelial cells of the renal tubules, congestion and occasional haemorrhages in the various tissues. Kidneys showed the most severe lesions. Immunoperoxidase staining revealed the presence of *B. melitensis* within the infiltrating macrophages and the epithelium of renal tubules, ureter, urethra and urinary bladder. Most extensive distribution was observed in the urinary bladder. *Brucella melitensis* was successfully isolated at low concentration (3.4×10^3 cfu/g) in the various organs of the urinary tract and at high concentration (2.4×10^8 cfu/mL) in the vaginal swabs of all infected goats. Although *B. melitensis* was successfully isolated from the various organs of the urinary tract, it was not isolated from the urine samples that were collected from the urinary bladder at necropsy.

Conclusion: This study demonstrates the presence of low concentrations of *B. melitensis* in the organs of urinary tract of pregnant does, resulting in mild histopathology lesions. However, *B. melitensis* was not isolated from the urine that was collected from the urinary bladder.

Keywords: Histopathology, Immunoperoxidase, *Brucella melitensis*, Urinary tract, Goats

Background

Brucellosis is a zoonotic disease that causes chronic debilitating disease in humans and major economic losses to livestock farmers [1, 2]. Caprine brucellosis is caused by *Brucella melitensis*, which has been recognized as the most pathogenic species of the Genus *Brucella*. It is least host-specific and is associated with most cases of human brucellosis [3]. As an intracellular parasite, the bacterium is able to manipulate the host's immune system and flourishes within the professional and non-professional phagocytic cells. Thus, it can replicate within these cells since it is protected from the humoral antibodies and antibiotic treatments [4, 5].

In some cases, infected goats and sheep appear healthy with no apparent clinical sign but usually become

* Correspondence: mzamri@upm.edu.my
[1]Research Centre for Ruminant Diseases, Faculty of Veterinary Medicine, Universiti Putra Malaysia, 43400 Serdang, Selangor, Malaysia
[4]Department of Veterinary Laboratory Diagnosis, Faculty of Veterinary Medicine, Universiti Putra Malaysia, 43400 Serdang, Malaysia
Full list of author information is available at the end of the article

lifelong carriers that disseminate the disease [6]. Accurate detection followed by successful removal of carriers and infected animals are imperative to reduce the cases of brucellosis [6–8].

Brucellosis in animals has always been associated with the disorders of the reproductive and reticulo-endothelial systems [5] causing abortion and enlarged spleen and liver [1, 9, 10] and less frequently affecting the musculo-nervous systems [10, 11]. *Brucella*-induced urinary tract infection is considered extremely rare in animals and humans [12]. To the best of our knowledge, no comprehensive study was done to assess the lesions in the urinary system of female goats following infection with *B. melitensis*. Thus, this study was aimed at determining the distribution of *B. melitensis* and the associated lesions in the urinary tract of does following acute experimental infection with *B. melitensis* in the third trimester of pregnancy.

Methods
Bacterial inoculums

A local strain of *B. melitensis* that was isolated from an outbreak of caprine brucellosis in Malaysia was used in this study [13]. The isolate was cultured onto *Brucella* Agar (BBL™, UK) for 4 days at 37 °C and later transferred into *Brucella* broth (BBL™, UK) and was further incubated at 37 °C for another 4 days in an orbital shaker incubator (YIH-DER LM-510, Taiwan). The bacterial cells were then harvested following a series of washing with sterile PBS (pH 7.4) and centrifugation at 5,000×g, 4 °C for 10 min each cycle. The final pellet was then diluted in sterile PBS to a final bacterial concentration of 10^9 cells/mL using McFarland's Standard.

Preparation of hyperimmune serum against *Brucella melitensis*

The local strain of *B. melitensis* was grown in 35 mL of *Brucella* broth (BBL™, UK) in shaking incubator for 4 days at 37 °C. The bacterial concentration in the broth was determined using the standard total plate count method. The cells were re-suspended in sterile PBS to obtain a final concentration of 1×10^9 cfu/mL, were then killed by adding 0.5% formalin and were emulsified with Freund's complete adjuvant (FCA) (Sigma-Aldrich, US) at 1:1 ratio. One mL of the emulsion was injected subcutaneously into rabbits. Booster doses of the emulsified inoculums, prepared using Freund's incomplete adjuvant (FIA) (Sigma-Aldrich, US) were injected on days 14 and 21. Finally, the hyperimmune serum was harvested at 28 days post-inoculation. The Institutional Animal Care and Use Committee (IACUC) of Universiti Putra Malaysia approved this protocol (AUP No: R019/2014).

Animals and management

A total of 6 clinically healthy Jamnapari crossbred does of about 3–4 months pregnant were obtained from a farm with no history of brucellosis. They were subjected to the Rose Bengal Plate test (RBPT) and Complement Fixation test (CFT) to ensure the brucellosis-free status. The goats were then divided equally into 2 groups; the uninfected control (Group 1) and the infected (Group 2) groups. Does of Group 1 were exposed to 100 µL of sterile PBS via the conjunctiva sac. On the other hand, does of Group 2 were similarly exposed to 100 µL of the inoculums containing 10^9 cfu/mL of live *B. melitensis*. The infected does were kept entirely in a restricted and isolated housing facility while the control goats were kept separately in a raised house with slatted floor. All does were fed with Napier grass and supplemented with palm kernel cake at the rate of 400 g/animal/day while drinking water was available ad libitum.

Following the infection, the does were monitored twice daily for clinical signs especially abortion before they were euthanized 30 days post-inoculation. All euthanasia were carried out in an isolated area at a government slaughter house using the standard electrical stunning and exsanguinations protocol, where animals were unconscious following the stunning prior to exsanguination. Post-mortem was carried out immediately and the various sections of the urinary tract encompassing the kidneys, ureter, urinary bladder, urethra, urine and vaginal swabs were collected for bacterial isolation and identification, and for histopathology examination and immunoperoxidase staining. At the same time, urine samples were collected from the urinary bladder into a sterile bottle for bacteriological isolation. For comparison, the uterus and vaginal swabs were also collected and subjected to the same process. The Institutional Animal Care and Use Committee (IACUC) of Universiti Putra Malaysia approved this study (AUP No: R019/2014).

Histopathology

The formalin-fixed samples were processed in tissue processor (Leica TP 1020, Germany) and Tissue Embedding Console System (Leica EG1150) before they were embedded in paraffin wax and sectioned using the rotary microtome (Leica Jung Multicut 2045, Germany) at 4 µm thick. The mounted tissue sections were stained with Harris' haematoxylin and eosin (HE). The slides were viewed under light microscope (Nikon Eclipse 50i, Japan) installed with Nikon imaging software (NIS-Elements D 3.2, Japan). The histological changes were noted and scored as 0: none, 1: 30% affected, 2: 30–60% affected and 3: > more than 60% affected [3]. All evaluations were duplicated and 5 microscopic fields of each slide were randomly selected for lesion scoring. The scores were reported as the average value of each lesion and average value for overall scoring.

Immunoperoxidase staining

The formalin-fixed, paraffin-embedded sections were fixed on Poly-L-Lysine (Sigma- Aldrich, USA) coated microscope slides. Then they were subjected to deparaffinization and rehydration before antigen retrieval was done in citrate buffer for 10 min. Indigenous peroxidase was inactivated using 3% hydrogen peroxide followed by protein block with 5% bovine serum albumin for 15 min. Rabbit hyperimmune serum was used as the primary antibody at 1:100 dilution, incubated overnight at 4 °C. Then, secondary antibody, the goat anti-rabbit IgG (Abnova, Taiwan) diluted to 1:500 was poured and incubated for 30 min at 37 °C. All slides were developed with DAB Chromogen (Dako, USA) and counterstained with Harris' haematoxylin, dehydrated and mounted. Control sections used normal rabbit serum as primary antibody. The slides were viewed under light microscope (Nikon Eclipse 50i, Japan), which was installed with Nikon imaging software (NIS-Elements D 3.2, Japan). The presence and distribution of IP staining were scored as 0: none, 1: focal, 2: multifocal and 3: diffuse [14]. All evaluations were done in duplicate and 5 microscopic fields were randomly selected for lesion scoring. The scores were recorded as average value of each distribution and intensity.

Bacterial isolation from tissues

The tissue samples were flamed and then placed into sterile zipper plastic bags to minimize contamination. Then, sterile PBS (pH 7.4) was added into the zipper bag at tissue to PBS ratio of 1:2. The samples were then pounded using mortar and pestle. The resultant mixture was used for bacterial culture and extraction of bacterial DNA. The urine samples (4–5 mL) were collected using needle and syringe into a sterile tube and immediately transported to the laboratory. About 10 μL of the tissue mixture and urine sample was cultured onto *Brucella* agar that was pre-added with *Brucella* Selective Supplement (Oxoid, England) and incubated at 37 °C for 10 days. Bacterial colonies that appeared small, rounded, smooth and translucent, glistening and bluish were highly suggestive of *B. melitensis* [11] and were confirmed using PCR. The results were presented as percentage (%) of positive samples over total number of samples.

Bacterial DNA extraction

The bacterial DNA was extracted according to the manufacturer's recommendations (NucleoSpin® Tissue DNA Purification Kit, Macherey-Nagel, German). The extraction was initiated by adding 75 μL of the processed tissue with 25 μL of Proteinase K solution and 180 μL of lysis buffer (Buffer T1) followed by rigorous vortex

before incubation at 56 °C for 3 h to lyse the samples. The mixture was vortexed regularly during the incubation period. Then, 200 μL of Buffer B3 (Lysis buffer) was added, vortexed and incubated at 70 °C for 10 min. This was followed by adding 210 μL of absolute ethanol into the mixture and vortexed. The solution was transferred into tissue columns in collecting tubes and centrifuged for 1 min at 11,000 x *g*. The flow-through was discarded before the silica gel within the tissue column was washed twice; first by adding 500 μL of Buffer BW followed by centrifugation and later 600 μL of Buffer B5. Then, the mixture was centrifuged at 11,000×*g* for 2 min to remove residual ethanol. The tissue columns were transferred into 1.5 mL micro-centrifuge tubes and 100 μL of pre-warmed 70 °C of Buffer BE was added and left at room temperature for 1 min. The elution containing highly pure DNA was obtained following centrifugation at 11,000×*g* for 1 min. The DNA was stored at -20 °C until used.

Polymerase chain reaction

The bacterial colonies and DNA extracts were used as templates for confirmation of *B. melitensis* using the forward P1 (5'-CATGCGCTATGTCTGGTTAC-3') and P2 (5'-AGTGTTTCGGCTCAGAATAATC-3') primer sequences that amplified the fragment at 252 bp [15]. The PCR was performed in 25 μL reaction mixture that contained 2.5 μL of 10× buffer, 3 mM MgCl2, 400 μM dNTPs, 500 nM of each primer, 1.5 U Taq polymerase (MBI Fermentas, Lithuania) and 1 μL of purified DNA or bacterial colony mixed with 1 μL of DNAzol® reagent (Thermo Fisher Scientific, USA). The PCR amplifications were performed in a Master Cycler Pro S (Eppendorf, Germany) in 34 cycles with an initial denaturation at 95 °C for 2 min and denaturation step for 1.15 min at 95 °C. The annealing, extension and final extension phases were set at 57.1 °C for 2 min, 72 °C for 2 min and 73 °C for 5 min, respectively. The PCR products were mixed with 1 μL of loading dye and were electrophoresed through 1% (*w/v*) agarose gel pre-mixed with RedSafeTM Nucleic Acid Staining solution (INTRON, Korea) in 1× TBE at 80 V (Bio-Rad PowerPacTM Basic, USA) for 45 min. Five μL of 100 bp DNA marker (GeneDireX®, Taiwan) was run simultaneously. The bands were documented using the gel documentation software called GeneSnap®, UK.

Results

Histopathology changes and IP staining

Infected does displayed mild glomerulonephritis with neutrophils, glomerular congestion and mild renal tubular necrosis (Fig. 1a). Haemorrhages and foci of inflammatory reactions were occasionally observed in the interstitium. Immunoperoxidase staining of the kidneys

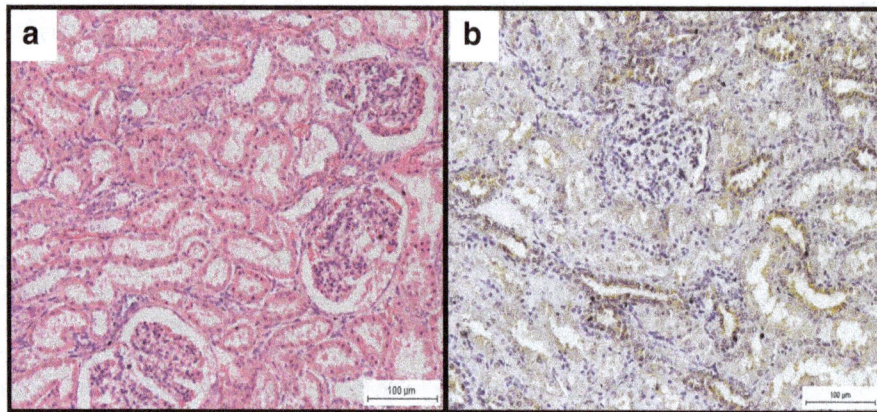

Fig. 1 a Moderate congestion of the glomerulus and mild glomerulonephritis with infiltration of mainly neutrophilic cells. H&E, × 200. **b** Diffuse and moderately strong immunoperoxidase stain reactions in the epithelial cells of the renal tubules and in the cytoplasm of inflammatory cells infiltrating the glomeruli. IHC, × 200

revealed strong to moderate staining (Fig. 1b). Strong reactions were observed in the cytoplasm of the inflammatory cells infiltrating the glomeruli and renal tubules, particularly the distal convoluted and the collecting tubules. Milder immunoreactions were noted in the epithelial cells of the proximal convoluted tubules and occasionally in the lumen of renal tubules. *Brucella melitensis* was isolated from 3 of the 6 (50%) kidney samples at an average rate of 3.9×10^3 cfu/g of tissue compared to 4 out of 6 (66.7%) kidney samples that were positive PCR (Table 1).

There was also mild inflammation in the ureter (Fig. 2a) with macrophages in the lamina propria and connective tissue stroma. The immunoperoxidase revealed positive staining, particularly within the macrophages and the epithelial cells (Fig. 2b). Again, *B. melitensis* was successfully isolated from 3 out of 6 (50%) of the ureter samples at the rate of 2.9×10^3 cfu/g of tissue compared to 4 out of 6 (66.7%) of the ureter were positive PCR.

All infected does had cystitis, characterised by intense perivascular inflammation with predominantly macrophages (Fig. 3a). The immunoperoxidase staining revealed immunoreactions within the transitional epithelial cells as well as in the cytoplasm of the macrophages (Fig. 3b). The bacterium was isolated from 1 out of 3 (33.3%) bladder samples at the rate of 4.2×10^3 cfu/g of

tissue while PCR was 66.7% (Table 1). Similarly, the urethra of all infected does showed massive infiltration of mainly macrophages at the submucosal and perivascular regions (Fig. 4a). The immunoperoxidase stained the transitional epithelial cells and the cytoplasm of macrophages (Fig. 4b). Attempts to isolate *B. melitensis* from the urethra yielded 2 out of 3 (66.7%) at an average rate of 2.6×10^3 cfu/g of tissue while PCR revealed 100% positive results. In comparison, *B. melitensis* was isolated from 2 out of 3 (66.7%) vaginal swab samples at a higher concentration of 2.4×10^8 cfu/mL but isolation was unsuccessful from any of the urine sample. The control uninfected goats revealed generally normal histological features with no inflammatory reaction and positive IP staining while *B. melitensis* was not isolated from any organ.

Lesions and immunoperoxidase scorings

None of the infected pregnant does of Group 2 exhibited clinical signs following experimental infection. However, 4 kids were eventually delivered weak by the infected does and none survived the first month after birth. Necropsy revealed no obvious gross lesions in the urinary system. Nevertheless, histopathological examinations revealed notable microscopic changes and immunoperoxidase staining in various sections of the urinary tract of the infected goats of Group 2 (Table 2). The average

Table 1 Rate of isolation and average concentration of *Brucella melitensis* in the various organs of the urinary tract of pregnant goats following acute infection

Group/Organs	Kidneys	Ureter	Urinary Bladder	Urethra	Average
G1	0/6 (0%)	0/6 (0%)	0/3 (0%)	0/3 (0%)	0%
G2	3/6 (50%)	3/6 (50%)	1/3 (33%)	2/3 (67%)	50%
	$[3.9 \times 10^3]$ [a]	2.9×10^3 [a]	$[4.2 \times 10^3]$ [a]	$[2.6 \times 10^3]$ [a]	$[3.4 \times 10^3]$ [a]

[a] unit = cfu/g tissue

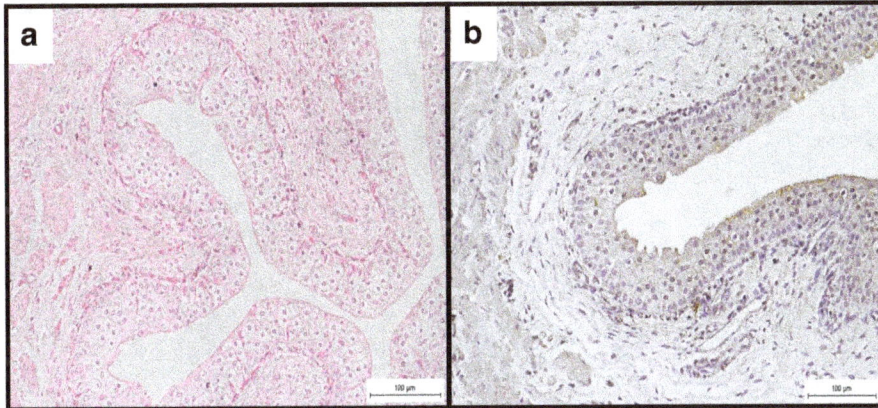

Fig. 2 a Mild congestion and ureteritis characterized by infiltration of macrophages in the connective tissue stroma. H&E, × 200. **b** Positive immunoperoxidase stain reactions in the cytoplasm of the epithelial cells of the ureter and within the infiltrating macrophages. IHC, × 200

lesion score for kidney was significantly ($p < 0.05$) higher (score 0.61 ± 0.28) than the urinary bladder (score 0.31 ± 0.15). However, the immunoperoxidase staining was significantly ($p < 0.05$) higher in the urinary bladder (score 2.01 ± 0.07) than the kidneys (score 1.33 ± 0.13) and gradually but significantly ($p < 0.05$) decreasing from urinary bladder to the urethra. The uterus of the infected goats showed significantly ($p < 0.05$) most severe histological lesions but IP distribution score was similar ($p > 0.05$) to those of urinary bladder (Table 2). None of the control uninfected goats of Group 1 showed clinical signs, gross and histopathological changes, and immunoperoxidase staining.

Discussion

There is a lack of information describing the pathological lesions and distribution of *B. melitensis* in the urinary tract of goats. This study revealed that the most common infiltrating inflammatory cell in the organs of urinary tract is the macrophage [16] while *B. melitensis* was present mostly within the cytoplasm of these macrophages. These are in agreement with earlier studies involving other organs, particularly organs of the reproductive tract [3, 14, 17]. Studies on *B. abortus* have reported its ability to reside and replicate in the macrophages [18] while hiding from the humoral immune responses and the effects of antibiotic treatments [5]. More importantly, the bacterium manipulates the macrophages by turning them into reluctant factory for massive replication of *Brucella* [19]. Apart from that, macrophages are unwilling agents of dispersal, responsible for the widespread dissemination of the bacterium [3, 20]. Furthermore, this study has proven that *B. melitensis* can invade non-phagocytic cells such as the epithelial and fibroblast cells [18, 21].

Brucella melitensis has been detected in the kidneys of West African Dwarf goats where the antigen was found mostly in the epithelium of renal tubules and glomeruli [14]. Similarly, *B. ovis* was successfully cultured from the kidneys and the urinary bladder of infected stags [15].

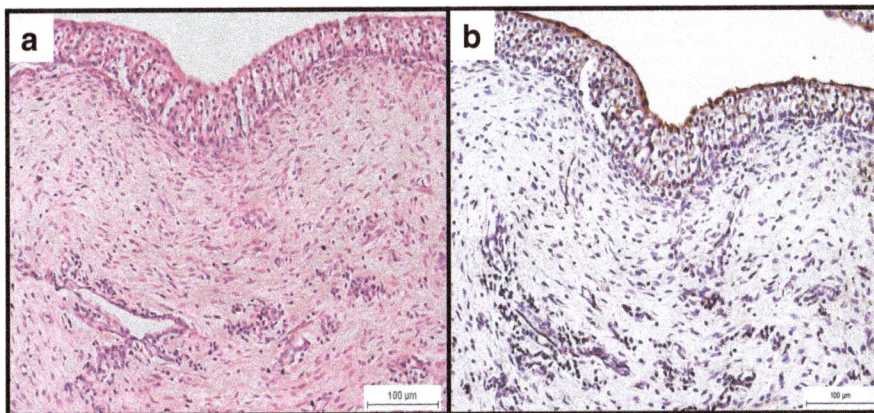

Fig. 3 a Cystitis with macrophages and few lymphocytes in the connective tissue layer of the urinary bladder. H&E, × 200. **b** Strong golden brown immunoperoxidase staining observed intracellularly in macrophages and in the transitional epithelial cells of the urinary bladder. IP, × 200

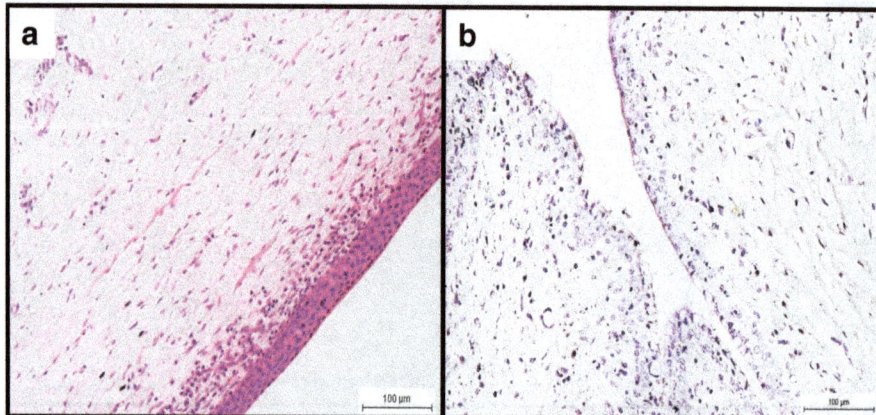

Fig. 4 a Infiltration of few macrophages at the perivascular area and the submucosa of urethra. H&E, × 100. **b** Positive light golden brown immunoperoxidase staining observed in the cytoplasm of the macrophages and epithelial cells of the urethra. IP, × 100

However, both reports did not mention the presence of *Brucella* in the urine. Furthermore, the concentrations of *B. melitensis* isolated from the various organs of the urinary tract in this study were relatively low compared to the reproductive tract. This might be the reason for the absence of *B. melitensis* in urine. Furthermore, immunoperoxidase staining revealed positive staining within the macrophages and relatively mild stain in the urinary epithelial cells. Therefore, the low level of *B. melitensis* within the epithelial cells of urinary tract was not enough to be excreted into the urine although excretion of *Brucella* in urine of infected animals has been occasionally reported [22]. Similar involvement of human urinary tract in brucellosis has been reported but the involvement is considered rare and almost always occur together with the reproductive system [12, 23].

Immunoperoxidase staining is a tool for detection of *B. melitensis* in tissues. It is highly specific and capable of showing the distribution of *Brucella* in affected tissues [3]. Using immunoperoxidase, *B. melitensis* has been shown to have tropism for the macrophages and the epithelial cells of urinary tract. Furthermore, polymerase chain reaction (PCR) has been used lately for antigen detection in infected tissues with high specificity and sensitivity [15, 22, 24]. Nevertheless, bacterial isolation is still the irrefutable method to confirm the presence of the pathogen thus, considered the gold standard for diagnosis of brucellosis [10, 24, 25]. Our attempts to isolate *B. melitensis* from the various organs of the urinary tracts were successful while PCR is deemed useful in detecting nucleic acid fragments of the bacterium [15, 22, 24, 25].

Conclusions

In conclusion, acute infection of pregnant goats by *B. melitensis* in this study led to mild lesions in the organs of the urinary tract. Low concentrations of *B. melitensis* were found within the macrophage and epithelial cells. However, it was not isolated from the urine samples that were collected from infected urinary bladder.

Abbreviations
CFT: Complement fixation test; cfu/g: Colony-forming unit per gram; cfu/L: Colony-forming unit per litre; DAB: 3.3'-Diaminobenzidine; DNA: Deoxyribonucleic acid; FCA: Freund's complete adjuvant; FIA: Freund's incomplete adjuvant; HE: Haematoxylin and eosin; IACUC: Institutional Animal Care and Use Committee; IgG: Immunoglobulin G; IP: Immunoperoxidase; PBS: Phosphate buffered saline; PCR: Polymerase chain reaction; RBPT: Rose Bengal Plate Test

Table 2 Average histopathology and immunoperoxidase scores (mean ± SE) in the various ogans of the urinary tract of pregnant goats following acute experimental infection with *B. melitensis*

Organ	Histology Score (Mean ± SE)	IP Score (Mean ± SE)
Kidney	0.61 ± 0.28[a]	1.33 ± 0.13[a]
Ureter	0.21 ± 0.15[b]	0.47 ± 0.18[c]
Urinary bladder	0.31 ± 0.15[b]	2.00 ± 0.07[b]
Urethra	0.21 ± 0.68[b]	0.13 ± 0.07[d]
Uterus	0.84 ± 0.33[c]	1.80 ± 0.42[c]

[a,b,c,d]Different superscripts represent significant (*p* < 0.05) difference of data within the respective column

Acknowledgements
The authors would like to thank Dr. Annas Salleh, Dr. Nur Adza Rina Mohd Nordi, Mrs. Latifah Hanan and Mrs. Jamilah Jahari of the Histopathology Laboratory, Faculty of Veterinary Medicine, Universiti Putra Malaysia for their technical assistance.

Funding
The FRGS Grant 07–03-11-1026FR of the Ministry of Higher Education Malaysia and the Universiti Putra Malaysia IPS Grant 9468500 funded the study.

Authors' contributions

MM and NNS collected and analysed data, and drafting of manuscript. SKB and HH designed the experiment and revised manuscript. TT revised the manuscript. MZS designed experiment, analysed data and revised manuscript. All authors read and approved the final manuscript.

Consent for publication

Not applicable.

Competing interests

The authors declare that they have no competing interests.

Author details

[1]Research Centre for Ruminant Diseases, Faculty of Veterinary Medicine, Universiti Putra Malaysia, 43400 Serdang, Selangor, Malaysia. [2]Department of Veterinary Pathology & Microbiology, Faculty of Veterinary Medicine, Universiti Putra Malaysia, 43400 Serdang, Selangor, Malaysia. [3]Puncak Jalil Veterinary Clinic, Taman Puncak Jalil, 43300 Seri Kembangan, Seri Kembangan, Selangor, Malaysia. [4]Department of Veterinary Laboratory Diagnosis, Faculty of Veterinary Medicine, Universiti Putra Malaysia, 43400 Serdang, Malaysia.

References

1. Seleem MN, Boyle SM, Sriraganathan N. Brucellosis: a re-emerging zoonosis. Vet Microbiol. 2010;140:392–8.
2. Bamaiyi PH, Hassan L, Khairani-Bejo S, ZainalAbidin M, Ramlan M, Adzhar A. Prevalence and distribution of Brucella melitensis in goats in Malaysia from 2000 to 2009. Prev Vet Med. 2015;119:232–6.
3. Xavier MN, Paixao TA, den Hartigh AB, Tsolis RM, Santos RL. Pathogenesis of Brucella spp. Open Vet Sci J. 2010;4:109–18.
4. Celli J. Surviving inside a macrophage: the many ways of Brucella. Res Microbiol. 2006;157:93–8.
5. Christopher S, Umapathy BL, Ravikumar KL. Brucellosis: review on the recent trends in pathogenicity and laboratory diagnosis. J Lab Phys. 2010;2:55–60.
6. Corbel MJ. Brucellosis in humans and animals. World Health Organization. 2006; http://www.who.int/csr/resources/publications/Brucellosis.pdf.
7. Kahl-McDonagh MM, Ficht TA. Evaluation of protection afforded by Brucella abortus and Brucella melitensis unmarked deletion mutants exhibiting different rates of clearance in BALB/c mice. Infect Immun. 2006;74:4048–57.
8. Gorvel JP. Brucella: a Mr "Hide" converted into Dr Jekyll. Microb Infect. 2008; 10:1010–3.
9. Traxler RM, Lehman MW, Bosserman EA, Guerra MA, Smith TL. A literature review of laboratory-acquired brucellosis. J Clin Microbiol. 2013;51:3055–62.
10. Bamaiyi PH, Hassan L, Khairani-Bejo S, Zainal Abidin M. Updates on brucellosis in Malaysia and Southeast Asia. Malaysian J Vet Res. 2014;5:71–82.
11. OiE. Bovine 355 brucellosis. OiE terrestrial manual; 2009. http://www.oie.int/fileadmin/Home/eng/Health_standards/tahm/2008/pdf/2.04.03_BOVINE_BRUCELL.pdf.
12. Stamatiou K, Polyzois K, Dahanis S, Lambou T, Skolarikos A. Brucella melitensis: a rarely suspected cause of infections of genitalia and the lower urinary tract. Braz J Infect Dis. 2009;13:86–9.
13. Plumeriastuti H, Zamri-Saad M. Detection of Brucella melitensis in seropositive goats. Online J Vet Res. 2012;16:1–7.
14. Emikpe BO, Sabri MY, Ezeasor CK, Tanko PN. Immunohistochemical detection of Brucella mellitensis and Coxiella burnetii antigens in formalin-fixed tissues of west African dwarf goats. Arch Clin Microbiol. 2013;4 https://doi.org/10.3823/270.
15. Ridler AL, West DM, Collett MG. Pathology of Brucella ovis infection in red deer stags (Cdervus elaphus). NZ Vet J. 2012;60:146–9.
16. Ahmed MO, Elmeshri SE, Abuzweda AR, Blauo M, Abouzeed YM, Ibrahim A, Salem H, Alzwam F, Abid S, Elfahem A, Elrais A. Seroprevalence of brucellosis in animals and human populations in the western mountains region in Libya, December 2006–January 2008. Eurosurveillance. 2010; 15: pii:19625. Available online: http://www.eurosurveillance.org/ViewArticle.aspx?ArticleId=19625.
17. Grilló MJ, Blasco JM, Gorvel JP, Moriyón I, Moreno 380 E. What have we learned from brucellosis in the mouse model? Vet Res. 2012;43 https://doi.org/10.1186/1297-9716-43-29.
18. Vitry MA, Hanot Mambres D, Deghelt M, Hack K, Machelart A, Lhomme F, Vanderwinden JM, Vermeersch M, De Trez C, Pérez-Morga D, Letesson JJ, Muraille E. Brucella melitensis invades murine erythrocytes during infection. Infect Immun. 2014;82:3927–2938.
19. Poester FP, Nielsen K, Samartino LE, Yu WL. Diagnosis of brucellosis. Open Vet Sci J. 2010;4:46–60.
20. von Bargen K, Gorvel JP, Salcedo SP. Internal affairs: investigating the Brucella intracellular lifestyle. FEMS Microbiol Rev. 2012;36:533–62.
21. He Y. Analyses of Brucella pathogenesis, host immunity, and vaccine targets using systems biology and bioinformatics. Frontiers Cell Infect Microbiol. 2012;2:2.
22. Moshkelani S, Javaheri-Koupaei M, Rabiee S, Moazeni M. Detection of Brucella spp. and Leptospira spp. by multiplex polymerase chain reaction (PCR) from aborted bovine, ovine and caprine fetuses in Iran. Afr J Microbiol Res. 2011;5:4627–30.
23. Uncu H, Demiroğlu YZ, Gül U, Güvel S, Turunç T, Cokaloğlu S, Arslan H. A case of brucellosis presenting with urinary tract infection. Mikrobiyologi Bulteni. 2006;40:275–8.
24. Smirnova EA, Vasin AV, Sandybaev NT, Klotchenko SA, Plotnikova MA, Chervyakova OV, Sansyzbay AR, Kiselev OI. Current methods of human and animal brucellosis diagnostics. Adv Infect Dis. 2013;3:177–84.
25. Yu WL, Nielsen K. Review of detection of Brucella sp. by polymerase chain reaction. Croatian Medic J. 2010;51:306–13.

Permissions

List of Contributors

Mona Saleh, Gokhlesh Kumar and Mansour El-Matbouli
Clinical Division of Fish Medicine, University of Veterinary Medicine, Veterinaerplatz 1, 1210 Vienna, Austria

Saleh Al-Quraishy
Zoology Department, College of Science, King Saud University, Riyadh, Saudi Arabia

Abdel-Azeem Abdel-Baki
Zoology Department, College of Science, King Saud University, Riyadh, Saudi Arabia
Zoology Department, Faculty of Science, Beni-Suef University, Beni-Suef, Egypt

Sergio Migliore, Salvatore La Marca, Vincenzo Di Marco Lo Presti and Maria Vitale
Istituto Zooprofilattico Sperimentale of Sicily "A. Mirri", Via G. Marinuzzi 3, 90129 Palermo, Italy

Cristian Stabile
Centro Veterinario "L'arca", Via V. Mazzini 112, 92013 Menfi, Italy

Anke K. Wiethoelter and Richard Malik
Faculty of Veterinary Science, The University of Sydney, Sydney 2006, NSW, Australia

Siobhan M. Mor
Faculty of Veterinary Science, The University of Sydney, Sydney 2006, NSW, Australia
Tufts University School of Medicine, 145 Harrison Avenue, Boston 02111, MA, USA

Amanda Lee
New South Wales Department of Primary Industries, Woodbridge Road, Menangle 2568, NSW, Australia

Barbara Moloney
New South Wales Department of Primary Industries, 161 Kite Street, Orange 2800, NSW, Australia

Daniel R. James
Small Animal Specialist Hospital, 1 Richardson Place, North Ryde 2113, NSW, Australia

Jean-Pierre Legroux
Clinique vétérinaire La Toison d'Or, Dijon, France

Lénaïg Halos and Marielle Servonnet
Merial, Lyon, France

Gilles Bourdoiseau, Luc Chabanne and Magalie René-Martellet
University of Lyon, VetAgro Sup – Veterinary Campus of Lyon, Marcy l'Etoile, France
EPIA (Epidémiologie animale Unit), INRA, Saint Genès Champanelle, France

Jean-Luc Pingret
Scanelis, Colomiers, France

Gad Baneth
Koret School of Veterinary Medicine, Hebrew University, Rehovot, Israel

Veronika Merino
Kuskaya: An Interdisciplinary Training Program for Innovation in Global Health, School of Public Health, Universidad Peruana Cayetano Heredia, Av. Honorio Delgado 431 San Martin de Porres, Lima, Peru

Christopher M. Westgard
Kuskaya: An Interdisciplinary Training Program for Innovation in Global Health, School of Public Health, University of Washington, Seattle, USA

Angela M. Bayer
Division of Infectious Diseases, David Geffen School of Medicine, University of California, Los Angeles, California, Los Angeles, USA
Unit of Epidemiology, STD and HIV, School of Public Health and Administration, Universidad Peruana Cayetano Heredia, Lima, Peru

Patricia J. García
Unit of Epidemiology, STD and HIV, School of Public Health and Administration, Universidad Peruana Cayetano Heredia, Lima, Peru

Peter Damborg, Arshnee Moodley, Bent Aalbæk and Teresa Pires dos Santos
Department of Veterinary Disease Biology, Faculty of Health and Medical Sciences, University of Copenhagen, Stigbøjlen 4, 1870 Frederiksberg C, Denmark

Luca Guardabassi
Department of Veterinary Disease Biology, Faculty of Health and Medical Sciences, University of Copenhagen, Stigbøjlen 4, 1870 Frederiksberg C, Denmark
Department of Biomedical Sciences, Ross University School of Veterinary Medicine, Basseterre, West Indies, St Kitts and Nevis

Gianpiero Ventrella
Department of Veterinary Medicine, Università degli Studi di Bari, Strada P.le per Casamassima Km 3, Valenzano-Bari 70010, Italy

Yongjie Feng, Yaoyao Lu, Longxian Zhang and Yurong Yang
Laboratory of Veterinary Pathology, College of Animal Science and Veterinary Medicine, Henan Agricultural University, Zhengzhou 450002, People's Republic of China

Yinghua Wang
Center for Animal Disease Control and Prevention of Henan Province, Zhengzhou 450002, People's Republic of China

Martina Crnogaj, Iva Šmit, Ivana Kiš, Jelena Gotić, Mirna Brkljačić, Vesna Matijatko Nada Kučer and Vladimir Mrljak
Clinic for Internal Diseases, Faculty of Veterinary Medicine, University of Zagre b, Zagreb, Croatia

José Joaquin Cerón, Camila and Peres Rubio
Department of Animal Medicine and Surgery, Faculty of Veterinary Medicine, University of Murcia, 30100 Espinardo, Murcia, Spain

Liping Yu, Xiaorong Zhang, Tianqi Wu, Jin Su, Yuyang Wang, Yuexin Wang, Baoyang Ruan, Xiaosai Niu and Yantao Wu
Jiangsu Co-Innovation Center for Prevention of Animal Infectious Diseases and Zoonoses, College of Veterinary Medicine, Yangzhou University, Yangzhou, Jiangsu 225009, China

Sonia Boughattas, Aarti Sharma and Marawan Abu-Madi
Department of Biomedical Science, College of Health Sciences, Biomedical Research Center, Qatar University, Doha, Qatar

Jerzy Behnke
School of Biology, University of Nottingham, University Park, Nottingham NG7 2RD, UK

M. Atlija and J. J. Arranz
Departamento de Producción Animal, Universidad de León, Campus de Vegazana s/n, 24071 León, Spain

B. Gutiérrez-Gil
Departamento de Producción Animal, Universidad de León, Campus de Vegazana s/n, 24071 León, Spain
Instituto de Ganadería de Montaña, CSIC-ULE, 24346 Grulleros, León, Spain

M. J. Stear
Institute of Biodiversity, Animal Health and Comparative Medicine, University of Glasgow, Bearsden Road, Glasgow G61 1QH, UK

J. M. Prada
Institute of Biodiversity, Animal Health and Comparative Medicine, University of Glasgow, Bearsden Road, Glasgow G61 1QH, UK
Department of Ecology and Evolutionary Biology, Princeton University, Princeton, NJ 08540, USA

M. Martínez-Valladares
Instituto de Ganadería de Montaña, CSIC-ULE, 24346 Grulleros, León, Spain

F. A. Rojo-Vázquez
Instituto de Ganadería de Montaña, CSIC-ULE, 24346 Grulleros, León, Spain
Departamento de Sanidad Animal, Universidad de León, Campus de Vegazana s/n, 24071 León, Spain

Michael S. Kent and Allison Zwingenberger
Department of Surgical and Radiological Sciences, School of Veterinary Medicine, University of California, Davis, CA, USA

Jodi L. Westropp
Department of Medicine and Epidemiology, School of Veterinary Medicine, University of California, Davis, CA, USA

Laura E. Barrett
William R. Pritchard Veterinary Medical Teaching Hospital, School of Veterinary Medicine, University of California, Davis, CA, USA

Blythe P. Durbin-Johnson
Department of Public Health Sciences, University of California Davis, Davis, California 95616, USA

Paramita Ghosh
Department of Urology, University of California, Davis, School of Medicine, Sacramento, CA, USA
Department of Biochemistry and Molecular Medicine, University of California, Davis, School of Medicine, Sacramento, CA, USA
VA Northern California Health Care System, Sacramento, CA, USA

Ruth L. Vinall
Department of Urology, University of California, Davis, School of Medicine, Sacramento, CA, USA
Department of Biochemistry and Molecular Medicine, University of California, Davis, School of Medicine, Sacramento, CA, USA
Department of Pharmaceutical and Biomedical Sciences, California Northstate University College of Pharmacy, Elk Grove, CA, USA

Michèle Bergmann, Theresa Englert, Bianca Stuetzer and Katrin Hartmann
Clinic of Small Animal Medicine, Centre for Clinical Veterinary Medicine, LMU Munich, Veterinaerstrasse 13, 80539 Munich, Germany

Jennifer R. Hawley and Michael R. Lappin
Center for Companion Animal Studies, Department of Clinical Sciences, College of Veterinary Medicine and Biomedical Sciences, Colorado State University, Fort Collins, CO, USA

Boris Fuchs, Barbara Zimmermann, Petter Wabakken and Alina L. Evans
Faculty of Applied Ecology and Agricultural Sciences, Hedmark University College, Campus Evenstad, N-2480 Koppang, Norway

Jon M. Arnemo
Faculty of Applied Ecology and Agricultural Sciences, Hedmark University College, Campus Evenstad, N-2480 Koppang, Norway
Department of Wildlife, Fish and Environmental Studies, Swedish University of Agricultural Sciences, SE-90183 Umeå, Sweden

Set Bornstein
Department of Virology, Immunobiology and Parasitology, National Veterinary Institute, SE-75189 Uppsala, Sweden

Johan Månsson, Olof Liberg and Håkan Sand
Department of Ecology, Grimsö Wildlife Research Station, Swedish University of Agricultural Sciences, SE 73091 Riddarhyttan, Sweden

Jonas Kindberg
Department of Wildlife, Fish and Environmental Studies, Swedish University of Agricultural Sciences, SE-90183 Umeå, Sweden

Erik O. Ågren
Department of Pathology and Wildlife Disease, National Veterinary Institute, SE-75189 Uppsala, Sweden

Kgomotso Sako
Section of Pharmacology and Toxicology, Department of Paraclinical Sciences, Faculty of Veterinary Science, University of Pretoria, Private Bag X04, Onderstepoort 0110, South Africa

Vinny Naidoo
Section of Pharmacology and Toxicology, Department of Paraclinical Sciences, Faculty of Veterinary Science, University of Pretoria, Private Bag X04, Onderstepoort 0110, South Africa
University of Pretoria Biomedical Research Centre, Faculty of Veterinary Science, Private Bag X04, Onderstepoort 0110, South Africa

Ilse jv Rensburg
University of Pretoria Biomedical Research Centre, Faculty of Veterinary Science, Private Bag X04, Onderstepoort 0110, South Africa

Sarah Clift
Section of Pathology, Department of Paraclinical Sciences, Faculty of Veterinary Science, University of Pretoria, Private Bag X04, Onderstepoort 0110, South Africa

Anna Bajer, Ewa J. Mierzejewska, Katarzyna Tołkacz and Renata Welc-Faleciak
Department of Parasitology, Institute of Zoology, Faculty of Biology, University of Warsaw, 1 Miecznikowa Street, 02-096 Warsaw, Poland

Anna Rodo
Department of Pathology and Veterinary Diagnostics, Warsaw University of Life Sciences-SGGW, 159c Nowoursynowska Street, 02-766 Warsaw, Poland
Lab-Wet, Veterinary Diagnostic Laboratory, ul. Wita Stwosza 30, 02-661 Warsaw, Poland

Antonio Bosco, Maria Paola Maurelli, Davide Ianniello, Maria Elena Morgoglione, Alessandra Amadesi, Giuseppe Cringoli and Laura Rinaldi
Department of Veterinary Medicine and Animal Production, University of Naples Federico II, CREMOPAR Campania Region, Naples, Italy

Gerald C. Coles
University of Bristol, School of Veterinary Sciences, Langford House, Bristol BS40 5DU, UK

Jianhua Liu, Lianrui Liu, Di Tian, Wenyu Li, Lixin Xu, Ruofeng Yan, Xiangrui Li and Xiaokai Song
MOE Joint International Research Laboratory of Animal Health and Food Safety, College of Veterinary Medicine, Nanjing Agricultural University, Nanjing 210095, People's Republic of China

Lingjuan Li
Henan Muxiang Veterinary Pharmaceutical Co., ltd, Zhengzhou 450000, People's Republic of China

Veronika Kovacova, Hana Bandouchova, Vladimir Piacek and Jiri Pikula
Department of Ecology and Diseases of Game, Fish and Bees, University of Veterinary and Pharmaceutical Sciences Brno, Palackého tř. 1946/1, 612 42 Brno, Czech Republic

Jan Zukal and Markéta Harazim
Institute of Vertebrate Biology of the Czech Academy of Sciences, v.v.i., Květná 8, 603 65 Brno, Czech Republic
Institute of Botany and Zoology, Masaryk University, Kotlářská 267/2, 611 37 Brno, Czech Republic

Natália Martínková
Institute of Vertebrate Biology of the Czech Academy of Sciences, v.v.i., Květná 8, 603 65 Brno, Czech Republic
Institute of Biostatistics and Analyses, Masaryk University, Kamenice 126/3, 625 00 Brno, Czech Republic

Alexander D. Botvinkin
Irkutsk State Medical University, Krasnogo Vosstania street 1, Irkutsk, Russian Federation 664003

Oleg L. Orlov
International Complex Research Laboratory for Study of Climate Change, Land Use and Biodiversity, Tyumen State University, Volodarckogo 6, 625003 Tyumen, Russia

Department of Biochemistry, Ural State Medical University, Repina 3, 620014 Ekaterinburg, Russia

Alexandra P. Shumkina
Western Baikal protected areas, Federal State Budgetary Institution "Zapovednoe Pribaikalye", Baikalskaya st. 291B, 664050 Irkutsk, Russia

Mikhail P. Tiunov
Institute of Biology and Soil Science, Far East Branch of the Russian Academy of Sciences, Pr-t 100-letiya Vladivostoka 159, 690022 Vladivostok, Russia

Victor R. Simpson
Wildlife Veterinary Investigation Centre, Chacewater, Truro, Cornwall TR4 8PB, UK

Damer P. Blake
Pathobiology and Population Sciences, Royal Veterinary College, Hawkshead Lane, North Mymms, Hertfordshire AL9 7TA, UK

João Xavier de Oliveira Filho, David Emílio Santos and Neves de Barcellos
Department of Animal Medicine, Universidade Federal do Rio Grande do Sul (UFRGS), Agronomia, Av Bento Gonçalves, 9090, Porto Alegre, Rio Grande do Sul 91540-000, Brazil

Marcos Antônio Zanella Morés, Raquel Rebellato, Jalusa Deon Kich, Maurício Egidio Cantão, Catia Silene Klein, Arlei Coldebella and Nelson Morés
Embrapa Suinos e Aves, Concórdia, Santa Catarina 89700-000, Brazil

Roberto Maurício Carvalho Guedes
Preventive Veterinary Medicine Department, Veterinary School, Universidade Federal de Minas Gerais, Belo Horizonte, Brazil

S. Jo Moore, Catherine E. Vrentas, Soyoun Hwang, Eric M. Nicholson and Justin J. Greenlee
USDA, Agricultural Research Service, National Animal Disease Center, Virus and Prion Research Unit, Ames, USA

M. Heather West Greenlee
Department of Biomedical Sciences, College of Veterinary Medicine, Iowa State University, Ames, USA

Teresa Maria Punsmann, Lucie Marie Grimm, Carolin Reckmann, Cornelia Schwennen, Matthias Gerhard Wagener and Martin Ganter
Clinic for Swine, Small Ruminants and Forensic Medicine, University of Veterinary Medicine Hannover, Foundation, Hannover, Germany

N. N. Shaqinah
Research Centre for Ruminant Diseases, Faculty of Veterinary Medicine, Universiti Putra Malaysia, 43400 Serdang, Selangor, Malaysia

M. Mazlina
Research Centre for Ruminant Diseases, Faculty of Veterinary Medicine, Universiti Putra Malaysia, 43400 Serdang, Selangor, Malaysia
Department of Veterinary Pathology & Microbiology, Faculty of Veterinary Medicine, Universiti Putra Malaysia, 43400 Serdang, Selangor, Malaysia

M. Zamri-Saad
Research Centre for Ruminant Diseases, Faculty of Veterinary Medicine, Universiti Putra Malaysia, 43400 Serdang, Selangor, Malaysia
Department of Veterinary Laboratory Diagnosis, Faculty of Veterinary Medicine, Universiti Putra Malaysia, 43400 Serdang, Malaysia

S. Khairani-Bejo and H. Hazilawati
Department of Veterinary Pathology & Microbiology, Faculty of Veterinary Medicine, Universiti Putra Malaysia, 43400 Serdang, Selangor, Malaysia

T. Tiagarahan
Puncak Jalil Veterinary Clinic, Taman Puncak Jalil, 43300 Seri Kembangan, Seri Kembangan, Selangor, Malaysia

Index

www.ingramcontent.com/pod-product-compliance
Lightning Source LLC
Chambersburg PA
CBHW082024190326
41458CB00010B/3265